Predatory Bender

America in the Aughts

A Story of Subprime Finance

by Matthew Lee

with a non-fiction advocates' afterword

INNER
CITY
PRESS
1919 Washington Ave
Bronx NY 10457
InnerCityPress.org

ISBN 0-9740244-1-4   Printed in the United States of America

Cataloging-in-Publication Data is available from the publisher on request

Library of Congress Control Number: 2003111283
(with *Predatory Lending: Toxic Credit in the Inner City*)   Cover design by Janine-Marie Boulad

This is a creative work: resemblances to non-public figures, locales or institutions are coincidental. Subprime consumer finance firms of the type depicted herein *do* engage in hard-selling, bait-and-switch, and also pack insurance on such dubious collateral as beds, ice chests and fishing rods. One company, Citigroup, whose chairman was asked about just such practices during an open meeting at Carnegie Hall, stated as this went to press (September 2003) that it had just "ceased offering optional personal property insurance in connection with its secured personal loans." Call it the power of the pen, or of persistence. Predatory lending continues in the United States, and even worse globally: including by CitiFinancial, HSBC's Household, AIG, GE and others. What follows, however, is a creative work: resemblances to non-public figures, locales or institutions are incidental.

For information on Inner City Press reading group guides, as well as ordering for use in educational institutions, contact editor@innercitypress.org. A portion of the sales from each copy of this book goes to the Fair Finance Watch, which advocates for consumers' and human rights.

I want to join Fair Finance Watch and receive a 10% discount on this and all subsequent orders. Enclosed is my contribution of: $100 - $50 - $30

Name
Address
City/State/Zip
Daytime Phone
E-mail

Make check or money order payable to:

Inner City Press, PO Box 580188, Mt. Carmel Station, Bronx NY 10458

CONTENTS

Part One: Pennies a Day

Part Two: The Cracker Jackal's Play

Part Three: The Rate of Exchange

About the Author

Matthew Lee is a public interest lawyer, growing out of community battles in the South Bronx of New York City to fix abandoned buildings before they were demolished or sold. He has been awarded Bronx Council on the Arts prizes for fiction and poetry. He has been involved in seeking accountability from banks and other corporations since the early 1990s, on issues of branch closings, redlining and then predatory lending. He now does this work globally through the Fair Finance Watch and its Human Rights Enforcement Project.

Part One: Pennies a Day

1. Jack in The Bronx

The West Farms Mall was built in the former South Bronx in the second year of the new millennium. While ostensibly the fruit of three decades of community struggle, the land beneath the mall was owned by Anguilla-based EmpiBank. The anchor tenant, too, was a part of Empi's empire: a storefront office of the high-rate lender EmpiFinancial. Jack Bender had worked for EmpiBank on the outskirts of Charlotte, North Carolina, the so-called Queen City. He was offered the position of deputy branch manager for EmpiFinancial in The Bronx and he took it.

"I'm tired of Bubba-land," he said. "I'm not *like* those people."

And so it was that Jack Bender parked his Ford Taurus under the towering halogen lights that late-May dawn, fumbling with his keys to open the storefront of EmpiFinancial.

It was Jack's custom to come to the office an hour early, alone. He poured himself a cup of yesterday's cold coffee, slipped into the machine a dry filter-bag and pushed the orange "On" switch. Jack used this silent hour to review the promissory notes his staff had managed to cajole from South Bronx residents the day before.

Bertha Watkins had agreed to pay twenty-four percent interest for a $2,500 loan to buy a new bedroom set at the Sicilian Furniture outlet on 161st Street. Gina had creamed her for credit insurance too. Two hundred dollars a month, prepaid, to protect a garish canopy bed that EmpiFinancial would never foreclose on because it couldn't be re-sold. People who buy pseudo-mobster furniture want it new. The point was to have the trappings of the nouveau riche; pre-owned (the euphemism for used) defeated the whole purpose.

Jack nodded as he reviewed Gina's handiwork. She was getting more and more vicious, which was just what EmpiFinancial liked in its employees. Vicious and smiling. Jack closed his eyes and pictured the closing:

"This way if you die, Ms. Watkins, you can rest easy that no one will come repo your beautiful new bedroom set. This protection, this peace of mind, costs only pennies a day."

Jack chuckled, lighting his first unfiltered cigarette of the day. Pennies a day was the classic phrasing, impervious to challenges from state attorneys general, or from Bush II's Federal Trade Commission, if for some reason they freaked out and sued. Any dollar figure was composed of pennies, wasn't it? EmpiBank's chairman, Sandaford Vyle, was paid pennies a day -- 63,562,600 pennies a day, to be precise. Jack had calculated it. $232 million a year, all told. Divide by 365, multiply by a hundred and you had it. Vyle was paid just pennies a day.

Jack'd always been good at math. Growing up in Charlotte with his daddy in jail, Jack got the best SAT scores in the school district's history. He could have gone to one of the UNCs, joined a frat house and guzzled beer straight from the keg. Instead at a teacher's suggestion he chose to pay out-of-state rates at SUNY Oswego. He'd been born in Bubba-land, as he called it, but he was not of it. He'd only returned after his mother had both her breasts chopped off in a failed attempt to stop the metastases that wracked her. He visited her -- the titless wonder, he called her, but never to her face -- in the hospital, then in a sort of halfway house for the dying where she languished for six and a half years. It had given Jack time to get married, have a kid and get divorced. He worked his way up from repo man to manager of a Charlotte EmpiFinancial office. A month after he watched his mother buried in the red clay of the cemetery across from the Waffle House, Jack'd been offered a promotion to start-up EmpiFinancial's South Bronx office. He rented a Ryder trailer and left the next day.

After a month in a Comfort Inn out by Co-op City, he'd found a two-bedroom on Olinville Avenue. This was not the South Bronx, he'd been assured. It was a white working-class neighborhood. In the days after he signed the lease he realized that he was one of only two white people living in his building. But so what? One of the ways in which he wasn't a Bubba was that he didn't care about race. He noticed it, but he didn't care. The color he cared about was green. Bertha Watkins might be a two hundred and fifty-pound African-American matriarch (this was Bender's assumption, the way his mind worked). But so what? She'd pay for the four posts of her canopy bed -- handcarved in Malaysia -- just as good as the next person. I have a dream, Jack thought: a dream that one day we will all be equally in the corporate spell, equally marching in the integrated army of corporate control, selling and buying and paying and dying. Jack was lighting cigarette number two when Gina came in, her shoulder-length dark hair not as neat as usual, an expression that Jack pegged as doped-up on her face.

"Gina, baby," Jack said, standing up from his desk. "I like the way you reamed this Bertha Watkins. The credit insurance on the mobster bed is priceless."

Gina smiled but inside she cringed. Jack had a beer belly, a comb-over and the remnants of a Southern drawl. Popped blood vessels made his cheek bones red, whether from drink or disease, Gina didn't know or care. Within EmpiFinancial the name they'd given Jack was The Cracker. Gina'd driven Interstate 95 to Delray Beach for spring break, sure. But to be working for The Cracker was not what she'd expected when she'd paid to attend EmpiFinancial's seminar at the Courtyard by Marriott conference center by LaGuardia Airport. "The sky's the limit," the trainer'd said. "You'll be sellin' a good product -- always remember that we have a product that people want -- and you'll be getting EmpiBank stock options that have never decreased in value. Never! Some say Sandy Vyle made a deal with the Devil, but me, I don't care." The trainer jangled his gold Rolex watch -- Patek Philippe, perhaps: from the audience it was hard to see -- and clicked to the next slide of his PowerPoint presentation. How after a year selling personal loans EmpiFinancial would train them down at its corporate campus in Baltimore to take the Series Seven, so they could pitch variable annuities to retirees. "You'll be workin' for Wall Street," the trainer said. "The sky's the limit."

That EmpiBank was based on Anguilla -- to Gina it sounded like a kind of lizard -- was not explained. Gina figured it was just smart tax planning. Who wanted to work for a company that was a sucker for the government anyway? If they didn't know how to manage their own money, what would they pay you with? Gina paid for the seminar, she got caught up in it like at a Baptist revivalist meeting -- and now here she was, smiling at a cracker with a comb-over about a loan to a functionally-illiterate welfare mother.

"We can flip her in a month," Gina said, going to the coffee station and filling her cup. "There's no way she can afford the monthly payments. She'll be back in here before summer's out and we can rip her on the refinance too."

"That's my girl," Jack said. Gina left the coffee station without even putting in the non-dairy creamer. She didn't want Jack to get within five feet of her. Vinny'd been rough last night but at least she'd felt something. The sky was the limit.

* * *

Jack watched Gina's ass as she walked to her work-station. Gina wore pants but they fit her well. Some off-the-rack crap from T.J. Maxx. He watched the crack of Gina's gym-firm ass and thought idly of his ex-wife Diane. She'd had a nice ass too, but someone must have reversed her intestines because the shit that came out of her mouth -- well, when he found himself in handcuffs for having slapped her for calling him a pathetic excuse for a man, that was it. It was a Bubba-land ballet, and he didn't want to play. He'd just have to find a way to get visitation with his daughter. He'd have to pay the child support, and find a way this summer to drive down to North Carolina and pick Azalea up, Zalie, he called her, maybe take her to Rosarito Beach down in Mexico.

Jack was cosmopolitan, in his way. He liked to vacation as far south and west as his car would take him. Eighteen miles south of Tijuana lies Rosarito, beer cheapened by the collapsing peso, suspicious eyes dampened by NAFTA but still yet no extradition treaty for child custody, much less child support. He'd tell Diane he was only taking Zalie to Myrtle Beach, or maybe out to those South Carolina islands where they speak African gula. To get Diane to buy into it he'd just have to pay her a few more rounds of the inflated child-support while she screwed other Bubbas she picked up in Beefsteak Charlie's in Charlotte. Actually they had franchises of pseudo-European sidewalk cafés in Charlotte now, sandwiches with snooty Italian names sold to get-over MBAs from New York and Chicago. It was still Bubba-land. Jack lit ciggie number three. He was glad he didn't have breasts so he couldn't get cancer there like his momma did.

* * *

The shit of it was, Bertha Watkins wasn't as stupid as they'd assumed. She came in just before lunch, a healthy-looking black woman with hair that had freshly been curled. She was pointing at her Note and Security Agreement, bitching about the credit insurance.

"I talked to a lawyer," she said. Jack thought: storefront shyster waiting for lead paint braindead babies in front of Lincoln Hospital. And Bertha wasn't as heavy as he'd imagined. For a moment he pictured her on the four-post bed.

"I want this charge taken off right now," Bertha demanded. "Mista Le-vine" -- she said it like a vineyard, like a fine wine, Jack immediately thought, Micah Levine -- "he said yer company's bein' sued for loan-sharkin', that the govahment's all over yer ass. So y'all just cancel the charge or I'm gonna--"

"Calm *down*, Ms. Watkins," Jack said. "That credit insurance there, it's just to help you. To give you security."

"I want it off," Bertha said.

Jack heard the elevated train rumbling out on Southern Boulevard, wondered whether Bertha had driven here or taken the Two Train, straight from Micah Levine's storefront on 149th Street and Morris Avenue. Micah has a garish electronic sign in front, scrolling again and again, "Have You Been Hurt?" in English and Spanish.

"Did he charge you for his advice?" Jack asked.

"What?"

"Did Mister Le-vine -- you know, your loi-ah -- did he charge you, to get you all fired up like this?"

"Who the *hell* do you think you're speakin' to?"

"'Cause it's all legal, and Mister Levine knows it. The moment you sign the documents, it's an enforceable debt. The insurance is pre-paid, ya know what I mean? It's become part of the loan. Now if there's any problem paying it, we can always extend the terms--"

"Y'all are no better than the Mafia."

Jack didn't disagree. But it was all legal. And with a few dozen more Berthas, Jack would get a nice quarterly bonus and he'd be driving cross-country with Zalie, or at least talking gula and picking up muted Dianes on the nineteenth hole. He smoothed down his hair and again heard the elevated train.

"I'll be back," Bertha said.

"Your payment's not due 'til the end of the month," Jack called after her.

"What was *that* about?" Gina said, coming out of the bathroom fresh from her lunchtime line of coke, her little pick-me-up, stronger and more reliable than Vinny but not an entirely satisfactory replacement.

"It's the lady you screwed over yesterday," Jack said. "She done got herself a loi-ah." Jack laughed. This was the way he could bond with Gina, he figured. They were united in sophisticated loan-sharking, lording their knowledge of the finer points over the vast unwashed of their South Bronx catchment area.

"D'ja cancel the insurance?" Gina asked.

"Hell no. Why'm I gonna give up good clean money that you earned -- that *we* earned -- just 'cause the lady has second-thoughts in the morning?" Gina looked at him strangely. "They always do," Jack added, thinking of Diane, hoping for Gina.

"Am I gonna get written up?"

"Not unless she calls Home Office in Baltimore and makes a complaint. Even if she does, we're only doin' what they tell us to do, right?"

Gina shrugged and licked a last grain of cocaine off her top lip. A white mustache like in the "Got Milk?" commercials. The Nuremberg trials were a long time ago.

"Most of 'em don't complain," Gina said hopefully.

"Most of 'em don't even know what the hell they signed," Jack said. "We gotta sell the insurance to meet our quota. Don't let this lady and her loi-ah make you gun-shy. Are you getting soft or something?"

"No, it's you--" Gina started to say, then stopped. Sexual put-downs would just make Jack more pushy. Gina was still dreaming of the Series Seven test, selling annuities and mutual funds, the whole aura of Wall Street. She didn't need some bogus complaint from a canopy bed.

"I'm gonna write down exactly how the closing went," Gina said.
"You do that."

2. Penny Zade

And here's how it went:

Bertha Watkins never *intended* to come to EmpiFinancial. Where she went was to the enticing showroom of Sicilian Furniture, which was located on 161st Street where Third Avenue wiggles, right in front of the abandoned courthouse. You passed it on the bus -- bedroom sets in fake rooms with mirrored walls -- and you couldn't miss it, especially not with the "E-Z Credit and Lay-Away" banners that flapped in the breeze.

Easy Credit was an attractive come-on in the South Bronx, as anywhere else. (In the second year of the millennium Argentina found out just how low those first free hits can take you, but that's another story.) Bertha Watkins stood looking in through the window until she saw the four-post bed she wanted: carved wood all glazed with varnish, a fluffy pillow and everything except insect netting but you could buy that elsewhere, later, when the bugs got worse when school got out.

The man in Sicilian Furniture -- a real Italian, he -- let her lie down on the bed, bounce around a bit, stare up at the discolored ceiling tiles on which water dripped until the roof was fixed.

"Tell me 'bout the easy credit," Bertha said, still bouncing.

"It's through a major bank," the man said. "EmpiBank -- ever heard of it?"

Of course she had. They ran ads on TV showing thin yuppies, some of them Asian, drinking cappuccinos in SoHo's narrow streets. Or maybe that was Volkswagen -- it was hard to tell the ads apart. They had a new slogan, "Live richly." Like on this four-post bed. "Where do I sign?" Bertha asked. And that's where Gina came in.

"I'll just fax the form up to their branch on 174th--"

"I'll take it there myself," Bertha said. "I want this bed today. I wanna sleep in it tonight." What was the point of E-Z Credit if you had to wait? And how Easy was it, then, if they had to check your credit history?

The Sicilian called EmpiFinancial and Gina answered the phone. "Tell the Cracker we got a live one."

"I'll be right there."

Gina liked to go out and do these deals herself, while the pot was hot, while the borrower was still staring at the trinket of their eye, looking right past the fine print and all the predatory niceties. Gina showed up with her clipboard, didn't disagree when Bertha said, "You're from EmpiBank, right?" Let her think it was a bank. For some reason people assumed that banks wouldn't screw you, at least not as badly as they could. Bank are regulated, right? They're insured by the government. They don't come after you with a baseball bat, don't break thumbs or knees to collect on loans. According to television they help yuppies drink cappuccino and live richly.

Gina used her cell phone to call in to the office, reading off Bertha's social security number digit by digit like some secret code. "Just a fast credit check," Gina told Bertha.

"I pay *my* stuff on time," Bertha said. But she was beginning to wonder if E-Z, in fact, meant Easy.

Bertha was known by Fair Isaac; Bertha was in and in deep with EquiFax. If Gina had wanted, she could have known everything that Bertha'd ever bought. But that wasn't the point. Bertha Watkins had a FICO score of 685: mainstream by any measure, "excellent" in Empi's matrix. At any conforming lender, the lady could get a mortgage at six percent, in the post-September 11 economic downturn. She'd pay twenty-five percent interest on this bed. You want Easy? You want to bounce on the four-poster tonight? You live in the South Bronx? You're gonna pay. And then there was the insurance.

Gina closed her eyes and tried to remember what if anything had been said about insurance. She hadn't used the word. "You'll want protection, of course" -- that's how she'd said it.

Bertha was lying back on the bed, watching the uncomfortable suckers on the BX 55 bus driving by. "Protection for what?" Bertha asked. Perhaps she meant "from what."

"In case something happens, you get sick or disabled or... whatever. God forbid." Gina liked to use religion with these people.

She didn't just mean "minorities" -- that's what she called them -- but even the white folks in the Bronx. Most of the people of pallor here were Catholic: Irish or Italian. There were Jews too, of course. The Bronx was or had been famous for that. But they weren't buying mobster furniture.

Bertha didn't answer.

"It's just pennies a day," Gina continued with her pitch. "You won't have to pay anything, not anything at all, today. It'll just be part of the loan. And the bed will be in your apartment before the sun goes down."

That closed the deal. The Sicilian was nodding too. He had three undocumented Mexicans out in the one-ton truck, ready to deliver this termite-fodder to anywhere in a ten-mile radius.

"Tonight," he said. "You'll be on that bed." He wondered, with who?

"It's a walk-up," Bertha was saying as she signed the contract.

"We're used to it," Mister Sicily said.

"Hey this is almost five thousand bucks," Bertha said, looking up. "In the window it says nine ninety-nine--"

"That's without the mattress and stuff," Sicily said.

And without the insurance and finance charges, Gina thought.

Somewhere Micah Levine was thinking:bait and switch. Actually Micah was picking a jury on 161st Street and the Grand Concourse, just eight blocks west, in the case of a baby whose forehead was pierced with forceps by a Filipino doctor-trainee who'd worked forty hours straight -- but that's another story.

Bertha'd already signed the form; Gina was reaching to take her clipboard back.

"You should change that sign, then," Bertha said.

Mister Sicily didn't answer. He and Gina exchanged a wink.

"I want it tonight like you told me," Bertha said as she went out the door.

Oh I'll give it to you, Sicily thought. Gina was already thinking about the next deal. If her numbers were good enough maybe they'd let her take the Series Seven even faster than they'd promised at the Courtyard by Marriott.

* * *

And here's the part that neither Gina nor Jack had been able to see:

Bertha Watkins had three kids now but she'd used to have four. Actually she was never sure how to answer that question, "How many kids do you have?" She'd *had* four: four live infants had come out of her womb, the first three the normal way then the last by vicious C-section named after some Roman following which she'd tied her tubes. And they'd been beautiful babies, all of them, but especially the last one, her daughter Penny. Duwon and Shaniqua and Starquaisha loved her too, their baby sister, with the pink elastics they called "thingies" tying her hair into pig tails, beating on her stroller's table. "Juice, mamma," she'd say and it sounds like "Jews."

Penny was almost three years old when Bertha got her tubes tied. Four was enough, and Arthur'd died by then, after a lobe-and-a-half of his lung were cut out from smoking Pall Malls every day of his life. Arthur Watkins, the money-makin'-est brother in the Concourse Village Houses. They'd had to move out of those buildings, too, after Arthur died. They were like a co-op, the maintenance didn't go down even when your income did. Bertha fled the free market to a City-owned building on 149th and St. Ann's, crack vials in the stairwell but only two fifty-nine a month, exactly one third of her SSI check. That's where Bertha headed from Sicilian Furniture, and it's where the bed would be heading tonight, to apartment 4B with its panoramic view of the youth prison and the new auto parts store.

Her three oldest kids all started at P.S. 277, a block south on St. Ann's, some Spanish name over the door but they all liked their teachers. St. Mary's Park was right across the street and Bertha could keep her nightgown on, under a raincoat, when she walked 'em to school, get the lady across the hall, Mrs. Morales, to watch Penny for her. She'd given her first three children African-style names, New Afrikan, Nouveau Afrikans, just as Arthur's wanted it. Arthur Watkins sounded like an accountant from London -- his parents down in Tennessee had wanted to give him that leg up in life. "They'll never know you're black," they told Arthur when he signed up for the Army. "When you get back and you apply for a job, or for a mortgage or whatever, they'll never know you're black from your name and you'll do better." When Arthur was in the Army he kept thinking they'd send him to Iran to free those white ambassadors, those "America Held Hostage Day 421" people, but it never happened. He did push-ups and shot pool at a series of Army bases and then came back to Knoxville, having acquired an unfortunate taste for horse which they hardly even had in his hick hometown and so he'd come to New York and got a job with the MTA. It had a different name back then, "Surface Transit" -- whatever they called it, he was a bus driver and he made damn good money. When he met Bertha at the club on 149 and Walton he fell in love and his first son was conceived. He'd had enough of taking on the white man's names and so he called the kid Duwon; he looked like a boxer in his double-thickness pampers, like a young Joe Frazier. "*Smokin'* Joe!" Arthur'd say, taking Duwon at five up to the park by Yankee Stadium for "road work," some slow jogging once around the cinder track. Then two daughters in a row -- two more African names -- and then the last one, their miracle girl, that Bertha'd insisted on calling Penny, after some damn movie she'd seen. Arthur insisted that she at least have a neo-African middle name: they'd chosen Zade, pronounced Zah-day like that sultry Nigerian singer Sade. And then for Arthur the coughing up of blood, the bored doctors in Lincoln Hospital, morphine like the horse from his Army days and then darkness.

They say tragedies come in threes. Arthur's one-and-a-half lung-lobes were enough for Bertha but like they said in old newsreels on PBS, time marches on. Through the MTA Arthur had not only health insurance but also death insurance, a death benefit to be used for a grave-plot and ceremony. "Any religion you want," they'd told her and so she'd listened to that "dust to dust" and "he was a family man" from an oily Spanish priest she barely knew, the fancy black car like the Mayor's driving through the rain all the way out to St. Raymond's Cemetery, by the highway by the Throgs Neck Bridge just before you'd get to Queens. The people from Concourse Village had given her three baskets of fruit, as if when your husband died all you'd want was a banana and some fuzzless peaches. They'd been nice at Concourse Village but there was no way she could afford to live there anymore.

Two months after they moved to 149th Street Penny got sick. She was only four so she couldn't quite describe what was wrong, if she even knew. Bertha thought it was a cold. She boiled water tinged with Vicks Vap-o-rub and held Penny up over it, breathing the green air into her lungs and it seemed to be working. And then one night when Bertha was watching a rerun of In Living Color on Channel 11 the WB, Penny rolled out of bed and onto the floor and her eyes wouldn't close and she gurgled and choked and Bertha's mind froze.

"Get up!" Bertha yelled to Duwon, poking him in the side, up on his top bunk in his boxer shorts with his poster of Tyra Banks. "Your sister's sick!"

Duwon jumped down from his bunk and looked at Penny. His face went flat. "Call the ambulance momma" he said and she did, dialing

9-1-1 and screaming at the monotone operator who kept asking about symptoms when there was no time to waste, no time at all, Time-as-she'd-known-it was ending. Finally Bertha ran down the stairs with Penny in her arms, out onto 149th Street flagging down a gypsy cab without even the plastic divider, unlicensed, driving the five blocks west to Lincoln Hospital. She tried to pay him but he wouldn't take money. He drove away after he dropped her. Maybe he didn't want to be part of a police report, maybe he was a good Samaritan. His car smelled of pimp oil and had a cardboard evergreen swinging from the rear view mirror that Bertha could still remember. There were bums sleeping in the Lincoln Hospital waiting room but they showed her right in, through the swinging doors with Penny in her arms -- Penny who had not breathed for ten minutes now, Penny who was frozen, looking more and more like a doll, eternal. Finally they pried Penny out of Bertha's grasp and put her on a raised-up cot behind a curtain but Bertha could still see: they tried two charges of electricity but that was it, they pronounced her dead.

The minutes and hours and days and weeks that followed Bertha no longer remembered or wanted to remember.

A month-and-a-half later she got a call from Micah Levine -- he trolled the death records of Lincoln, especially for kids, and made his cold calls himself. "You may have been a victim," he began. "Your daughter, I mean. And sorry for your loss. But Lincoln Hospital is on the state's watch-list for malpractice and negligence -- a woman was given the wrong medicine just last week, and a guy had an operation and the doctor left his Macintosh iPod right inside him -- so I'll like to come by and discuss your case, or to see if you have a case, whenever it might be most convenient for you."

What's an iPod, Bertha wondered, after her first wave of disgust at this ambulance-chaser had died down. "I'll come to your office," she finally said. Duwon came with her; the girls stayed at home with Mrs. Morales drawing pictures.

Micah was a white man but hardly albaster: he had dark hair, lots of it, and could pass for Hispanic. "This is your son?" Micah asked, thrusting out his hand so his suit-sleeve pulled back showing a wrist with some hair and a thick gold bracelet. Duwon'd already learned that you called this cheddar, this gold false or real, this metal you managed to grab with a gun or a law license.

Bertha nodded and waited. She told her story for the umpteenth time, she signed a form so that Micah could review Penny's medical file.

"Maybe we can sue Vicks" was all that Micah came up with. He said he had a whole library on Lincoln's negligence but since Penny'd been dead on arrival, and since you couldn't sue the ambulance since she'd taken a gypsy cab, their only case if they had one was against the manufacturers of Vap-o-Rub.

"Screw it," Bertha finally said. Some things were fate, you just had to live with them. But despite herself she'd gotten to like Micah. He was a greedy bastard but he did nice things for no apparent reason, like bringing Duwon a baseball glove and taking him to sit in the bleachers at Yankee Stadium, even after they'd decided that she had no case. Maybe he was interested in her, Bertha thought, laughing at the idea of this mousse haired Jew climbing the dirty stairwell with fresh-cut flowers from the Mexican's shopping cart down in the Hub. Maybe he liked her like that. He didn't seem to know what he was doing, and she wasn't in the mood, not in this lifetime, for real romance at this point but he'd become a friend and a bit something more. And so Bertha called him about the bed, about the contract she'd signed as she bounced there on it; he promised to come by and take a look at her copy of the loan documents, he'd bring a new DVD video game for Duwon, too, and probably his circumcised penis, his curved Sim-City with Peyronie's syndrome in his sharp-creased loose-fit Italian pants.

There's a beer from Italy called Peroni -- Micah knew this but Bertha didn't, and Bertha didn't care.

Actually they hadn't *given* her a copy of the contract, there in Sicilian Furniture -- Gina took both copies with her, on her clipboard. But when the delivery arrived, Bertha refused to accept it until she got a copy. And so they gave her one. After the bed was in place (she watched the Mexican carry her old mattress down to the sidewalk, then throw it on the vacant lot next door, rev their truck north over pot-holed St. Ann's), Micah arrived. He played three games of Sim City with Duwon on the WebTV. Bertha always sent her daughter next door to Mrs. Morales' when Micah came; she didn't need those confusions, about whom he was coming to see. There was perverts of every race, of course, but the white man seemed sicker than any other. Finally Micah sat down and read the fine print, sipping from time to time the Peroni beer he'd brought with him.

"This was a bait and switch," he muttered. "Unfair and deceptive practices act, Truth in Lending--"

"You sayin' I don't got to pay?"

"You shouldn't have to pay *this* much," Micah said. "Especially the insurance -- they charged you the whole premium up front, you know that?"

"What's that mean?"

"They're charging you interest on money you don't even owe them yet," Micah said. "It'd be like you decide to pay Con Ed for your electricity bill for next year, except you don't actually pay them -- they charge you now, and charge you interest, all the way until you actually use the lights you've already been paying for."

"So what'do I do?"

"Tell 'em cancel the insurance."

Duwon threw down the joy-stick of the WebTV.

"What'd I tell you about that?" Bertha demanded. But by then Micah had already picked it up, and he and Duwon proceeded to play three more games while Bertha put the sheets and blankets on her new four-poster bed and Micah dreamed, perhaps, of bouncing on it but got scared for his car and so he left.

"I think he like you," Duwon said and watched to see his mother's reaction.

Bertha scoffed and told him to go wash up then go to bed. They'd brought the bunk bed with them from Concourse Village, despite the bad karma. But tonight the girls would sleep with their mother in the four-poster bed. Penny Zade would have fit, too.

3. Elizabeth or the Apocalypse

In Midtown Tom Bain watched or played at watching the Bloomberg machine because that was his job. He was a stock analyst whose beat was the euphemistically-named field of "specialty finance," otherwise known as subprime lending or, less politely, loan-sharking. Bain tracked publicly-traded loan sharks and issued research reports on their future prospects under different interest-rate scenarios. Bain had concluded that the Federal Reserve's interest rate moves had little impact on the loan-sharking field. The customers were not, the catch-phrase went, "interest rate sensitive." In his off-hours Bain didn't attend to the Wall Street niceties: the subprime customers were desperate, or ignorant; in any event, they didn't rush out to refinance when the Fed lowered rates, as it did after the September 2001 plane-bombing of the World Trade Center. Bain had used to work there, across the street from the Towers in Seven World Trade.

The building didn't get hit by a plane but it collapsed nonetheless. By then Bain was in his studio apartment in Battery Park City, watching the chaos and breathing the dust. He drank three six packs of beer that day, and now had gone back to smoking pot, taking crystal meth and ecstasy, partying away the few hours he was not glued to his Bloomberg screen. He could get married later. The women he'd met in business school were a bunch of infertile sharks; the bimbos in the Wall Street bars, the so-called networking parties, cared more about your stock options than your dick size, much less your sense of humor.

Bain would take them out to fancy dinners -- Windows on the World had used to be his trump card, leading to the full Greek sodomy sixty-nine, just like blow-dried Mister Trump must get -- but he hadn't found a marriage prospect in this way and didn't expect to. He was sowing his wild oats although he was now thirty-six and was starting to lose his hair, *a little light on top* he'd whisper as he leaned down in front of a mirror. Other than that he was a healthy specimen: smooth-skinned and moussed in his striped Oxford shirts, he was a hunting machine and he aimed to maintain it. He checked the stock price of the maker of Rogaine from time to time but held off from buying it. To order the stuff, even over the 'Net, would be conceding too much.

He thought about his girlfriend from college, Elizabeth Bullard, who hadn't cared about money at all -- she read Emily Dickinson for fun, for God's sake. She'd gotten married then divorced and now lived in Greenwich, Connecticut. Once a week or so Tom thought about calling her and trying to revive things. But it was probably too late. He was at the tail end of being a young Turk and it was already too late.

Sometimes Tom took crystal meth at lunchtime. Maybe Al Qaeda would blow the whole thing up, the whole island or the whole country, and none of it would matter anymore. For now he analyzed EmpiFinancial's tracking stock, breaking out its fundamentals from those of its EmpiGroup parent, and issued reports touting its business model as positively Darwinistic. Elizabeth would have liked that phrasing. And so again he thought of calling her. Anything to avoid ending again at midnight standing naked in front of the plate glass window of his living room waiting for Al Qaeda's planes to give his life meaning.

This afternoon, though, he couldn't get naked, couldn't take drugs, had to put on his tie and squint his eyes like any other Midtown wolf. Empi's chairman Sandaford Vyle was presenting, as they called it, at the Securities Industry Association's 21st Annual conglomerates conference. They'd be a Q&A and Bain was expected to ask a question about EmpiFinancial, whether the same model could work equally overseas as it did in the United States. Maybe Bain would get to take a trip to kick the tires of Empi's 200 percent interest rate loans on bicycles in India. Bain traveled three or four times a month, always first class. Since "The Event," he'd gone to Birmingham, Alabama, to spot-check AmSouth Bank's home equity loan portfolio and meet -- which meant drink with -- its risk-management staff. He'd gone to Charlotte, North Carolina, where he snorted six lines of coke in an absurd skyscraper with a guy who issued lines of credit to payday lenders. He'd interviewed a wannabe loan-shark in Cincinnati, who spent half his time ranting about riots and ingrates and Over-the-Rhine. Pittsburgh, where you could smoke in the airport and the steel industry had apparently entirely disappeared. His next step was Southern California, where many loan sharks liked to put their headquarters, million dollar *faux* Mediterranean villas with home-offices with maps full of pushpins on the wall. Maybe he'd do some surfing, in the three-foot waves of Laguna Beach. But now he had to mock-grill Sandy Vyle, issue a glowing report and then get high.

Since the collapse of Seven World Trade Bain had been working out of temporary digs in one of the dozen faceless office blocks on Park Avenue north of Grand Central Station. The street was wide and filled with well-tailored despair. The SIA conference was in the amphitheater of the building that used to be Bankers Trust, before BT got taken over and most key functions moved to Frankfurt. Globalization cut both ways -- witness EmpiGroup's tax-dodge shift to Anguilla. Sandy Vyle spent three months a year down there, getting as sun-burnt as a blood-red beach ball. He must have just returned, because up on the stage, standing alone at the podium with a white wall behind him, he looked to be on fire. Vyle wore a bright yellow tie and one half-expected him to pull a tropical drink out from under the podium, a daiquiri with a turquoise paper umbrella, some houseboys and a native girl physical therapist. Vyle was bioviating about EBIDA -- Earnings Before Interest, Depreciation and Amortization -- as Bain walked in. Tax wasn't mentioned; taxes had been evaded a long time ago. Bain hadn't missed much. He found a seat near the front and loosened his tie so he could speak when the moment came.

Vile as yet had no successor. He thought he would live forever and perhaps that had been arranged down on Anguilla. Perhaps he was video-taping corporate pep-talks for the next decade, doing an as-told-to memoir with some sycophant journalist, buying spare organs in Chile and keeping them on ice. In business school, Vyle was all that Bain had wanted to be. He was a case study: the hard-charging Brooklyn-born hard-lender who now ruled Wall Street from a tropical tax haven. Now Bain no longer knew what he wanted to be when he grew up -- he'd have a pension by then, an investment secured against all but a dozen Al Qaeda attacks. He'd worked on a boat once, the summer between his freshman and sophomore years, before he met Elizabeth, and he supposed he could do it again if Al Qaeda destroyed his nest egg's value.

Vile was racing through the consumer finance numbers. Delinquency rates had been stemmed, Vyle said, and more and more sales finance contracts were being converted into home equity loans, the hammer of the threat of foreclosure, the very definition of having them by the balls. Bain jotted down the phrase about sale finance conversions -- *that*, he would ask about. He'd seen the term in Empi's Form 10Q's but had never been sure what it meant.

When the Q&A came, Bain asked the question. Some in the audience laughed, that the supposedly-expert analyst didn't know this basic scam.

"I'm glad you asked, Tom," Vyle said, smiling hearty and false. Vyle had a photographic memory for the stock analysts who covered Empi: he knew where they lived, and you knew what that meant. "These are, you know, private label cards, loans made through retailers, all at twenty-plus-percent interest but what's *most* promising is our demonstrated ability to convert these loans into liens, to lower the rates slightly in exchange for a mortgage on the borrower's house." Vyle smiled contendedly. He was still a walking, or limping, encyclopedia of consumer finance terminology. EmpiFinancial had been his first business. He'd bought it near bankruptcy for a song and used it as his base to build his empire. Vyle was sure he could still sell a loan, glazed with credit insurance like gravy, at any of EmpiFinancial's two thousand storefronts from coast to coast. "Crazy Sandy," he could see it now: "No money? No problem! Only pennies a day!" The phrase had been his invention. He should have trademarked it like that basketball coach who now owned the phrase Three-Peat™ for the next forty years.

Bain's face was turning red; he regretted now asking such a rudimentary question in this public forum. So he tried to make it seem like a set-up: "But how can you include in next year's projections this same rate of conversion? With the economic slow-down eventually the pool of home equity will be--"

"It's all explained in the footnotes," Vyle cut in. "We've stress-tested our model under more than sixty-four scenarios. I'd happy to speak with you off-line, Tom."

"That'd be--"

But Vyle had already pointed to the next questioner. And soon Bain would be high and naked, waiting for Elizabeth or the Apocalypse.

* * *

Seated in the front row but not on the stage at the SIA slam-jam was Robert Rudehart, ex-Secretary of the Treasury, emaciated New Democrat extraordinaire, the public face for Empi's vicious lending. He'd helped get Clinton elected, by timely expressing Wall Street's confidence in the corn dog's genius. He'd lent to Asia and screwed it all up then run away and been on the cover of Time. Now he got paid more then Jason Giambi to use his government connections to cover Empi's ass. Soon he could write a book like Jack Welch, if he wanted. But for what? Words could only tarnish his sage reputation. George Soros was a billionaire who hawked his books in Barnes & Noble -- Rudehart didn't need it. Maybe Soros felt guilty. If so he should go lie on a bed of nails, Rudehart thought. Rudehart drank Cristal with rappers in the trendiest spots of asbestos SoHo, getting-off on the smell of so much lithe young flesh right there for the taking, but not needed -- only the gym, only the StairMaster, only the live-forever shakes of ginseng and lemon grass.

The red-faced analyst made Rudehart laugh. Who was _he_, to question Sandy Vyle? They play-acted accountability, these Q&As for wannabe MBAs, but everyone knew what the analysts would write. The business model was perfect and the stock was a buy, a strong buy, like ambrosia heroin you had to have it in your portfolio or you'd die. The red-faced analyst looked like he was going to puke and this, Rudehart liked. Rudehart was down to three percent body fat, from a mixture of tofu and Tai-Bo. He could get Billy Blanks to train him and he could probably get Billy Blanks to do other tricks for him, if he wanted to. Everybody had his price. Even Rudehart, the best-paid showdog on The Street.

* * *

Bain stumbled toward the door, some sour bile at the base of his throat. In the foyer he ran into a colleague, Steve Silvestri from Bear Stearns' mortgage desk. Steve the Sleaze they called him, for the way he accepted numbers at face value for an extra tip under the table. Steve had praised Mercury Finance right to the end; he'd called Conseco - Green Tree a home run, until the CFO was indicted and the stock tanked.

"Bain, you look sick," Steve the Sleaze said, not a bit concerned.

"Yeah I'll catch you later Sleazer -- I feel like I'm gonna boot."

"Cognac for breakfast'll do that... What the hell were you *thinking*, in there?"

"It's our job to ask questions."

"It's our job to *read* -- yeah, even the footnotes -- before we ask questions. You're losin' your touch, Bain."

"I'm losin' my *lunch*." But he hadn't eaten any, so transfixed had he been by his Bloomberg and his thoughts of Liz and Emily Dickinson, a lesbian two-way across the ages complete with javelin, some black-and-white collective memory the photographs of which were probably copyrighted and the user-fees securitized, the structure deemed bullet-proof and timeless by the trained paid eye of Steve the Sleaze.

"See you in Malibu?" Sleazer asked. That was the subprime conference they'd all been invited to.

"Have surf board and condoms, will travel," Bain said, rushing past Steve and out onto Park Avenue.

4. Money-makin' Micah

From the West Farms Mall Bertha Watkins took the Two Train south past the ticky-tacky houses of Freeman Street, the crazy corner on Simpson where you're two feet away from the judo loft, then the old vaudeville theater on Prospect that was now a discount store, underground after Jackson Avenue and off she got at 149th Street. They were tearing up the intersection of The Hub, where Third and Melrose Avenues meet; all the traffic was rerouted, so Bertha could walk in the middle of the street up the hill to Courtlandt, down the hill again to Morris. Micah's storefront was as blinking as ever. Through the vertical venetian blinds she could see Micah, leaning back in his puffy expensive chair. Across the desk from him was a man in blue workman's clothes with his arm in a sling.

"Mister Levine is meeting with a client," Micah's secretary told her. She probably didn't know that they were friends, actually friends, that she wasn't just another longshot client trying to make money off a dead kid. Fine. She waited.

Finally Micah came out, shaking the workman's unslinged hand. "I'll write them a demand letter," Micah told him. "If they won't settle we'll sue their asses off... Oh, Bertha, I didn't expect--"

"They wouldn't cancel nothing. The guy said it was totally legal, I just have to pay. Cracker guy they got running the office. Like loans from the Klan if ya axe me."

"Did you tell them you have counsel?"

Bertha laughed. "Yeah. The guy axed how much you're chargin' me."

Micah glanced over at his secretary, then gestured for Bertha to come into his office. Then he stopped. "Let's go get something to eat." Bertha followed him out onto the sidewalk. An ambulance went screaming by, pulling into the driveway of Lincoln Hospital. "We can drive up to Arthur Avenue," Micah said. "Maybe we'll drive by these loan sharks' office and put the fear of God into 'em."

Micah left his BMW parked in the municipal lot between Morris and Courtlandt. He paid the attendant extra to keep an eye on it. Some might call it extortion but Micah called it smart. He got the best cases because he was right across from Lincoln's slaughterhouse. You wanna catch grouse you gotta get in the swamp. A hundred a week to keep his car unscathed was worth it.

They drove up Morris, behind the Melrose and Jackson Houses, turned east on 161st Street. Micah turned on his CD player. He was still listening to Steely Dan's Two Against Nature: it reminded him of his early twenties, of being the coolest guy in his law school class, getting high and acing torts. They'd called him The Snake for at least two reasons. The lyrics on this one were all about middle age despair but he could ignore them and just sing along.

Bertha thought the music was fruity. Not fruity like a wine, or like the mango Italian ice the Mexicans sold on rolling carts, but fruity like homo, pseudo-pop high-pitched voices: white man's music.

"Duwon's gettin' into trouble with his English teacher," Bertha said. Micah put the CD on pause; he wanted to hear that song again, Janie Runaway, he liked it.

"What kind of trouble?"

"She says he didn't do a paper but he says he did. She don't like nothing that he writes. Says it's too raw. Least that what Duwon tells me."

"Nothing wrong with raw," Micah said, thinking that might make a good lyric beginning. "Nothing wrong with raw at all."

Bertha was waiting for something more than that.

"Maybe you should go in and talk to the teacher," Micah said. "Don't they have a PTA or something?"

"That won't do no good. That's just some political shit, to collect ballots for the school boards. Nah, those teachers don't stay in the school not one more minute than they got to. Two forty five they're pullin' out in their cars, down to the Bruckner and they're gone."

Micah didn't respond. Even if it wasn't what Bertha meant, he felt implicated in this view of white professionals in The Bronx. They come in to make money then they leave. Probably like the guy Bertha called the Cracker, up at EmpiFinancial; like most of the doctors in Lincoln; like most of the lawyers whose storefronts encircled the hospital; like the police captains who surveilled the whole chaos keeping score. Micah wanted to turn the music back on but resisted the impulse. "They must have parent - teacher nights," he finally said.

"Yeah I'll look into it. It's up here, in the new mall."

Micah turned east on 174th Street, then left across traffic into the mall's parking lot. There was EmpiGroup's red logo; two storefronts down was a Rent-A-Center, its window filled with sofas and stereos and a dozen other overpriced, never-to-be-owned things. There was talk of a nationwide class action and Micah wanted a piece.

"That's the guy," Bertha said. The cracker had just come out of the office, like a rat out of his hole, walking toward the three-stand food court at the center of the mall. Bertha rolled down her window.

"Remember me?" she shouted.

Jack turned and looked. The loud-mouthed bitch was in a BMW. Maybe she was the wife or girlfriend -- Christ, maybe the mother -- of a drug dealer, Jack thought. Micah's car had tinted windows, so Jack couldn't see who was in the driver's seat. Maybe this was a drive-by. Maybe *this* was why Empi couldn't get anyone else to run their office in The Bronx. The driver's side door opened and Jack recognized the guy in the flashy suit who got out. Micah-the-Shyster Levine, who ran his ads on Bronx cable television, "Have you been hurt? *Llame* 1-800 Micah-Law."

"This is my loi-ah," Bertha shouted, getting out of the car. Jack was tempted to turn back into his storefront and lock the door. But what was Micah gonna do -- shoot him down with an Uzi like some kind of Israeli mercenary? Like a hijacker in Entebbe, gunned down on the asphalt of a mall instead of an airport?

"I ain't got no fancy law degree," Jack said, directing his exaggerated Bubba-drawl at Micah. "But where I'm from, a deal's a deal."

Micah was in his element now. In his loose-cut suit and his shiny car, he felt like Al Pacino in Scarface. "Ever heard of unconscionable?" Micah asked Jack.

"That's a three dollar word that only the shysters use," Jack said. "We can extend the loan, that's what I told the lady. But you can't just break a deal. You sign, you pay."

"Live richly," Micah muttered. He got mailers all the time from EmpiBank, asking why he as a professional didn't want to consolidate all his accounts and pay his bills online. But they'd give his info to the IRS. So Micah kept most of his money in cash and real estate. Liquid, he called it. Juice.

"I'm putting you on notice," Micah said. "We intend to sue on this loan."

"Good fuckin' luck," Jack said. "Now if you excuse me, I'm gonna go get me one of them three-meat tacos."

But when the moment came, Jack didn't have a stomach for it. He didn't like this fucking Micah but if it was up to him he'd just cancel the insurance. Even without it they'd ripped Bertha good. But the loan had already been entered into EmpiFinancial's proprietary computer system known as Monstro -- Bertha's whole history of debt, the interest-rate points over prime and the terms of the insurance contract. Jack would need approval from above to change anything now, and he'd never get it from Home Office. Even the watered-down hot sauce hurt his gut. The fix was in.

Micah wondered if Bertha was disappointed. He was a lawyer, not a hit-man. The Cracker for all his crackerdom had stood his ground. Now Micah'd actually have to find a cause of action in all the fine print. He'd try the state attorney general first. That guy was always looking for publicity.

* * *

120 Broadway had been covered with dust on September 11 -- probably some DNA in it too, if you thought about it -- but since then it had been steam-cleaned and re-wired with T3 lines. Ernest Swanker spent most of the work-week here; he only went up to Albany when he had to testify to the state legislature, or in the months before the election, to show he was an Up- as well as Downstate guy. He was the up of the down: he was the patrician defender of the downtrodden. He lived in Riverdale in the northern-most Bronx, with a well-coiffed wife and two well-coiffed children who went to Horace Mann and a well-coiffed future, especially with all the money his daddy'd made in real estate. He was a populist crusader -- even Barron's called him that -- whose initial campaigns were funded by a slumlord's rent roll. Well, the Kennedys' were bootleggers, Swanker told himself. At least slumlording was legal.

He even sometimes sued for rent overcharges, just to prove he wasn't in anyone's pocket. He could have been on Wall Street but now he was Wall Street's nightmare, digging into stock analyst conflicts, overvalued shares and misleading 10Ks, stepping into the void left by Bush II's SEC. He was Ernest Swanker and his next stop was Washington, with the *faux*-fur pelts of corporate hides on his walls. A new Teddy Roosevelt. Not as hearty, perhaps, and with no taste for hunting. But he knew a photo-op when he saw one.

Swanker was the type of rich good-looking Democrat who became all the rage when the unions stopped funding the party of the working man. Corzine, Edwards, that guy from Minnesota -- Swanker was right on their heels, not yet tainted by Washington gridlock. A sort of Abe Lincoln -- no one else had made the comparison but Swanker thought about it, studied every extant drawing of the bearded one hunched over his law books -- ready to run, for something, in 2012 or even 2008. He'd had a facelift before his first election and subtly dyed his hair. He'd do more as it became necessary. He was ready.

Swanker was ready when Micah Levine asked for fifteen minutes, to talk about predatory credit insurance. It sounded dry to Swanker -- he appraised each issue as to how it would play in a headline and this one was too long -- but he agreed to meet Micah, in his official NYS van on the way to a talk at a synagogue in Williamsburg, Brooklyn.

"Yo know Al Qaeda was gonna blow this neighborhood up, right?" Swanker asked as they crossed the bridge over the East River.

"But it's mostly Puerto Ricans."

"Except south of Division Street. Then they decided on the World Trade Towers. Go figure." The van descended past Peter Luger's Steakhouse, past warehouses converted into yuppies' artist lofts. "If you're gonna pitch me you better hurry," Swanker said.

"A client of mine -- a friend, really -- showed me a contract for a personal loan she got," Micah began. "It's only $2,500, or five thousand all told--"

"It's not a mortgage?"

"No. It was a loan to buy a bed."

"Some bed."

"It's a four-poster, like with a canopy and all, anyway that's not the point. They charged her credit insurance, two hundred a month and all of it paid upfront."

Swanker whistled. "And what exactly was she insuring?"

"Purportedly" -- Levine talked like a lawyer and Swanker, being one, didn't object to these four-dollar words, inflation was rampant -- "it's so the company wouldn't foreclose on the bed, wouldn't come and repossess it."

"But who'd pay $2,500 for a used bed, even if it had *eight* posts?"

"That's my point. It's bogus insurance that has no benefit to the customer."

"So whatdaya want?" They were pulling onto Division Street and time was short.

"I think they do this all over the place. I mean, Upstate too."

Swanker smirked. Don't push my buttons. Still...

"So if you filed suit, or issued some scathing guidance, I could drum up a class action. We'd both look good--"

"And you'd make money--"

"Hey, I always donate right up to the limit. Even over it sometimes."

That was true. Swanker kept two sets of campaign finance books: one filed in Albany and the other in a safe in 120 Broadway, the code to which was kept in a separate wall safe in Riverdale, the key to which not even Swanker's wife had. Swanker The People's Candidate In Two Thousand and Eight.

"You got the documents?" Swanker asked.

"Right here."

Swanker saw the logo at the top of the contract and groaned. "Empi's not the right target," he said flatly.

Micah had anticipated this, and he had a slogan ready, a challenge. "Anyone can sue the small guys. It takes real balls, and real ambition, to sue the largest."

Yeah and a real political death wish, Swanker thought but didn't say.

"Gimme the copies, I'll think about it," Swanker said. "Now I gotta give a speech about the New Anti-Semitism."

"There's always a new flavor," Micah muttered. Then, louder, "Give 'em hell." He'd call a livery cab and pay forty bucks to get back to 149th Street. It'd probably be worth it. He made his campaign contributions to have access and now he had it. If Ernest Swanker would grow some balls they'd really be rocking. Janie Runaway: he hummed it in the back of the livery cab on the BQE.

5. Beam Me Up

"Diane, I got a *right* to see my daughter, ya know?"

Jack was toying with his cigarette, trying to keep his Kool. Without much success: "Yeah well I fucking *paid* you the child support... If the mail screws up it's not my problem... You know you could work more, right? Like a real *job* -- ever heard of it? Diane? Diane? Fuck!"

Jack slammed the receiver down and the phone fell on the floor. Gina and the rest of them were prairie-dogging, sneaking glances into his office which was really no more than a cubicle. EmpiFinancial believed in the open office plan; it was part of their cookie-cutter corporate culture. Jack could see his loan officers and they could see him. "What the *fuck* are you lookin' at?" Jack screamed at Maye, a trainee who kept forgetting to automatically include insurance in her loans. The policy was no personal calls but fuck it, he was the branch manager. And it wasn't like he was trying to set up a date to get laid. He wanted to see his daughter, that was it. He was getting an ulcer listening to bitches like Bertha Watkins all so he'd earn his bonus, his Rocopoly Money they called it, and be able to take Zalie away from Bubba-land and never bring her back, not ever. Fuck!

Gina had another sucker on the line: a bigger ticket item this time, a home equity loan secured by a two-family house in Tremont. The owners were a Spanish couple, Amado and Milagros Guzman; they'd both come in today for the closing. The wife looked to be in her late thirties, trim and pretty like a Cherokee squaw, Jack thought. The man looked older and in pain. A $64,000 refinance, consolidating credit card debts and a hospital bill for Amado. The guy said he worked construction but it couldn't be higher than mason tender, given the income he listed. Not in the union, that was for sure. They could have just blown off the hospital, Jack thought, declaring themselves indigent like half of the patients at St. Barnabas Hospital did. But they wanted to pay the bill. This type of rectitude was Empi's bread and butter. Milagros was working at a maid in Riverdale -- damn he'd like to see her in that uniform -- but they didn't list her income. In any case it wasn't enough. Now they were putting their house on the line, and Gina was packing the insurance with her "just pennies a day" sing-song. Jack almost felt sorry for them. But he felt more sorry for himself.

"Okay," Gina said, "the payment is thirteen hundred dollars a month."

"The money, it will be sent to the hospital? They keep sending us letters--"

"Yes Mrs. Guzman, as soon as you sign we'll send them the payoff. You just sign here... and here... and here."

Jack stood watching. Gina said Guzman like Scuz-mun. Not Gooz, that cooze. Jack needed booze. Neither Guzman read the documents before signing. Gina kept talking fast, distracting them whenever they looked at any page for too long.

"Your credit cards too, you won't have to worry about them any longer. Just one single payment. You can mail it to us--"

"We will bring it in," Mrs. Guzman said.

"That'll be fine," Gina said, rushing to collect the signed papers from Mr. Guzman. "You've done a smart thing."

Gina escorted them to the door, smiling and waving as she closed it behind them. Then she laughed. "They coulda gotten seven percent from a bank," she said. "FICO score of six-eighty, if you can believe it. Real moral people, pay their debts on time. But we've ripped 'em at fourteen-and-a-half percent."

"You'll go far," Jack said. The business was making him feel sicker than usual. It wasn't just the interest rates -- buyer beware, Jack bought into the whole Roman line that trickled down through Empi from Emperor Sandy -- but he was more and more queasy about the credit insurance. Down in Charlotte he'd tried to stop selling it but they sent down a re-education team. Their first meeting was over burgers and brew and Jack'd been honest, telling them he didn't believe in the product. After a beat they'd responded, "You're not paid to believe in the product -- you're paid to *sell* it!" And so he shut up and internalized the nausea. Or maybe it was just Diane, trying to squeeze an increase in child support out of him in exchange for visitation. A man had to do what a man had to do. "Go file the lien," he told Gina.

"But don't they have three days to pull out of the deal?"

"They won't," Jack said. "Go file it then take the rest of the day off. You earned it."

"I got a few prospects to visit anyway," Gina said.

"You wanna be a branch manager or something?" Jack asked. "You tryin' to replace me?"

"Oh, I'm aiming higher than that," Gina said. And then she went to stake Empi's claim to the Guzmans' house. The law called RESPA had a three day "cooling off" period, in which home mortgage borrowers could cancel a deal. But no one ever did. If they even tried, you just told 'em the lien had already been filed, and they'd still have to pay the appraiser's costs. Offer 'em a refi and rack 'em up for some more fees and points. It never failed. If only it was this easy with Diane.

While Gina was up at the county clerk's office, Jack got a call from his district manager Janet Peel. Janet was a decade older than Gina, not as attractive, no longer dreamed of getting a Series Seven. She wore boring business skirt-and-jacket combos; she had drab blond hair. You might pick her up and fuck her in a motel bar if nothing better came along, and then you might regret it, at least Jack thought. But she oversaw three branches in lower Westchester, two in Queens and this new Bronx operation. Jack'd met her in Baltimore at EmpiFinancial's "Beam Me Up" training, the required indoctrination before they let you run a branch. It was very rah-rah -- watery coffee at dawn, slide shows and break-outs and role-playing in clusters, all the jargon -- and by the end Jack wondered if this was a company or a cult. Religions held out visions of an after-life; with EmpiFinancial the rewards offered were all right here. Bonuses, stock options whose value went only up as Empi marched toward world domination. All of it fueled by ripping the customer for interest-rate points and useless insurance.

Of course the trainer didn't phrase it that way. The Customer is King, one of his PowerPoint slides said. *Yeah*, Jack thought -- like the idiot king in a Shakespeare play he read at SUNY Oswego, he couldn't remember the name any longer. At Empi's Baltimore corporate campus they made them all read and discuss a business management book full of pithy sayings like big hairy goals and the "tyranny of OR," as in either / or. Jack'd been high and had the clap when his SUNY class covered Kierkegaard, but he still remembered that title, *Enten Eller*, Either / Or. Empi eschewed such choices, saying you could always have both. You could still be moral while screwing-over the customer; you could make loans you *knew* couldn't be paid back yet still be safe-and-sound. Whatever. The moment you stopped believing, your career with Empi was over. And for Jack that moment approached.

"I got a call from home office," Janet told him. The pin heads in Baltimore. "They say the state A.G. is nosing around, asking about credit insurance." Jack waited. What did this have to do with him? "They asked about a loan you made, personal loan for five thousand, a Bertha Watkins. You know the one I'm talking about?"

"Bitch with a lawyer," Jack said. "Sorry -- lady with a lawyer. Don't worry. She signed. It's no problem." He paused. "Look, I was almost tempted to cancel the insurance. We're making enough money on that loan anyway. So if you gimme the okay to cancel it, there'll be no issue, right?"

Janet had heard this about Jack, had caught glimpses of it too: that he was a pussy when it came to putting and keeping the screws on the customer. There was a note in his confidential file on Monstro that he'd questioned credit insurance. Within EmpiFinancial this was heresy; it was not an honest mistake but a sin. A single rotten apple can spoil the whole barrel. Light the faggots.

"Don't cancel it," Janet said. "Home office is just gonna come up and do an audit."

Jack lit another cigarette, exhaled long, counted to three. He thought back to the show-down in the parking lot, that Micah Fucking Levine calling him out on the asphalt. He thought of the Come-to-Jesus meeting in that bar in Charlotte: you're paid to sell the shit, not believe in it. "The loan's perfectly good," Jack said, more to himself than to Janet. Now he wished he hadn't sent Gina up to file the lien before the three day waiting period ran. It was a bullshit violation, but the kind they could use against you. He wanted to call Gina on her cell phone, try to reach her before she filed the thing. "Look, I got someone in the office, I'll call you back."

"Audit starts tomorrow," Janet said. "Don't make me look bad. And do *not* --" she pauses for emphasis -- "cancel the credit insurance." Then she hung up.

The phone rang and rang and rang. Fucking Gina'd left her cell phone in her car. Jack had half a mind to drive up to the county clerk's, catch her while she waited in line. But fuck it. They'd be auditing him for personal loans, anyway, not real estate. And the violation, even if they found it, had nothing to do with Bertha Watkins' complaint. That fucking Micah was trying to bust his balls, and Janet was playing right along with him, trying to cover her ass. It was a regular anatomy lesson. But he'd come out of it standing tall, Jack told himself. If worse came to worst he'd blame it on Gina. It'd serve the uppity bitch right anyway.

* * *

Jack Bender sat in his Ford Taurus on Olinville Avenue drinking his third forty-ounce Olde English of the night. He didn't want to go upstairs and sit in his apartment alone. If he didn't watch himself he'd called Diane again and yell and then he'd never see Zalie. Any threat he made would show up in an affidavit, "termination of parental rights," whatever they called it. So he drank beer, this pseudo-medieval brand he'd taken a liking to since moving to The Bronx, and thought about the audit that would start tomorrow. He kept his shit in order. Of course, they could always find something, if they wanted to screw you. He started the car, drove down to Pelham Parkway, through the Zoo and south again on Southern Boulevard. Maybe he'd go into the office, make sure things were shipshape, shred what he could. EmpiFinancial made sure that every office had a shredder -- that too was a part of their corporate culture. Any loan document you were going to throw out, even a draft, should be shredded they told you. In practice no one did it. But the machine would come in handy now, on the night before the audit.

Jack pulled into the parking lot of the West Farms Mall. The lights in EmpiFinancial were off as they should be. Rent-A-Center was still open; there was an employee inside talking to a woman over the counter. Jack laughed. Rent-A-Center was one step below EmpiFinancial: people would rent a couch or a television set, pay more in five months that the Goddamn thing was worth and they still wouldn't own it. The mangers might extract "couch payment" -- they'd ask customers to sleep with them, to forget a month's rent on the VCR. You came in for household comforts and you left as a prostitute, a comfort woman. If it was in you...

The thought distracted Jack and he didn't even turn off the car. He pulled out again, heading east this time on 174th Street, over to Boone Avenue, an industrial street by the Bronx River. Sometimes there were whores here, real whores. If not he could go to Hunts Point. In the aftermath of Nine Eleven, a woman near here died of anthrax; the streets were full for two days with government men in astronaut suits. Then nothing. Jack cruised slowly down Boone until he saw a cluster of high-heeled women on the corner of Jennings Street. Jack rolled down his window and pulled to a stop. The cluster turned out to be three women, only one of whom was looking at his car. Young-looking woman, white she seemed, under the street light.

"You wanna go out?" she called over to him. He smiled, screwing the cap back on his forty. She came closer. Not bad-looking. Not bad at all. Jack didn't usually have to pay for it but The Bronx was different and tonight was an exception. He needed to cool his nerves before the audit tomorrow. So why not?

"Forty dollars the whole thing," the woman said. Jack was opening the passenger's side door. He didn't like to talk business in the street. "Get in," he said.

"Yes or no," the woman said. "Forty bucks. I don't got time to waste."

"Sounds okay," Jack said. The woman was still at his window, not crossing to the car's other side.

"It's in advance," she said.

Jack had never seen this protocol and he was beginning to get second thoughts. But three fourties of beer and the thought of couch payments had fogged his mind. "Cash on the barrel," he muttered, opening his wallet, counting out a twenty and two tens.

When he looked up, there were three figures at his window. All women, but two of them had something shiny in their hands. A gun, he thought, dropping the money to his knees and putting the gear in "Drive." They were trying to car-jack The Cracker.

"Stop!" a woman yells. "Get out of the car with your hands up!"

What the fuck? Then Jack saw what the other woman was holding. A police badge. He thought of ramming the car forward anyway but didn't want to die. "Alright, alright," he slobbered. He turned off the car and stepped out, blinded by a bright light. And then he got his disclosure: "you have the right to remain silent," the bitch told him. "If you cannot afford a lawyer one will be appointed to represent you. Anything you say can and will--"

"I get it," Jack said. He watched TV. This Miranda bullshit was like the fine-print consumer disclosures in the loans Empi made. Boilerplate words whose subtext was "you're fucked, you've fucked up, the recitation of this mantra is proof that this rape is voluntary." Jack stared at his wrists and the handcuffs as they drove his car away.

* * *

In the lock-up at the 48th precinct Jack had time to read-up on Operation Losing Proposition. The Billionaire Mayor was cracking down on quality of life crimes, like his helmet-haired Republican predecessor. They took your car and put you through the system; they published your name in the newspapers if they could. Name and shame. But Jack had a problem: the audit started tomorrow.

"Look I gotta get out here," he called out through the bars to the cop dozing on a chair outside the cell. "I'm serious, I got a big fucking problem at work tomorrow and--"

"Shoulda thought a that 'fore you went cruising for whores," the cops said. "Now shut the fuck up or I'll put you in the other cell."

With the animals, the implication was. Jack wondered who he could call. Not Gina, no way, not her. Not Diane -- it's just be more ammo against him in the child custody case. He'd just have to wait it out, hope the audit went okay in his absence. What would they say when he didn't show up? He'd leave them a message that he was sick. Or that he had a family emergency down in North Carolina. Maybe they'd never find out. He cursed Micah Fucking Levine, and Gina for fucking Bertha Watkins so bad. He'd have to pay six hundred bucks to get his Taurus back. Just pennies a day, if you looked at it that way.

6. The Axe Must Fall

Nicole Nour was writing the stock market round-up, in the Journal's temporary office on Avenue of the Americas. They'd been at the World Trade Center, all evacuated fifteen minutes before the first Tower fell. Now they were still in this faceless rent-a-space while Dow Jones shook down the city for rent abatements, threatening to move the newsroom across the Hudson to New Jersey. They'd never do it. How could you be the Wall Street Journal and be based in Exchange Place in Jersey City? But the Mayor had a soft spot for financial news so he was coming through with the tax-free bonds. The Journal'd be almost rent-free for the next decade. *Bisma Allah.*

Nicole Nour was a Muslim herself. An upper-class Egyptian, to be sure. And so not an Arab. Even her hair was uncovered; other than her last name no one would ever know. She'd made up her first name, not from self-hatred she told herself and not even to get ahead, but because she liked it. Her parents -- well, her father -- had named her Nadia, but insisted on calling her Niki. She'd taken this one step further, to Nicole. If she got married and changed her surname too, that'd be that. Nicole Smith: she could pass for an American. Add Ana instead of silicone. It would sure make her waits in the airports more brief. But Nicole still liked her last name and her faith, loved them, actually, now more than ever, and hadn't met any man she'd like to marry. She wanted to become a managing editor. Then maybe, if she was still fertile, she'd have kids. Or maybe not. You couldn't get a promotion writing un-bylined markets round-ups. She needed to write a feature, Page One Above The Fold complete with a pencil-and-ink drawing, something at the cusp of human nature and the securities markets. You had to think these things up yourself. You had to develop sources, then something bad had to happen. For now she had to characterize an eleven point drop in the Hang Seng index overnight. "Careened?" "Slid down?" She'd used those all before. "Decayed," that was *le mot juste.* But the Journal didn't like to link markets and mortality. "Off eleven in heavy trading." That was bland enough. *Al-hamdulilla.*

* * *

Uptown Keith Mudnick, fresh off Amtrak's Acela service from Baltimore, was poring through Jack's files. Each had been entered into Monstro, but the underlying documents, the hard copies, were in the file cabinets behind Jack's desk.

"Where *is* Mister Bender?" Mudnick asked Gina.

"I don't know," Gina said. "He does this sometimes." Actually, he didn't. But Gina wanted his job. It would bring her the Series Seven all the faster.

At lunchtime Janet Peel came in. She'd retouched the blond dye in her hair. "Any problems, Keith?" she asked.

Mudnick didn't look up. He was more interested in Gina than Janet. "There's some things that don't make sense," he said. "I'll probably copy some of the docs and take 'em back to Baltimore."

"You took the train?"

He nodded.

"I'll drive you back to Penn Station when you're done," Janet said. "I can tell you how we've reduced delinquencies in the New Rochelle office."

Great, Mudnick thought. Just the kind of mundane crap he liked to hear about.

* * *

They'd transferred Jack from the 48th precinct down to the Bronx Criminal Court on 161st Street. In the lock-up they were all together: gang bangers, rock-slingers, drunken hobos, pimps and short-eyes. Jack kept his mouth shut and his back against the wall. He'd already smoked or given out all his cigarettes. He hadn't called anyone, so he couldn't post bail. Hopefully they weren't in the mood to fuck Johns this afternoon. He could tell them where he worked -- that he had "ties to the community" and all -- but then that'd go into a file somewhere and they'd call Baltimore, or EmpiGroup downtown. He'd take his lumps, for his idle hunger for a hump. Fuck.

Finally they called him out, into a windowless courtroom no more than twenty-foot square. The judge on the bench was white, looked mean, didn't even look up. "Bender, Jack. Number 21-38-003. Solicitation of prostitution."

In the front row Jack saw the woman who'd offered the date, who'd asked for the forty dollars. She was in a uniform now. At least she *was* good-looking. He didn't have to be ashamed about that on top of everything else.

"No priors," a black woman at a cheap podium said. "It was a one-time thing -- right, Mister Bender?" She was looking at him and then he understood: she was his lawyer. Either Legal Aid or an 18-B, assigned to his arraignment.

"Strictly one time," Jack stammered. "In fact, I wasn't even thinkin' of it, until the lady--"

"That's enough, Mister Bender," the judge said. Now the judge was looking at him. Cold lifeless eyes like planets or marbles. "You offered money for sex, isn't that correct?"

"She asked for it," Jack said, turning to point at the front row.

"Are you saying you're *innocent*?" The judge was smiling, and the black woman was shaking her head at Jack. She leaned over and whispered, "Don't say you're innocent. Then you'll go back into lock up. Just say you did it, you'll probably only have to pay a fine and go to John School."

"Do you need a moment, Ms. Thompson?" the judge asked.

"No, your Honor, I think it'll all in order. My client pleads guilty, with the understanding that--"

"Is that true, Mister Bender? Do you admit offering money for sexual relations with Officer O'Flaherty?"

Jack stood mute. So she was Irish.

"We'd consent to a five hundred dollar fine and probation, your Honor," the black lady said. "He'll also be paying to get his vehicle back."

"Pay to play," the judge said. "Are you agreed, Mister Bender?"

Now Jack nodded. It was all moving so fast.

"Then tell us how it happened," the judge said smiling.

Jack looked at the black lady. "Do I have to?" She nodded. Jack spoke as softly as he could. "I was driving home from-- I was driving and this young lady, she offered--"

"She called you over? Or did you stop your car and--"

Now Jack understood the game. "I stopped the car. It was all me. I don't know what I was thinking. I took forty dollar out of my wallet--"

"Forty dollars for *what*, Mister Bender?" The judge waited.

"For sex," Jack whispered. "I'm sorry, it was for sex." Jack felt like there was a whole audience behind him in this windowless room, a whole Yankee Stadium, Diane with a microphone, Gina and Janet Peel, all of them. His lawyer looked like Bertha Watkins. This was his come-upance, he thought. Screw the poor and they'll screw you right back.

"Okay Mister Bender, it's five hundred dollars and six months probation. If in that period you commit any crime -- misdemeanor, violation, any breach of the peace whatsoever -- you *will* serve time in jail. Do you understand?"

Jack nodded, feeling almost like he was going to cry. He wanted out of here. He wanted his Taurus back. He wanted to see Zalie, drive south all the way into Mexico, find the fountain of youth, anything.

"I can't *hear* you, Mister Bender."

"Yes," Jack said.

"Thirty days to pay or we'll issue a warrant. Next!"

It was already dark when Jack Bender staggered out onto 161st Street. There were cops and crooks lounging around in front of the building smoking. It was Crime and Punishment on Viagra. They did arraignments all night long in The Bronx. The Dunkin' Donuts across the street was still open, but Jack needed something stronger. He went into a bodega on Sheridan and bought a forty-ounce Olde English. Something to take the edge off on the Two Train back up to Olinville Avenue.

The train was already turning the corner at Simpson Street by the judo loft when Jack remembered that he should at least check the office. It was probably already too late. But maybe from the state of the office he'd get an insight into how the audit had gone. Jack got off at the 174th Street station, walked down the urine-smelling stairs and over to the mall. He needed his Taurus back. He did not like riding the subway at night, or even evening, with people staring at him.

The Rent-A-Center was still open -- no surprise there, couch payments were going on apace with no problems from the law, the cops would never run a sting there, the customers had enough of an Operation Losing Proposition as it was. But the light was on in EmpiFinancial too. Jack stood at the glass door and peered in. Gina and Janet Peel were inside -- and they were sitting at *his* desk, making themselves at home in *his* cubicle. A coven of bitches. Jack opened the door with his key and they looked up.

Janet spoke first. "You really screwed up this time, Bender," she said. Gina looked happy.

"Look, I'm sorry, something came up--"

"Don't bother. It's not just that you were missing in action today. Keith Mudnick said he found all kinds of irregularities. He took a lot of files back to Baltimore with him. As of now, I'm running this office."

"Whatdaya mean?"

"You're suspended," Janet said, looking to Jack like a clam, a shell he'd like to crush. Jack felt the effect of the beer. He was suddenly tempted to tip over the file cabinets in the office, to put his fist through the computer screens, reach in and pull the guts out of Monstro's database.

"That's what Mudnick said?" Jack asked.

"Yeah. After he called home office."

Actually, it had been Janet who'd talked Mudnick into authorizing this fast suspension. In the car on the way to Penn Station, while Jack had been waiting to be arraigned, Janet had alluded to a pattern of problems she'd been having with Jack, how they were consistent with the confidential write-up on Monstro.

"He's constantly trying to undermine the line staff," Janet said. "He tells them to go light on insurance, sometimes not to write it at all. I don't know *why* he was made a branch manager."

"He made money in Charlotte," Mudnick said. He'd read his Monstro too. "He was sub-par on insurance, but he made up for it with sales finance conversions. He signed up jewelers and pawn shops -- he would have signed up a liquor store if they'd let him."

"Up here insurance is the only way to make money," Janet said. "With interest rates capped at twenty five percent it's the only way. So if he won't sell the insurance he's going to bring *my* numbers down."

Mudnick didn't care one way or the other. But that the branch manager hadn't even come in to work on the day of the audit was a bad sign. Sign of a bad conscience, or of what the H.R. department called a problem with substance abuse. H.R. didn't like heresy about credit insurance either. Janet floated the idea: "I think we should suspend him."

"Fine," Keith said. "Just document your reasons for the file. We don't want Bender trying to sue us."

"It's mandatory arbitration, right?" Janet asked. "I mean, he couldn't really sue us."

"Whatever. Just cover your ass with paper."

Janet didn't like the phrase but she liked the result. "Remember to tell them how things are going in New Rochelle," she told Mudnick as they approached Penn Station.

"Yeah," Mudnick said. Before the train reached Trenton he'd drunk three beers in the café car and he'd forgotten all about it.

"So you better clean your stuff out," Janet was saying. Gina had moved back to her cubicle; Jack thought he heard her humming.

"This is bullshit," Jack said. "I give up my job down in Charlotte, come to start this two-bit office -- and now I'm fired?"

"Suspended," Janet corrected him. She noticed he said Charlotte like "Shah-lit."

"The guy didn't even finish the audit yet."

"He saw enough. Don't make this ugly. Just pack your stuff. When they finish going through the files they'll call you. Or I will."

"I'm not fucking takin' this lyin' down," Jack said.

"I'll need your keys too," Janet said.

"Yeah, bullshit!" Jack shouted. It was now that he tipped over a file cabinet, then another. It surprised even Janet, who was not without experience with the one-two punch of suspending then firing people. She'd been trained to do this, down at Empi's ashram in Baltimore. So she knew what to say.

"Don't *make* me call the cops," she said. She was hoping that Gina would do just that, dial 911 from her cubicle and get this out-of-control Cracker locked up.

Jack didn't have much in the office. He took his rolodex, and he took some of his loan files for good measure.

"Those are company property," Janet said. But she didn't try to grab 'em. Jack could slap both of 'em silly right here in the office. Take 'em next door to Rent-A-Center and lay 'em out over a couch. Gina first, and Janet sloppy seconds. The bitches. He'd call Baltimore himself, tomorrow.

Jack picked up the cardboard box he'd thrown his shit in and then remembered: he didn't have a car anymore. He'd be a mark on the train, drunk and carrying an open cardboard box. He'd like to ask for a ride but it'd be too pathetic. Fuck 'em. He'd find a gypsy cab out on Southern Boulevard.

As he opened the door, he turned back toward Janet. "You're gonna regret this, you bitch," he said.

Janet smiled, angry now. "Whatever happens," she said slowly, "you'll never work under me again."

"In your dreams," Jack slobbered. "I was *never* under you."

"Good-bye," Janet said with finality, locking the door behind him. He'd like to put his fist through the glass front door, set off the alarm, pour gasoline through before the cops showed up. Oh yeah -- and a match. They were four blocks south of Tremont, where a Cuban immigrant killed eighty-nine people in 1987. Happy Land Social Club. They'd promised a community center for Hondurans, since most of the dead came from there. They never built it. Talk was cheap, Jack thought as he squinted into the traffic for a gypsy cab. How would he see Zalie now? How would he get his car back from the city? Fuck Bertha Watkins in her four-post mobster bed. Maybe Gina'd get suspended too, unless the audit was just a set-up. Jack again felt like crying; again he felt like having another beer. He'd get these bitches back. He just didn't yet know how.

7. "yoU aRe been roBbeD" (Follow the Bouncing Fax)

Keith Mudnick watched the flames from the oil refineries through the train's smoked glass. Then there was marshland, the dead zone between Wilmington and Baltimore. What a joke Wilmington was, Mudnick thought. Almost all Fortune 500 companies were incorporated there, because the judges did as they were told and the taxes were low. EmpiGroup had gone them all one better: it paid no taxes at all in Anguilla, though it had voluntarily built a courthouse there and drafted the island's corporate bill of rights. That they still kept a back-office in Baltimore was a patriotic anachronism. Keith's days with Empi at least in the U.S. were numbered and he knew it.

Baltimore's Penn Station was small but refurbished; on the sidewalk outside three African American girls who looked about twelve were panhandling. "Mister do you got a dollar?" He shook his head. Beggars in New York were more violent, but they were older too. There was something Third World about this Baltimore streetscape, something Anguilla like: the Charles Street bridge was being rebuilt, just a few rusted girders and all-night traffic flares. He'd parked his car in the lot on St. Paul's Street and was glad to find it with its windows intact. He'd lived in Fell's Point because he'd seen the neighborhood with its cobble stone streets and crab houses on TV. The vomiting frat boys from Johns Hopkins and Towson he could handle. But desperate junkies stealing his hub cabs had driven him to the suburbs, to a shingled Cape Cod out on 83 in Lutherville.

It was hot, it was too hot, and he decided to have a final beer before driving home through Hampden. The Club Charles was open, its walls blood-red through the cigarette smoke. This was Ground Zero, such as it was, of Baltimore's white counter-culture. MBAs who tracked stocks for T. Rowe Price came at night to The Chuck to flaunt their tattoos and earrings, to assert that they might be *in* the Bloomberg world of arbitrage but they were not *of* it. Mudnick ordered a micro-brew on tap and scanned the crowd looking for fresh meat like that Gina in The Bonx. All the women seemed spoken for; they all appeared to be speaking to someone else not him. The jukebox played late-stage bubbly B.B. King and Mudnick lit a smoke. He was at a crossroads, over the railroad crossing. That Jack Bender was a poor fuck, there was no question about it. Janet Peel had a hard-on to get him fired and that was just what would happen. Mudnick would play along because who gave a fuck, anyway? Empi's structure was military -- Vyle had never served his country but he'd read Carl von Clausewitz and Sun Tzu and quoted from them often -- Janet out-ranked Bender and that was that. Mudnick finished his DeGroens and went out to his car. There he found the left side window smashed and his radio gone. He regretted the beer, regretted society's rules and this town. The City That Reads, they called it -- city of Mencken and Poe, city of Babe Ruth and T. Rowe Price, and this is what it had come to. Charm Fucking City, Mudnick thought, pulling out through the canyons of boarded-up brownstones toward Hampden. Fuck EmpiFinancial, fuck Jack Bender and fuck this town. He'd apply for a job in Empi's Emerging Markets before summer was out.

* * *

The gypsy cab dropped Jack Bender on Olinville Avenue, not in front of his building but two doors down. There was a huge SUV double-parked, a wild-haired kid with a Walkman taking orders for drugs from the driver. Jack took the first of the cardboard boxes out, balancing it on the roof of a parked car. He put the second box on top. As the gypsy cab drove off Jack heard a voice from behind.

"Get that shit the fuck off my car." It was the wild-haired teen's boss, a fat man in his late forties with a gold chain and an eye that had gone all white -- a violent man, clearly, not a man to be trifled with. Jack picked up his boxes but still the man wouldn't let them go.

"If my shit is scratched you gonna pay." Jack nodded, trying to walk by the man without looking into his eye. "Yo what's in there," the man demanded.

"Jes papers," Jack mumbled. He could run for his building's entrance, but he'd have to put down the boxes to take his key ring out of his pocket.

"Lemme see." The guy took the top box and there was nothing Jack could do about it, he was holding the bottom box with both hands. He could try to kick the guy in the balls but he still had to live around here, at least for now.

"I tole you, it's jes papers."

The guy was flipping through the files, shaking the box around. Some of the files fell out on the sidewalk. There was dog shit from people's pit bulls that they walked without leashes.

"Boring pinhead shit," the guy said, throwing the box on the ground. As Jack stooped down to pick it up the guy added, "Don't be *touchih*my car, ya hear?" Jack's mouth had gone dry and he didn't say anything. He tried not to think anything either. He'd moved here for this job and now he'd been suspended and he lived on a block with drug dealers and had to take their two-bit pay-back for a whole history of slavery and the guy wasn't even black, a fat Puerto Rican in a t-shirt treating him like a punk. There. If you confronted your fears you could see that they weren't so important.

Jack didn't stop at the mailboxes; he went straight to the stairs and felt short of breath as he climbed them. Someone had urinated on the second floor landing and it got on Jack's shoes. Just two more flights then he could let it all hang out; he could scream then draw up a plan to do battle. Janet Peel was a bitch and she should get fired or worse. The fat Puerto Rican he didn't have time for. Hopefully the cops would get him first and he could try that act up in Ossining until he got cut and his other eye turned white. Oracular Michael Jackson, Victor Fucking Jara except with eyes cut out instead of tongue.

It was quiet in Jack's apartment and it depressed him, the pornographic rap music coming up from the street, the fridge empty except for a week-old quart of now-flat beer. He'd like to sit down and watch the tube, just entirely space out but it was eleven o'clock, only bullshit local news and reruns of sitcoms, ESPN was covering some golf tournament and who gave a shit about golf anyway? That's how they marketed Charlotte: year-round golf, they claimed, though in winter the fairways were frozen. Jack could give a fuck about golf. He lit a smoke and breathed it deep. Smoking in Charlotte was like breathing or fucking -- everyone did it, whatever they said in church on Sunday. The first avowed atheist he'd met was his twelfth grade English teacher Mr. Cromartie. People called him a fairy; perhaps as revenge he talked a lot about some crazy German whose name he couldn't spell who wrote about the Overman. Cromartie'd talked Jack into applying to his alma mater, SUNY Oswego. He said that fat black weatherman and a bunch of businessmen had gone there. Well it was time for good ole Jack to go beyond good and evil. He'd plot and get revenge and then go steal Zalie from his cunt of an ex-wife and he'd start a new life where no one could treat him like a punk -- he wouldn't want his daughter to see how they played him. Mr. Cromartie neither, may his played-out ass rest in peace at last. Jack would set things right and then he'd start over.

* * *

Gina was in the office running the numbers for a sadistic EquityPlus loan when the fax came through. She was expecting a pay-off order, maybe a credit check, but the typeface was wrong. Cut-out letters glued askew to spell out words, in the kidnapper's style that some cutting-edge advertising campaigns used. "yoU aRe been roBbeD," it began. Janet Peel is a bitch and a thief and she should die, it concluded. Gina stifled a laugh and thought immediately of Jack. How stupid could that Cracker be? She looked at the small print at the top of the fax to see where it came from. Kinkos, it said, with a 718 number. Jack Bender drunk in an outer boroughs Kinkos. The fax was signed with some weird name, "Tariq Noor," whoever the hell that was supposed to be. Gina thought of just putting the page on Janet's desk but then she thought better. With Jack out of the picture she'd be named branch manager all the faster. She opened the Monstro program on her computer and found Janet's home number. Screwing the Guzmans could wait. Now was the time to screw Jack.

But Janet'd already gotten a call. Two, in fact: from the EmpiFinancial offices in New Rochelle and Jackson Heights, Queens. The fax had been sent to all six of the offices she oversaw, and who knew where else.

"He's not going to get away with this," Janet told Gina. She was thinking clearly and she already had a plan. "Can I pick you up at the office? It won't take long but there's something we need to do."

Vinny was playing softball or said he was. Anyway the pot was hot for promotion. "Sure," Gina said. "I'll just finish structuring this EquityPlus loan while I wait."

Jack was an impotent fuck but a threat was a threat. Janet picked up Gina and the fax -- she'd taken to calling it a death threat -- and drove to the 48th precinct, under the Cross-Bronx Expressway. This was Bronx Borough Command; this was the homicide unit, the chief of detectives, the all-night cells.

"My life has been threatened," Janet announced to the cop behind the desk.

"By who," the cop asked, "your husband? A mugger?"

"A fax," Janet said, holding the page between her thumb and index finger like it might have fingerprints on it.

The cop stared at the lettering and shook his head. "A real pro," he muttered. "So you wanna file a complaint?"

"Definitely. Right now. Tonight." Janet paused. "I feel in danger."

"You're Janet Peel I take it."

Janet scowled. "Where's your commanding officer? We need to find where this came from as soon as possible."

"While the fax machine's still hot," the cop said. Janet couldn't tell if he was joking or not. "Wait here."

The cop who came out looked tired or high. His eyes were red and his shield said O'Brien. "We'll take down a complaint, lady," he said. "You wanna know where it came from, call Kinkos."

"But you'll come with us, right?"

O'Brien shook his head slowly, as if it might hurt if he did it full-strength. "We got, you know, real crimes around here lady. Not fax crimes, not virtual crimes -- real blood and guts raping and shooting and arson."

"This is a *death* threat," Janet insisted.

"If you read it that way. It says you *should* die. I mean I know it's not a nice thing to hear but hey, we all do die in the end, know what I'm saying? Now the *bitch* part..." O'Brien smiled at his own joke.

"Come on," Janet told Gina. "We'll find the Kinkos and prove it was --" she stopped and thought the better of it -- "we'll find out who sent it. Maybe on the *day shift* over here they'll take this more seriously."

"Yeah, the fax investigation unit comes in at nine," O'Brien deadpanned. Gina wanted to laugh but it was Wall Street she wanted, not the cement-ceilinged world of law enforcement.

"We've got all the employee photos on Monstro," Gina reminded Janet in the car. "If we take Jack's picture we could just ask them, was he here."

"You know it's him, right?" Janet asked.

"Who else? But he's dumber that I thought."

"Not me."

On Kinkos' web site it was easy to trace from which office it had come. Not Brooklyn, thank God. Gina laughed that Jack had been so lazy he'd faxed from Kinkos' one and only office in The Bronx, an incongruous 24-hour a day storefront on Webster Avenue across from Fordham University. During exam season it was busy; the rest of the year it sat empty at night, a clear misstep in Kinkos footprint. Kinkos' error was Gina's convenience: she'd had her résumé typeset there.

Behind the counter was a thin black man with a neatly-trimmed Afro named George. He had a name tag on, immediate first-name basis, another customer-centric corporate culture driving the surnamed competition into the sea.

"Did this come from here?" Janet demanded, holding out the fax but not letting it go. George looked at the number at the top and nodded.

"That's our machine, yeah. What's the problem? It's not legible?" Then he looked closer, the cut-out letters reminding him of some movie, he couldn't remember which one.

"It was sent less than two hours ago." Janet looked around the storefront. It wasn't hard. There was only a fat woman in an overcoat who looked homeless sheafing through papers without faxing anything. "Would you remember who sent it?"

George shrugged and wondered if he was supposed to protect the privacy of the customers. He didn't remember anything about it in the manual they'd made him read. They didn't give much training because most people didn't stay working here too long. After two years they gave you a stock option. Maybe it was three years.

Now the blonde lady had a photograph out. White man that George might have seen somewhere, yeah maybe it was tonight, he wasn't sure.

"Was this man in here?" the lady asked.

"I can't say."

"You don't know?"

George glared. "What are you, the police?"

"My life has been threatened, from this very store, so I want--"

"Lemme check the time." George looked at the top of the fax again. Nine fifty-one. He turned to the computer terminal, punched in the time.

"Someone sent like a dozen one-page faxes," George said. "He paid in cash. No credit card for--" he looked at the fax again -- "Tay-Rick Noor."

"But you remember him, right?" Again the lady was pointing at the photo.

"That's not too good a picture," George said.

"Could it be him?"

George shrugged. "Sure, could be."

Janet was on overdrive; she didn't know who to call. "How late do you work here?" she asked.

"Until seven. It's a twelve hour shift at night."

Janet nodded and took her cell phone outside. The persistence of slavery did not cross her mind. She could call EmpiGroup downtown but they wouldn't know her from Adam, or Eve. She dialed Mudnick's cell. He'd know what to do.

In Lutherville Mudnick answered "yeah." He'd cut his hand sweeping glass shards from the car. He was in no mood for jokes. Janet read from the fax, said she was at some photocopy place in The Bronx, needed Empi Security, somebody to take an affidavit. To Mudnick it seemed ridiculous, but he gave her the number of the security office in Midtown. Mostly they went out to protect busted-open ATMs until the cops came. Faxed death threats would be a welcome change of pace. Mudnick put a Lean Cuisine Chinese dinner in the microwave, still cursing the inflated price of replacement auto glass. And between this nuking of food and the two air-conditioners, BG&E -- Baltimore Gas and Electric -- was killing him   As someone apparently wanted to literally do to Janet Peel.

It was three a.m. when Empi's deputy chief of security and head of Black-Ops arrived at Kinkos. Chuck Stewart was a notary, he carried a gun; he'd stopped at White Castle on his way here and now he belched. Janet'd already primed the witness and George signed the form Chuck put in front of him. Brother to brother.

"Like I told you, it *could* be him. I'm not totally sure."

"It says 'on information and belief.' Don't worry about it."

George shrugged. They should have trained him better. Anyway he'd be out of here when school started in September, if the financial aid came through for City College. Fordham was too expensive. Though when he looked at the student term papers he photocopied their shit didn't look any better than his, shit all of it, make-work theses, collated feces. Just four more hours. Time to re-stock the toner.

* * *

Janet arrived at the precinct at nine -- she'd hardly slept -- and demanded to talk to the captain, the chief of detectives, someone in authority. They gave her another sleepy-looking Mick. McBride this one was called.

"EmpiBank, eh?" McBride said, looking at the affidavit. "You guys don't miss a trick."

At least he hadn't said *gals*, Janet thought. "So are you going to arrest him?"

"Usually we like to investigate before we do that."

"Here's the fax -- the death threat -- and here's a sworn statement that Jack Bender was the one that sent it," Janet said. "There's nothing to investigate." She handed McBride another piece of paper. "And here," she said, "is Jack Bender's address. He's probably there. He's out of work. That's why--"

"Okay lady," McBride cut her off. "I'll make a few calls then we'll probably pick him up. Unless you guys fired some Arab guy called Noor--"

"It's Bender," Janet said. "He'll stay in jail, right? I mean he's threatened my life...".

"He'll probably get bail, and not too high a bail at that. D'ya really think--"

"The man is insane," Janet said. "I think I need police protection."

McBride laughed at that. Witness protection program, he wanted to say. But he was too near retirement to take the chance of a complaint. Nineteen of the required twenty years. "You could get an order of protection," he said. "But that'd be civil. You'd have to file your own case. Or get EmpiBank to do it -- it's not like they don't have enough lawyers."

"Will you call me when you've picked him up?"

Why not, McBride thought. Maybe he could go work for EmpiBank, as security or maybe even a loan officer -- what the hell did those people do anyway -- once he served out this last year. He took her phone number and his copy of the fax upstairs. Use of interstate communications to convey death threats -- maybe it was even a felony. The poor fuck, McBride thought. Though he could see why someone might want to kill this Janet Peel.

* * *

It was two in the afternoon and Jack was already thinking of having a beer when they knocked on his door. Jack looked out through the peephole and saw a florid red face, not unlike his own but with a blue hat on top of it.

"Open up! Police!"

Jack turned to the bedroom to put on his pants but their knocking got louder. "Open the fucking door or we take it down!"

"All right! Take it easy!" Jack opened the door still in his underwear and the next thing he knew they'd knocked him on the floor and had a gun in his face.

"Jack Bender? Eh-Kay-Eh Tay-rick Noor?"

"Th-that's me," he stammered. "The first one I mean."

"You're under arrest for aggravated harassment by means of interstate commerce and related charges. You have the right to remain silent--"

But Jack'd heard these words before.

8. Power of the Press

Sandy Vyle felt crucified on the buzzword of the early Aughts: accounting irregularities. Ever since Enron imploded these grandstanding jackasses wouldn't accept anything at face value. Vyle didn't like to read the newspapers but today he had copies of a particular Journal article in three formats. Hard-copy, e-mail and print-out. They called it Heard on the Street but the bitch that'd written this one was just filling in on that column while the real guy, the real set of ears who knew better than to trifle with Sandy, was on vacation in Tuscany. Nicole Nour -- what the hell kind of last name was that? Maybe she was Muslim and wanted to undermine the whole stock market, some Al Qaeda fifth column in the fourth estate repeating gossip from unnamed analysts and giving him *agita*. Vyle doubted this but it might be a good spin. The insidious decay in confidence in corporate numbers. Go to Anguilla and count the loans yourself you bitch, he thought, popping another Rolaids and chewing it with his ten thousand dollar false teeth.

Rudehart came in, thin and fruity -- that's how Vyle pegged him -- and plopped down his copy of the article on Sandy's king-sized desk.

"Fuck the Journal," Sandy said. "We'll pull our ads for a few weeks, see how they like that."

Rudehard shook his head, barely perceptibly. "If we respond it just gives it more play. Anyone who knows anything knows this reporter's a rookie."

"Joe Schmuck investor reading the Internet doesn't know that," Sandy said. "They're in their chat rooms jacking each other off and the next thing you know, our stock price is trimmed a buck-fifty."

"I took some notes," Rudehart said -- he always did, he would have done it in PowerPoint except that Sandy hated technology. "Nothing that she said, even if it *were* true, is criminal. It might not even violate SEC rules."

"The SEC is not our problem," Sandy said, thinking of all the money he'd given Bush II, how a single call to Bush's drawling chief of staff could solve any problem with federal regulators. "Take Swanker, for example -- that cocksucker *lives* for shit like this."

"I can handle Swanker," Rudehart said. "I know his type." And he did.

* * *

Nicole Nour was walking on air -- she wished the World Trade Center had never been blown up, not least because today she could float through the Winter Garden collecting the accolades of analysts who'd forget her tomorrow. The Journal's temporary digs on Canal Street kept you out of the action. She'd returned some e-mails with pithy false modesty but now headed to Midtown to meet with her source for the story. "An analyst of EmpiGroup's stock," she'd called him. There were dozens, probably hundreds, who fit that bill. The Heard on the Street column was like the Post's Page Six. You could run blind items, not-for-attribution dirt, the kind of bar- bathroom banter that actually moved stocks. She was new at this so she was paranoid and full of herself: she'd arranged to meet Bain at a soon-to-be-closed coffee shop off Times Square. "No one will recognize me there," she'd told Bain. Bain laughed. He didn't even know what she looked like. She'd never been on CNBC, never been on Bloomberg's feed. He'd told her the flaw that he'd seen in Empi's numbers just to get revenge. It wasn't just the way Vyle'd shamed him at the SIA -- Bain took pleasure in hammering the companies he covered, off-the-record of course. His bosses didn't care one way or the other, as long as he gave them a heads-up so they could trade on the dirt. This time he hadn't. His nights of naked condominium desolation were bleeding over into his days. Maybe he should join Al Qaeda. He wanted darkness and death. Elizabeth or the Apocalypse.

They bought their coffees -- Bain a French vanilla, Nicole a thick Turkish in honor of the Middle East -- and carried them up to a plywood-floored loft.

"My editor wanted more proof," Nicole began.

Bain shrugged. Nour was younger and prettier than he'd expected. He was already her source -- now he wanted to be her horse, by force if necessary, a vicious Wall Street coupling. He gathered his thoughts. "It's right there in the numbers, you can see something's missing."

"Empi says it's credit derivatives, off-balance sheet action that no rule requires them to disclose." Nicole wasn't in the market for men --

she had a career to develop, Goddamn it -- and the Bain was red-haired and goofy, probably volunteered with the National Guard on the weekends, a real G.I. Joe.

"The rules are changing," Bain said as Bogart as he could. "After Enron it just won't work when the numbers don't add up."

"Hey, I wrote the story, didn't I? You don't have to sell me. But if you come up with anything else, will you bring it to me first?" This was a trick they were taught at the Journal: always ask for an exclusive, always imply you won't cover it if anyone else has it. Sources were so desperate to be in the Journal -- either their name or their sly stock-moving dig -- that they usually went along.

Bain nodded; he was bluffing. It wasn't every day that he found an error in an earnings report. If not an error at least something that didn't add up. "I've got more," he said darkly. He liked this dark-haired filly with the full fire-power of the Journal behind her. It was an aphrodisiac, this power to kick Sandy Vyle in his steel balls anonymously and get away with it.

"You have it with you?"

Bain shook his head. He had nothing. "I'm getting all my ducks in a row," he said.

Forget the National Guard, he probably mock-hunts on weekends, Nicole thought. Even back in Egypt, at first chaperoned then under a nine o'clock curfew -- ten during their Agami and Zamelek Island summers -- she'd met false *machos* like him. She knew his type and didn't like it.

Actually Tom Bain *had* gone hunting last month, a whisky-fueled male bonding frenzy on a gator farm in the Cajun bayou. Ten analysts from his firm had flown to New Orleans, took limousines a hour south to get primal with thousand-dollar shotguns and a toothless trainer who told them war stories and offered to order whores from the next town over. Bain had been game but the other analysts were all married -- it's not that they wouldn't have fucked some French-speaking swamp girls, they just didn't want anyone to have the evidence over them. They changed firms constantly and even the implied threat of blackmail could be leveraged into millions of trading dollars. So they pretended to be chaste and instead got drunk. They lowered rotting chicken carcasses off their boats with strings, blasted the gators' heads off with shotguns when they broke the surface. The firm paid for the whole thing, thinking it made them all more bloodthirsty and brotherly.

Bain considered telling this story to Nicole, but he didn't know her like that -- hell, she might even be a vegetarian. Though Bain wondered what woman *didn't* like a man who killed gators with his hands, well at least with a shotgun that he held in his manicured hands. Then he remembered: Elizabeth didn't. Elizabeth who simultaneously lived in Greenwich and on some purist cloud. Well fuck her and her cobweb-filled nun's cunt. Bain would pursue this exotic cub reporter and soon not be nude in his condo alone at dawn. She wanted info, she wanted exclusives. He'd give her that and a bit more and it would all be different.

* * *

Swanker saw the story -- that's how he got most of his leads -- and he read it like some might read the Talmud, looking for secret meanings, for any slam-dunk case that Empi might settle quickly, another painless pelt to put on his résumé. Insufficient disclosure in financial statements... If he could just spin it into a case of investor protection, of defending the virtue of the market with a fast consent decree, maybe some chump-change fine to split with the other state AGs, he'd have a winner. Swanker wondered what if anything in the article had to do with what Micah Levine had told him. Micah was small fry: he could pay to play in New York State, but he couldn't project himself beyond.

Swanker was already tired of the Big Apple: he had bigger fruits to fry. Suing EmpiGroup could get him in the Journal, maybe even Sixty Minutes or Prime-Time Live. But Empi would have to agree to it, behind the scenes. It would have to be like kabuki theater, like a fixed fight where both pugs get the same purse. Forward-looking immunity for EmpiGroup; another notch in Swanker's belt. It was delicate but he knew who to call in Empi: Robert Rudehart, who'd been everywhere that Ernest Swanker wanted to be. Six years as a statesman on the national stage and then the gravy. Dinner in Riverdale with Carolyn and the kids; a walk on the terrace over the Hudson with Rudehart and the fix would be in. Micah Levine would cream in his jeans to attend, but what would be in it for Swanker? You didn't share access for free. Swanker'd heard of karma but he didn't believe in it. If what you put out came back to you then Swanker would be a defendant forever. No -- what you took in was always yours to be used. What you put out could only be used against you. A joint press release with Empi: from this Heard on the Street, that was Swanker's end-game.

Carolyn complained but he knew she would do it. Sun-dried tomatoes from Dean & Deluca; quaint Bronx olive bread from that place on Arthur Avenue. Dinner with an ex-Treasury Secretary? She'd be sure to charge the batteries of the digital camera. This was the reason she'd married Swanker. He wasn't much of a lover but he was ruthless and smooth in his work. She imagined herself a second Jackie Kennedy; she'd already scouted out townhouses in Georgetown, the Sidwell Friends Quaker school for the kids, all the trappings of the New Democrat aristocracy. Even the Mexican maid -- Millie still cleared the wrong forks at the wrong time, but she could be trained and she sure was cheap. Milly'd mentioned something about an injured husband; Carolyn had given her a few days off because that's what New Democrats did. But she'd dress Millie in black with a white apron on the night that Rudehart came. Something about it felt right so she gave Ernie the okay, as he'd known she would.

But Rudehart was flying to Mexico City, to visit the *cacique* from whom Empi'd bought a bank last year. They were still integrating NaraMex but EmpiFinancial was soon to begin an offensive south of the border.

"Don't drink the water," Swanker said, making a joke just a few decades out of date. Rudehart didn't laugh. He had a memory that would fill a ten-pack of CD-Roms: Jimmy Carter once mentioned Montezuma's revenge and triggered an international incident. This Swanker was rough around the edges. But he was open to learning, to bending over for EmpiGroup, and that was what was important.

"I'll call you when I get back and we'll pick a date," Rudehart said. "Don't do anything until then--"

"Of course not," Swanker said. He'd always wanted to meet Sandy Vyle but in a way the prospect frightened him. Vyle was like a bully in school, with none of Rudehart's social graces. This could wait. EmpiGroup wasn't going anywhere -- it didn't need to, since it had sanctuary on Anguilla.

"We can talk politics too," Rudehart concluded.

"I'd like that," Swanker said. Carolyn would too. The future was boundless.

9. The Night of the Zygote

Sublimation was Kurt Wheelock's favorite word: a touchstone or a lifeline it was what he needed to do. He'd never been to A.A. or N.A. or any of the A's except Fucking A but he *knew* that he was an addict, he had a penchant for addiction, obsession he sometimes called it or to put on a nicer gloss, focus. He needed something to focus on or he'd feel himself lethargic and thinking more than he should about death. The more arcane the subject the more it excited him. It was something to be cautious of or he'd end up in a cult. He almost had--

When they offered to let him move in he should have known. It began with an ad in the Village Voice classifieds. "Do you want to work for justice?" the ad had asked, and Kurt said yes. He'd gone to a storefront in Brooklyn and even then he should have known. A dozen twenty- and thirty-somethings much like himself were doing telemarketing into headsets -- how was this justice? They explained to him that social change had to fund itself, it had to be entrepreneurial, it had to be self-supporting. Hence their wholesale business selling heating oil and photocopy paper. Those who wanted to join the movement as organizers spent half their days as Willie Loman, saying "Whatever you're paying now, I can beat it," then hitting the lean streets of East New York and Bushwick identifying grassroots leaders whom they could manipulate without it showing. It was called the Federation of Community Organizations; FOCO was its acronym and he'd liked how it sounded Spanish, as he tried to convince people he was.

Kurt Wheelock had a file full of clipping about a Sandinista *comandante* named Jaime Wheelock -- "we're related," Kurt used to say, vaguely alluding to mortar fights with *contras* in the coffee groves of Esteli. His mother had long ago written Kurt off as crazy. "You're denying your past," she'd tell him. His father he hadn't seen in years and so perhaps he *was* this dashing Jaime Wheelock, the poet guerrilla with the Anglo name.

The problem as he got older was that fewer people around him gave a shit about Nicaragua. When the Sandinistas got voted out and America stopped paying thugs to blow up teachers, the lefties' focus turned elsewhere. He knew people who claimed that Slobodan Milosevic was a victim of The West; at a rally in defense of Iraq he'd attended he'd seen the succinct banner, "Civilization Is Genocide." Even

Kurt knew this was too far gone. When he spoke his mind at FOCO things had come to a head.

FOCO's founder Gene Ramos shared many of Kurt's proclivities, only larger and more malign. The last time Kurt had seen him, in the rent-controlled safehouse in Bushwick, he'd been alternating puffing on a Pall Mall and an oxygen tank. Gene spoke about the coming cataclysm in America then asked how many reams of copy paper Kurt had sold that day. "Write it down," Gene said, "write it all down." That was how they broke your will, with bed checks and accounting slips, the need to document and encrypt every cold call and bowel movement. "We need to know the people in our movement," Gene said. Kurt thought back to the Village Voice ad and felt vertigo.

Gene Ramos was not FOCO's founder's real name: the exposés pegged him as Jerry Dorden, a Lutheran, of Minneapolis. How and when he'd turned from common grift to revolution was not known. He began on the tip of Long Island's North Fork, urging migrant workers, Mexicans and Salvadorans who picked potatoes mostly, to form a union and fight for their rights. He claimed he knew Cesar Chavez; he claimed he knew Dorothy Day; he had an old radio over which he said he got instructions. When the Berlin Wall fell -- Kurt then had yet to see the Village Voice ad, and why the Berlin Wall fell was now a mystery -- Gene Ramos had to reinvent himself, welcoming Communism's fall as an opportunity for a "fuller and more robust liberation," as he called it. The first liberated zone, the new in the shell of the old, was this drafty Brooklyn storefront from which they hawked photocopy paper. Today twenty-two dollars a case -- tomorrow the world!

Perhaps it was like the Moonies. But the mere mention of religion would have set off alarms in Kurt Wheelock's atheistic head. It was subtle how FOCO drew you in, how they complimented your door-knocking and cold-calling style, scheduled face-time for you -- always past midnight -- with the wheezing Field Commander, offered to consider your ideas while they compiled a psychological study of your every weakness and Achilles' heel. Kurt's was obvious. He hated what he was, or more precisely, where he was from.

Their offer was simple: we'll pretend you're Kurt Wheelock of the Nicaragua Wheelocks; you can wear a ski cap and go on furloughs to the East Village or Spanish Harlem, as long as you return to the safehouse at night. They all had quotas for recruitment and that's where Wheelock drew the line. His doubts about FOCO were growing -- when his mother called it a cult he didn't disagree -- so he couldn't in good conscience troll for converts in the alternative bookstores of Avenue A. This made Gene Ramos mad. Re-education sessions were scheduled and then the hijackers blew up the Towers. For Kurt it was his salvation.

The Feds who'd ignored Gene Ramos and his FOCO for a decade staged a raid. Kurt had been out, thank God, getting day-old bread from the Pechter's bakery. When he came back he saw the swirling sirens and police tape; he saw Gene Ramos being carried out in his wheelchair singing "We Shall Overcome;" he ran to the subway and rode to the end of the line in The Bronx. Dyre Avenue, the sign said. He got out and walked around. It was almost suburban, Jamaican beef patty stores and three-family houses on all the side streets. It was then he decided to move to The Bronx, to forget FOCO and to sublimate -- that word again -- his sicko desire for justice into practical campaigns against corporations. He'd done the fundraising for some of FOCO's fronts so getting seed money was not a problem. He knew the Internet, too, so he could project the group as Actual and growing as soon as the domain name came through. WatchCorp, he called it -- WatchCorp dot org.

He designed the web site on his laptop in the uncomfortably plush apartment of his girlfriend Candida Azuela. She had seven rooms on Riverside Drive, bought by her doctor ex-husband, haunted by suicide attempts of which Kurt had known nothing when he'd first dallied with La Candida. What she lacked in candor she made up for in curves. Probably it was also because she was Spanish -- *latina*, she called it -- that he'd been attracted to her, when they first met in blue-lit club on the Lower East Side. She'd been wearing a baseball cap; they'd danced and drank and done what used to be called heavy petting. Then they'd taken a cab -- she paid -- north to the Upper West Side to continue the proceedings. They'd screwed for two days straight; Kurt left a late-night message on FOCO's answering machine saying he was hard at work on a hot prospect for recruitment. Candida was pretty and svelte, worked out in a glass-windowed gym on Broadway and 98th Street. Kurt was not without options, there were other women he could be with but it was Candida he'd chosen.

At first she placated him by speaking Spanish but then she grew tired. She'd had enough of rice and beans. Her Peruvian father'd been a super, raped her repeatedly in a boiler room in Queens. She wouldn't play Spic for anyone, least of all Kurt. Though she wanted to have a baby with him. Her clock was ticking and Kurt's genes seemed alright. For all his unkempt bluster he was blond, dirty blond. More importantly he was smart, even if he had played the flunky for that Brooklyn cult. The night Kurt showed up with that crazy look in his eyes, speed-dialing around the cable TV remote trying to find news of FOCO's fall, she thought it was a good sign. But when they ordered take-out Chinese she saw that nothing was different.

The Chinese man had come to the door -- no different than a billion other Chinese men, in Candida's view -- and Kurt had insisted on inviting him in. Kurt asked the delivery man what he got paid, whether he got to keep all his tips, whether he could afford to eat the food that he delivered. The man had grunted some replies and Candida had known that he thought Kurt was crazy. Hell, she *knew* Kurt was crazy. "I'm going to move to The Bronx," Kurt said after the man had left, with a twenty dollar tip (her money, not Kurt's).

"Give it time," Candida said. But she knew there'd be none. From one cult to another. Kurt was a junkie and she was wasting her time.

Physically-speaking it was Candida who was addicted. She worked as a part-time nurse at Metropolitan Hospital on the East Side; she snuck into the supply closet and took every controlled substance she could get her hands on. One thing you could say for Stewart was that he got the best drugs. But he was entirely disinterested in sex -- Candida firmly believed he was gay -- and so they got divorced. From a basement apartment in Queens to Riverside Drive: it wasn't bad. But her hands shook in the morning and Kurt's mindless hatred of wealth made her sick. "Wanna-be b-boy," she said in her head. And soon she'd say it out loud and her clock would tick past midnight.

It was Candida who bought Kurt the software, FrontPage Express from the Seattle robber baron. It was Candida who fucking supported him until the first two grants for WatchCorp came through. What hadn't she done for him? She'd let him fuck her up the ass, never saying what her father used to do. She was "there for him," like they say, in the only way she knew how. Still he cross-examined delivery-boys and spoke of moving to The Bronx. Kurt was an idiot, she'd concluded. He wasn't gay but he was an idiot.

FOCO's fall was recounted as farce in the paper of record. "Justice Mask Reveals a Cult, and Guns" the sidebar headline read. Gene Ramos was defrocked as a Lutheran check kiter; his followers were portrayed as dupes most of whom would not be prosecuted. Whew, thought Kurt. He could play dupe -- he had played it, even since he saw the Voice ad if not before. He had no interest in joining a cult deprogramming group. His focus, his addiction, was now EmpiBank.

"Why a bank?" Candida asked, though in a relative way she liked it, it sounded cleaner and more mainstream than targeting slumlords.

"People need loans to buy a house; developing world countries need loans... well, to pay back old loans," Kurt said. "Those bastards run the world but there's no oversight."

"And you're going to do it, baby?" Candida asked, trying to send the signal. They might scarcely know each other; they might have nothing in common; they might even hate each other -- but their sex togethr was always *muy bueno.*

"I'm gonna try," Kurt said. He missed the signal until Candida put her head in his lap. He had a whole theory about sublimating the sex drive into work, but with FOCO gone under it was time to let libido run.

They began in the kitchen -- Candida's whitefish spread from Zabar's made for a protein-filled lubricant -- and they moved into the bathroom, chromy and foamy and neurotically spotless as Candida kept it. Candida thought this might be the night of the zygote but when the moment came Kurt pulled himself out. He'd picked up this yen from porno films: they made coming inside too bland, no pay-off, no money-shot, no sense of conclusion. Candida smeared the stuff around as if she liked it. Maybe she could store some and inject it in, herself. The sun-dried madnesses of these Riverside Drive co-ops were many-hued, barely plumbed in film or sit com. Sizzling semen reheated by race hatred, creeping infertility and web sites under construction: this was the brave new world and Sichuan beef was only a phone call away.

While Kurt uploaded Candida cried.

Part Two: The Cracker Jackal's Play

10. Criminal Defense

They'd taken Jack straight to Bronx Criminal Court on 161st Street but they'd left him overnight and now there was vomit on his shoes and he'd been out of cigarettes for hours. He'd made the mistake of giving a smoke to the first and largest guy who'd asked. Thereafter shorter but equally threatening skels had made their demands. Back in Charlotte he'd chewed chaw but he had none with him now. He was sober, all too sober, but still he tried to blank his mind. Aggravated harassment was bullshit. Whether he'd done it or not didn't matter. People said things all the time. This was Janet Peel trying to take not only his job but his balls. Gina was probably in the picture too but only because she liked him, despite herself. She wanted his job too but hey who didn't.

His mistake was in saying that he already had a lawyer. They'd postponed his arraignment until Ms. Thompson was on -- "catching," as they called it, as if these unwashed accused were baseballs in a batting cage. The wait had given them time to find the other charge against him. When they hauled him blinking out into the windowless room Ms. Thompson shook her head. "Death threats?" she whispered. "I thought you were just a john."

"Not guilty" was all that Jack would say. He was learning quick in this Northern justice. Don't talk to the cops, don't talk to the judge; don't even talk to your lawyer. The ACD was the rub: adjourned contemplating dismissal meant that another arrest made the old charge live. Or was it another conviction? He asked Ms. Thompson and she shrugged.

"You can't plead to this," she said. "Otherwise you'll do time."

Lorraine Thompson didn't like not guilty. Sure she liked it at first, when a case began -- it was the only bargaining chip a defendant had. But if you couldn't end up pleading the thing out, you had to go to trial and that meant time and the state only paid forty lousy dollars an hour, twenty-five for out of court. Fucking beauticians made more than that, at least the ones who did conk perms for rap stars on 125th Street. She needed to get rid of this case and she thought she knew how.

"I have concerns," she told Jack, "about your income eligibility."

"Come again?"

"I think you're over-income. I'll work on your case then the state won't reimburse me. How much didja make last year?"

Bitch, Jack thought. "Hey I'm out of work, I jes got fired--"

"It goes on last year's income. You filed a 1040, right?"

Jack figured the game and made his play. "Look, just get me through this, this first appearance, whatever you call it, so I can get home. You don't wanna represent me after that, fine, I understand it."

"It's not that I don't *want* to," Lorraine said, though that's exactly what it was.

The judge came in and damn if it wasn't the same helmet-head as before. He looked twice at Jack as if he recognized him, then looked through the papers on his desk to find the chili pepper suppository he wanted to use on this white trash menace.

"I see that you're back, Mister Bender," he began. "I thought I warned you--"

Lorraine cut in. "My client vigorously denies these new charges, Judge Birnbaum."

"They always do," Birnbaum deadpanned. "But this is more serious than prostitution. Death threats?" He shook his head.

"It's nothing but a fax, it's signed with someone else's name--"

Birnbaum scoffed. "They picked him out of a line-up."

"They showed an overnight clerk a photograph, a single photograph. That's not a line up."

Birnbaum didn't like to admit it but that was true. The assistant DA who was catching was a spaced-out Asian man named Wing Tsai -- Birnbaum didn't know how to pronounce it so he didn't. Just as he hadn't said the crazy Arab name at the bottom of the fax.

"Do the People have any more evidence?" Birnbaum asked Tsai.

Wing had gone to CUNY and passed the bar exam on his third try just last May. It had taken them a year to let him represent the august People of The Bronx in this windowless room where the charges were mostly public urination, unleashed dog and fare beating. Wife beating was higher profile and was handled in a special courtroom down the hall. Tsai couldn't get his hands or mind around the file in front on him. A photo ID in a Kinkos? What the fuck *was* this?

"We think he's a danger," Tsai said without looking up. "We understand that the previously charge isn't at issue until he's convicted -- unless he's convicted -- but we think the two taken together militate for ten thousand dollars bail."

Birnbaum suppressed a smile -- rare for him -- at this Chink and his fancy "militate" and his request for a bail five times the size what was daily done in this courtroom.

"How 'bout it, Mister Bender?" Birnbaum asked. Jack looked at Lorraine Thompson -- he was surprised that she'd even known it was about a fax -- asking with his eyes, do I speak or do you? Thompson nodded and cleared her throat.

"My client has ties to the community," she said. Jack thought of the fat drug dealer on Olinville, of the wild-haired teen who should be here instead of him.

"Bail's not necessary to ensure his continued presence -- but if it *is* set, we'd suggest a thousand dollars." Jack thought of his car still in the pound, of Diane just waiting for him to be late with a child support check, of Zalie getting further away, further down the road to being a cracker slut one day like her mom.

"I can't," Jack whispered.

"You should count yourself lucky," Birnbaum said, "that I set bail at all. Two thousand. And you'll need the court's permission to leave the state, pending the trial." Birnbaum paused, smiled what seemed to Jack a sadistic smile -- Jack couldn't focus, now even if he paid he couldn't go down to Charlotte, couldn't see Zalie, was stuck here in this shit hole. Birnbaum continued, "And if and when you pay it and get out, Mister Bender, don't be sending any more faxes -- do I make myself understood?"

Jack woulda liked to punch him, but the court officers all had guns and the two thousand would be hard enough to come up with. Empi still owed him his last monthly Rocopoly bonus, it should have been mailed out before he got fired. That should just about cover his bail, though he could kiss his car goodbye. He wished Zalie were older than six so he could ask her advice. 'Cause other than her he had no one at all.

* * *

"So I guess this is it, Jack."

Lorraine Thompson was saying her farewell to the loser in lock-up. "I need to ask you a favor," he said.

Lorraine sighed. She liked to leave things polite with her clients when she dropped them -- today's deadbeat was tomorrow's drug defendant flush with cash -- but this Bender character was a little too pushy. Whoring then faxing death threats to his job. He'd come to no good end, she'd decided. She didn't respond. But neither did she call for the guards.

"The only way I can post bail is with my bonus check. It should be in my mailbox at my building already. If you could pick it up--"

"Don't you have any *friends*?" Lorraine asked like she was surprised but she wasn't. What kind of man cruised the South Bronx for whores?

"I'm new in town." Jack felt the moment, this last chance, slipping away. "The check should be for twenty five hundred clams. Post my bail and the rest is yours."

Lorraine calculated. Five hundred dollars for a couple hours' work? "You'll have to endorse it," she said.

"Get my keys from the property room," Jack said. "I ain't goin' anywhere."

Ain't *that* the truth, Lorraine thought. She went to get his keys.

* * *

Lorraine quickly scoped the whole drug dealing hierarchy on Olinville -- might be some good clients here -- and used the cracker's keys to open his bent metal mailbox. It was full of junk mail and an envelope from EmpiFinancial. Back in her car, on her cut-up naugahyde seats patched with duct tape, Lorraine ripped it open. Not a check but a letter. She read the legalese slow and easy. Since his employment had been terminated, it said, his severance would only be paid on conditions. There was a contract attached, a contract of adhesion they would have called it in law school: he'd agree to never sue about being fired, and not to "disparage EmpiFinancial or any member of the EmpiGroup family in any manner whatsoever." Hard ball, Lorraine thought. Only an idiot who was also desperate would sign this. But Jack seemed to fit both descriptions.

Back in the lock-up, Jack already looked haggard. She gave him the letter. She watched his lips move as he read it, or thought she did.

"They *owe* me this fucking money," Jack said without looking up.

"Possession's nine-tenths of the law," Lorraine said. "The question is, is there any other way you can post bail?"

Jack thought about it. Asking Diane for a loan was out of the question. His number two at Charlotte Empi, Eric Taylor, was a good ol' boy but at least on him the word "good" was literal. "Litch-ral," as Eric would say it. But he didn't have Eric's home number with him and he didn't want to call him at work and anyway two thousand bucks was a lot and Western Union was slow. "Fuck it," Jack said. "I'll sign it, you go to them and get the money and get me the fuck out of here."

"I'm not representing you on this, you understand that, right?" Lorraine didn't need a malpractice complaint and any lawyer who let a client sign this would be begging for one.

"Whatever," Jack said, signing the contract in the three places marked X. "Just go get the money. Maybe you could leave me a hundred bucks cash?"

Always backsliding. Still four hundred dollars wasn't bad. "Fine," Lorraine said. She wondered if EmpiBank had black lawyers to do foreclosures. Maybe she'd ask.

The postage-paid envelope wasn't returnable to the West Farms Mall but rather to EmpiFinancial in New Rochelle, the office Janet Peel worked from. Lorraine took the Bronx Rive Parkway to Wakefield, drove around under the elevated train, stopped in for some curry goat and rice and peas, Jamaican food made best up here. Then she crossed into Westchester County. New Rochelle was more abandoned than she remembered, an inner-ring suburb all fucked up, the American Dream gone sour. This was EmpiFinancial's bread and butter: working folks trying desperately to keep up with the television Joneses, paying hospital bills with home equity loans, buying their next used car when there was absolutely no other way to get to work. I better watch out, Lorraine thought -- at these 18B rates *I* could be coming to these loan sharks soon.

Janet Peel pegged Lorraine as a customer as she came in, X-rayed her bulky frame for her credit card debt, ready to consolidate, ready to boil all the fat off her bones and make soap -- when Lorraine pulled out the contract, handed it to Janet along with her card. Jacqueline Thompson, Esquire, Attorney at Law. Real gentry.

"Jack has a *lawyer*?" Janet asked. This was just what Mudnick had said to watch out for.

"I represent him in a criminal case," Lorraine said. She saw the name plate on Janet's desk and put two and two together. "You're the one he *allegedly* threatened?"

"He's crazy," Janet said. "Is he paying you or what?"

"I'm not at liberty," Lorraine began then stopped. She didn't have to tell this bimbo nothing. "He's signed, as you see. I've come to pick up the money."

Janet was surprised that he'd signed. Mudnick would be happy. They'd gotten rid of him, gotten a gag order and had him in jail, too. "I betcha he needs this for bail," Janet said, watching Lorraine's face for her reaction.

"Like I said I'm not at liberty," Lorraine said. She reached to take the contract back from Janet until she got the check.

"It takes a few days to process," Janet said, making it up. The two women tugged discretely at the contract, like this was a playground and Jack's gag order a toy.

"You don't get this til you pay," Lorraine said. Nine-tenths of the law and all that.

"Let me make a call," Janet finally said. She could have cut the check right then, but she wanted to keep Jack sweating in jail as long as possible. She'd had a dream last night that Jack'd been raped up the ass like they showed in the movies. It'd serve him right. Janet dialed Mudnick's number but got only voice mail. She pretended she heard him. "Okay," she said in the phone. "I'll calculate the withholding."

Now Lorraine was getting mad. If they withheld taxes on the money she wouldn't get shit. "He's no longer employed here," Lorraine cut into Janet's mock call. "And the contract doesn't mention withholding."

Janet wondered how far to push it, decided this was enough, this heffer being a lawyer and all. Anyway Janet had a training to attend tomorrow. "We'll be informing the IRS," she told Lorraine. What did Lorraine care? The check was payable at EmpiBank.

"Any branches near here?" Lorraine asked Janet. EmpiBank's branches were almost all in Manhattan, below 96th Street.

"There's one in White Plains," Janet said.

There was a word for this, that Lorraine tried to remember. Redlining, that was it. Refusing to lend or have branches in poor neighborhoods, "communities of color" as the politically correct called them. Lorraine still called it the ghetto, still listened to WAR and Sly and the Family Stone. Parliament Funkadelic. She had a tape in her car.

"I'll cash it," Lorraine said. And that was that: Jack was gagged. If he disparaged EmpiGroup they could sue him for damages. It wasn't Lorraine's problem. There was one piece of advice she would give him, however: if he wanted the case to go away before trial, he'd have to get some leverage over EmpiFinancial, put some pressure on this white Janet Peel, make her squeal and recant, take the fax and say she liked it.

11. "March Directly Toward Your Goal"

Other than porno, Jack wasn't much for the 'Net. He'd brought his America Online account with him up from Charlotte along with his clunky three year old laptop; he entered the local Bronx access number and limited himself to JPEGs. Amazing what they could get Asian girls to do with donkeys. Sometimes he thought that the photos were doctored, were air-brushed, computer-generated, like that big-titted action star that all the kids watched. Neither Monstro nor Empi's offices were even connected to the Web -- it kept the worker bees in their cubicles with their eyes on the prize, the shimmering sea of home equity than beckoned. But laid off and out on bail Jack had time for the 'Net. He had little else to do.

Jack knew his body and this is what he knew: after he jerked off he couldn't get hard for at least a half an hour. To kill the time he ran searches, finally arriving at a term that he liked: "EmpiFinancial and Scandal." There were squibs about tax evasion, the summary of a Wall Street Journal article for sale -- fat change, Jack thought, if you could see snuff films for free -- and finally this weird web site called WatchCorp, which outright accused EmpiFinancial of predatory lending. Jack had heard the term down in Carolina, read the term in the newspaper up here in New York. Whoever'd written this site didn't know the half of it. It was talking about interest rates when credit insurance was the ultimate fuck. It was the engine of Empi's profits, the practice that could not be questioned. He remembered how they cracked down on his in Charlotte, how he'd silenced his doubts to get the promotion back up North. But now what did he owe Empi? Nothing. He hit the "Contact Us" button and an e-mail form popped up. These fuckers probably didn't even have an office. But he was flaccid and had nothing else but time on his hands. And Lorraine'd said to raise the stake on Empi. And so he wrote:

"I just got fired by EmpiFinancial for refusing to break the law."

He stopped. That wasn't quite true, but it was just a web site anyway, right? He continued: "I have a lot of information I could share with you if you are interested. But you can't use my name I am being sued or could be sued so let me know if I can be anonymous."

Jack wondered how or if to sign his message, then realized that his e-mail was traceable. Bender74 at aol dot com implied that there were at least 73 other Benders who'd been roped in by the mundane sharks from Virginia, now headquartered on Columbus Circle near failure -- but it was time for a new name. He flicked through AOL -- five screen names per account -- and chose a new one. Jackal, he chose -- with no number afterwards because no one else had chosen this name for whatever reason. He'd be The Jackal not The Cracker and henceforth stalk EmpiFinancial until they paid him money, all the stock options they cancelled the day he was fired. He fired off the e-mail and found he was once against stiff.

* * *

Candida has gone to the hospital for drugs so Kurt was alone in his six tastefully-lit rooms with the e-mail came in. A guy called the Jackal offering documents to bring EmpiFinancial down. This was why he'd started WatchCorp, this was the promise of the Internet, the infinite promise of anonymous dirt. AOL offered profiles of its members but for Jackal there was none. Kurt popped open another bottle of hyper-caffeinated soda and responded:

"Absolutely, you can be anonymous. We never reveal our sources" -- Kurt paused and wondered who this "we" was, then went on -- "and we can report the information in a way that cannot be traced to you." Kurt remembered seeing an old fax machine in Candida's walk-in closet, under a pile of high heeled shoes of various heights -- she was like Imelda Marcos when you got right down to it -- and he went in to check. It was dusty but it seemed to work; at least it worked to run photocopies and so why then wouldn't it receive? Kurt typed in Candida's phone number, then set up the machine between the jack and the base of Candida's cordless phone. "Send whatever you can to this number," Kurt typed and then hit Send. He waited but there was no reply; nor did the fax machine ring.

Jack by this time was languishing in the seventh set of photos of the Asian Hijinx library, all thoughts of The Jackal and his cardboard box of docs far from his mind. In a way he was not even a mind at all, just a sewer system of blood vessels that filled up then drained. Sometimes he wished he'd never fucked Diane -- it would have saved him a lot of money and heartache, but then he wouldn't have Zalie either. He'd have to call Diane to explain the delay in her check. She'd threatened to garnish his wages -- the phrase made Jack think of parsley, the sprigs on the top of his steak with the speckled butter, so good -- but now there was nothing to garnish. He'd have to call Diane and the thought deflated him. Maybe he should just go down to Charlotte and pick up Zalie, before Diane caught wind of the fact he'd been fired. Maybe Judge Birnbaum would never figure out he'd left the state. Maybe he'd just keep running. In Charlotte he could probably stay at Eric Taylor's, or at a cheap motel far from Tryon's crossroads. But he didn't have his car... Then with a jolt he remembered: he had frequent flier miles from his last solo junket to Rosarito Beach. He'd flown into San Diego then taken the train to San Ysidro then a bus and got laid. He'd saved enough credit for a free flight to Charlotte, maybe even a one-way to San Diego or at least Tijuana. BJ in TJ, that had used to be his slogan. But if he used his frequent flier miles would the court system find out, and lock him up at the airport, either here or where he got off? Maybe that could be checked online but for now he had better things to do.

* * *

The trainer was trim; his hair cut short and prematurely gray. He'd flown on the shuttle from Boston with his boss to fine-tune EmpiFinancial's corporate culture, to seduce middle management with a glimpse of Sandy's hairy goals. Like JFK projecting a man to the moon, that was the model. Sure they had core values; sure they had a mission statement in their annual report. But the hairy goal was where the rubber met the road -- where the rubber met the sky, as Bernie's boss Martin Blowman quipped whenever possible. He'd probably stolen the phrase from another management book, from another trainer on another circuit. Like snake oil salesmen they traversed the nation and now the globe offering accounting tricks and tax shelter advice, dressed in a thin veneer of leadership development and group-think. It was post-industrial capitalism morphed into a religion long after the Death of God. There was no Supreme Being but there were nonetheless big goals. There was no creed but profit-maximizing litanies of values, slightly tweaked for every different tribe, whether they made weapons or SUVs, or, as in the case of EmpiGroup, simply lent to make these things possible. Bernie was like a priest in a sense; this was like a spiritual retreat though it took place in a conference center on the top floor of Empi's skyscraper in Queens.

"Shall we begin?" Bernie said, smiling lithe and deathless, feeling these people's hunger for profit, for promotion if not meaning, for the tricks that would make all their teams work more smoothly. That was the Gordian knot to be cut: to harness the primal greed of each of these into teamwork, through an innovative compensation scheme and a culture of surveillance. Bernie's boss in fact had designed EmpiFinancial's Rocopoly system. Lending officers at its branches got bonuses all together or not at all. This cut down on the risk of team members fighting over the same sucker, as you'd see in an electronics store. They would sink or rise together -- but individual statistics would be kept. Promotion would ride on these. It was just the right balance. He even had a PowerPoint slide on that: "Our associates are fiercely competitive yet support each other." Holding two thoughts at once: it was almost a new religion.

This was Gina's first time at the altar. She felt a thrill with all these laptops out, the smell of cologne and mousse. Janet'd invited her at the last minute, saying "if you're going to run the branch you should come to the training in Queens." They left Maye in charge back at the West Farms Mall. They'd lose some juice around the edges, some tack-on charges would be foregone, but Gina'd recoup them with her new-found knowledge. She opened her laptop like all the others, smiled over at Janet, exhaled.

"So what do we sell?" Bernie asked, and one by one a dozen hands went up. Bernie shook his head. "Don't wait, just speak. 'Try it and fast' -- does anyone know which company uses that slogan?"

"Three M," a broad-shouldered cannibal from the Hicksville office said.

"And what did they invent?" Bernie asked.

"Scotch tape," said one. "Post-it Notes," said another.

"That's it," Bernie said. "Branch and prune. It's harder in financial services, but if you find a new way to make money you need to let your colleagues know. We measure and reward sharing. Don't hoard your ideas 'cause there'll always be more." He paused. "How many of you have met Sandy Vyle?"

There was silence; there was desire; there were no takers. Even if someone *had* they wouldn't say it here. "I heard him speak in Baltimore," a woman finally said. Others shook their heads. That didn't count. Bernie had never met Vyle either -- his boss Blowman was schmoozing with him right now in Bronxville -- but it didn't stop Bernie from referring to Vyle by his first name.

"Sandy has a goal," Bernie confided. This was the hairy goal but Bernie didn't like to call it that -- then they'd have to pay licensing fees to the business school wonks who'd written that book. "Sandy wants EmpiFinancial to be number one or two -- and one is better -- in every market we serve. Sandy wants the customer relationships you create to last for life. We are part of the American Dream"™ -- Bernie's speech was faster, this was where you sold them, gave them purpose, some post-September 11 patriotism -- "and as our customers move up we want to be there for them, with the right product at the right time."

Gina was rapt then she thought of the Guzmans, signed up for a loan they could never repay. She thought of Bertha Watkins, paying more for insurance on her bed than in rent. Would these people move up? Gina doubted it. She wanted to sell Empi's other products, mutual funds and annuities, but it wouldn't be in West Farms. She was proud to be here but it was just a stepping stone. By next year the Series Seven;

the year after that, the world. Maybe she could be a stock analyst. She'd heard they made a lot.

"You have to have passion," Bernie said. "Success directly correlates to having passion. You have to build passion in your team, because without each other you are nothing. EmpiBank is respected worldwide -- but without you, Sandy couldn't do it."

He'd be just another loan shark in Brooklyn, Gina thought. He wouldn't have his name on a hospital wing and a concert hall. She wanted that but not by mattress work, not by a pre-nup marriage and a bunch of screaming kids but through her own labor. She felt three or more of the men sneaking glances at her and she liked it. Not to be tied down now but because it was a weapon she could use. Vinny was temporary; Vinny was good but he was expendable.

"Just as Sandy does, you need to picture where you want to be in five years." Bernie had closed his eyes and encouraged the others to do so. "What kind of car do you want?" Bernie said. "Where do you want to live? What kind of legacy do you want to leave? Inheritance and such?"

The last part Gina could give a shit about. But car? She could almost feel it now, the white leather of its seats under her thighs. There was an English accent in there somewhere, champagne dreams, maybe Australian. "Picture it!" Bernie shouted as if in a trance. "Form the vision then march directly to your goal!" Gina clenched her eyes and she could see a big house in Greenwich, on a street where the plebes couldn't even park. She would drive there tonight, slowing but not stopping, observing and recording every detail to fuel the steps of her great long march.

12. Blowman's Brain

When Martin Blowman passed security in Bronxville in his rent-a-car, pulled up the circular driveway to EmpiGroup's glass-walled retreat house, he was surprised to see only four limousines parked in front. Sandy'd said it would be one of his patented think-n'-stink sessions where they'd take Turkish baths and discuss global domination. But the world was getting smaller every day.

A light-skinned Caribbean woman with high cheekbones took his coat -- Sandy can still pick 'em, Blowman thought -- and told him to go directly to the bath house, "Mister Sandy" was waiting for him there. Blowman has wondered why Sandy set his pow-wows in this too-precious suburb and not in one of Empi's dozen skyscrapers in Midtown or Queens. For secret merger meets he could understand it: the Mexican *cacique* had come here to sell his bank, flew in his jet to the White Plains airport, fewer journalists and tipsters there. Let no one inside-trade except Empi itself. Maybe it *was* a merger that Sandy wanted to discuss. It was an honor to be summoned by the meanest man on Wall Street. Jack Welch of GE had gotten all the press, but Sandy had gotten and still got most of the green. Blowman was on the EmpiGroup board, got paid $50,000 for every meeting he attended, including the bacchanals on Anguilla. To see some rolls of fat was not too much to ask in return.

Through the steam Sandy looked sicker than Blowman remembered: an obscene pink beach ball in a towel far too small. There was only one other figure in the steaming pool and it looked like a boy -- a young Turkish houseboy, Roman somehow, I Claudius stuttering out his corporate dictates.

"You know Bob," Sandy said curtly. Now that Blowman was closer of course he recognized him. Clinton's troubleshooter, Clinton's slick-tongued liaison to Wall Street, Rudehart himself.

"Marty," Rudehart said, as if they'd just played tennis last week.

"Robert, uh, Bob," Blowman said.

Sandy stood up and Blowman looked away. "Don't just stand there -- get naked," Sandy commanded.

The dressing room was more spacious but had fewer mirror than the New York Yankees clubhouse -- Blowman should know, having been there during three of the last five World Series'. Blowman hung his suit then his shirt and his boxer shorts on a series of hangers. He'd like to wear swimming trunks but there were none to be seen. When in Rome.

Sandy and Rudehard had moved to the cold water now and they were both shriveled up. "Go in the hot first," Sandy said. "That's the only way to get the full effect." Sandy believed that these hot and cold treatments would keep him alive forever. At the last board meeting -- Rudehart had missed it, some secret mission in Cancun -- Blowhart had obliquely mentioned the best current thinking on the touchy issue of succession. He mentioned GE, what else: how Jack Welch had spent nine years evaluating candidates before deciding on the current what's-his-name. Sandy had exploded and said he felt better than ever. Blowman had made a mental note never to mention the topic again. Even if Sandy did look embalmed as he bobbed in the frozen pool.

The heat turned Blowman's skin an embarrassing red. He didn't want to complain; the money was too good. The ice water was both a shock and a relief. Then they got down to business.

"Bob got a call from the fucking A.G.," Sandy said.

"Ashcroft?" Blowman's brain was paralyzed or at least slowed by the transition from hot to cold.

Sandy laughed. That holy-roller had staked his whole future on Al Qaeda. "No. Swanker."

"That's not good," Blowman said. He'd read a profile of Swanker in BusinessWeek. "The New Crusader," they'd called him. A moniker more fitting for Ashcroft, if you were referring to the old time Crusades.

"Bob's gonna have dinner with him, feel him out. Worse case scenario we'll hire him, like we hired... well, Bob." Sandy laughed at his own joke and even through the funhouse water Blowman saw that Vyle belly jiggle. He'd flown down for this?

"We wanted to know if you've got any hooks in him," Sandy continued. Blowman didn't. But he was sure they could be gotten.

"I could ask my other clients," Blowman said.

"*What* other clients?" Sandy loved to insult people, especially those he could smash, which was nearly everyone. I'd like to see him naked in Harlem, Blowman suddenly thought.

"We're doing a training in Queens today," Blowman said to change the subject. "The finance company. Typical rah-rah stuff."

"The hairy goal bullshit? What a crock."

Blowman had a sound byte: "Hey, this is where we write the jingle. But someone's got to play it, you know? It's classical music, not jazz."

"It's schlock if you ask me," Sandy said. "How much are we paying you for those fucking trainings, anyway?" Blowman didn't answer and Sandy went on. "Whatever it is it's too much. When I first bought EmpiFinancial we didn't use that soft dick bullshit. It was fuck 'em while the stars were in their eyes, switch the docs on 'em, whatever it took, to make their lives better." Sandy was cold and nostalgic. Blowman glanced at Rudehart who shrugged. Neither of them knew much about EmpiFinancial. It had been Sandy's baby, his first public company, his stepping stone into insurance and then investment banking. It was the one Empi business that Blowman had never attempted to re-vision, to break apart and reassemble. It was Empi's dark closet, the engine of its profits; it was Sandy's dark domain. To Blowman it was sleazy but for fifty large a day who's counting.

Sandy had a bug up his ass about management theory: he didn't believe in it. He paid outside consultants to drown mid-management in it like Prozac. The recruits seemed to need it, or at least to have acquired a taste for all its trappings in B-school. Case studies, product imagineering and all the buzzwords. To Sandy, Clausewitz On War was enough. He'd tried to read The Prince but it left him cold. It was time to get out of the bath.

"Are you, uh, gonna make Swanker an offer?" Blowman asked Rudehart as they dried off. Sandy was getting a massage and would not be out for at least an hour.

Rudehart smiled, his Hollywood teeth gleaming, more confident now out of Sandy's presence, the statesman again, everything looking and feeling larger. "We need to see what he's got," Rudehart said.

"And how's Mexico going?" Blowman could never get a straight answer from Sandy, even at the board meetings.

"*Va bien*," Rudehart said, like it was a speech in Austin or Miami. "It was all tax free down there and we're getting ready to roll EmpiFinancial out through the NaraMex branches, starting in Baja California."

"They've got whale sighting trips there," Blowman said. Rudehart looked at him strangely. This was not a meeting of equals. Rudehart dropped his towel to make the point clearer.

"And how's Harvard?" Rudehart asked, as if Blowman was up to the moment on all things Beantown. "How's little Larry Springtime doing at the helm of John Harvard's ship?"

"He got a pie in the face the other day--"

"A pie in the mouth, more likely--"

--"from these ungrateful kids talking about minimum wage in the cafeteria there. But he's raising money, that's for sure."

"That's what they got him for." Rudehart paused, then continued as if talking past Blowman, as if talking to himself. "I could have had it, you know. It was mine for the asking. But I thought this opportunity... was interesting."

Yeah fifty million dollars a year more interesting, Blowman thought. What did a management consultant have to do to hit those big leagues? I could have been you, Blowman wanted to say but it was absurd. It was like they were still in sixth grade: who's is bigger. In this trio Blowman was low man on the totem pole. But everywhere else he walked tall. And that was probably enough.

Sandy waddled out with a turkey drumstick like Henry the Eighth and they both stopped talking. "You really got to try her," Sandy said, directing it at Rudehart. Blowman ignored it, thinking already of the shuttle flight back to Boston. Two of Al Qaeda's missile had flown from there, full of well-meaning people and a tank full of jet fuel. Now MassPort had freaked out and insisted you take off you shoes while the swabbed them. Sandy and Rudehart flew private jets so didn't notice. Blowman felt an absurd twang of class resentment, as of a millionaire for a Pharaoh. The biggest bank on earth and it was all built on smut and sleaze. Amazing, Blowman thought. This was the management book he should write, an exposé if he cashed in his pension for armed guards. The secrets of the Wall Street stars.

"I have to go," he said.

"Call in all favors on Swanker," Sandy said. "Collect all his I.O.U.'s and we'll stick them up his ass."

"Gently," Rudehart added and Sandy smiled. It was a pampered iteration of good cop bad cop and it made Blowman sick. If Bernie wasn't at the airport when he got there he'd just fly. He'd had enough.

*　*　*

Bernie was in a yellow cab -- a regular fucking pedestrian yellow cab -- stuck in traffic on the Grand Central Parkway. "Why doncha get off?" he suggested to the turbaned man in front. The man shrugged and obliged but the service road was hardly better. They passed a cemetery and Bernie turned the other way. He wondered if Blowman would look different, after a full day with Sandy. Bernie had taken to dreaming in PowerPoint slides; he believed what he said at these trainings. He liked the focus on organization over individual -- clockmaking over time-telling, as his slide on the topic put it -- because he'd been dealt a bit short in the field of charisma. There were people he could impress, like those drones in Queens today, but the most important people didn't even see him. It was a Darwinistic world where they took off your clothes and measured you before you even knew it happened. He had a slide on that too, a corporate adaption of Darwin. "Multiply, vary; let the strongest live and the weakest die." That one stuck in his throat so he usually just let the slide speak for itself. It was meant to refer to experiments and innovations -- like the Post-It Note or Marriott's entry into the airport and hotel businesses -- but his audiences usually read it literally, looking around at their colleagues sizing up whose cubicle they could take. If he'd been born earlier -- a half-dozen centuries, say -- Bernie could have been a Jesuit, written a treatise on purgatory, on unbaptized babies going to limbo and why that's okay, even almost poetic. Now he was left mouthing exegesis of the wisdom of Hewlett-Packard. "We exist as a corporation to make a contribution" -- what the hell did that mean? A contribution to the laser-jet reproduction of motivational speakers' calls to be more selfish? To dump the used-up parts in landfills in Asia, to leech their toxins into the water supplies of those who even *had* water in those countries? He had to cut his non-business reading back, Bernie decided. It was starting to interfere with his work.

13. Peeping Tom

Jack was raw as he rode the BX 12 bus through Bronx Park to Kinkos. This WatchCorp character, this Kurt if that was his real name, said he wanted documents. The stuff in Jack's cardboard boxes were mostly loan files, the last two dozen loans made in the office before the axe fell. Among them were the Watkins and Guzman files. They were run-of-the-mill EmpiFinancial loans but maybe this Kurt would go to town with them. Jack'd thought of calling Micah Levine but something about it rubbed him wrong. And he'd been rubbed enough. Let's see what these Internet jokers could do.

George was chilling listening to the latest Jay-Z joint on CD when the white man came in. He recognized the man, from the photo he'd seen. Had he seen him before that? He still wasn't sure. The two exchanged glances over the counter while George handed him the copy card.

"I don't know how to say this," George said, "but these people came in here the other night showing me your picture--"

It came together in Jack's head. "You're the one who signed the statement, the affidavit, whatever?"

George backed away from the counter so the man couldn't hit him. "It *was* you, right?" George asked.

Jack gathered his thoughts -- he felt so empty it was not difficult -- and decided to ask a question himself. It was based on something Lorraine Thompson said in court. "How many pictures did they show you?"

"Just one, man. Yours. It was three in the morning. If it *wasn't* you, you sure pissed those people off."

"Did you, like, give them any description before they showed you the picture?"

"Nah. They flashed the thing at me, then some kind of contract, information of disbelief, some shit like that. They said it was okay if I wasn't sure. I mean they didn't tell me what they were gonna do with it, I'm sorry if--"

"Don't worry," Jack said. He'd seen enough private eye movies to know not to show his cards. The kid had already done what he did. If he felt guilt there was no reason to piss it away. "Just remember what happened," Jack said. "Someday I might need you to testify--"

"I'll say it just like it happened," George said. He paused. "And yo -- whatever you're faxing tonight, it's on the house." George turned off the monitor that counted the number of copies made. Fuck Kinkos anyway.

* * *

Candida was red-eyed and desperately upbeat when the fax came through. Part of her liked it, that Kurt would use her home as his office. If only he was faxing out résumés instead of soliciting long blurry documents that would tie up her phone for an hour. The machine reminded her of Stewart and she wondered for the millionth time if perhaps they shouldn't have stayed together. Kurt was wilder; Kurt was more fun -- but Kurt made no money and was constantly judging her and her lifestyle, a hair-shirt when he had no right to be, as if he would have liked to live in a basement in Queens, turned pervert by hours greasy-handed with boilers like her papi.

"Kurt," she called into the kitchen where Kurt was playing with his laptop and stinking up the place with his roll-your-own smokes, "there's a fax for you."

Kurt hit the Save button -- he was dissecting and deconstructing EmpiGroup's Statement of Commitment to Customers -- and extinguished his smoke in the aerated tap water. He was going stir-crazy, on this blond wood kitchen table from Ikea. Maybe the Jackal was answering his call. He bent over the fax machine. They were loan documents, all right. They had the people's social security numbers on them, their interest rates and home addresses. "Mother *fuck*er," Kurt whispered.

There was no cover sheet, just the single I.D. line at the top, Kinkos. 718, the outer boroughs. Kurt hoped it was not Brooklyn. Sure a tree grew there -- but there were cops there too, and the ghost of Gene Ramos, FOCO's spies in every 'hood, or so Kurt imagined. He counted the pages backwards, wanting to read them in order, the first loan and then the refi, the flip, taking notes on a yellow pad, picking which documents he should scan and put on the 'Net, WatchCorp's first exclusive, incontrovertible proof that Wall Street was based on crime.

The first loan documents was from a couple named Guzman who lived on Park Avenue -- Kurt did a double-take, thinking of the condominium canyons north of Grand Central, then looking closer and seeing it was Park Avenue in The Bronx, a number in the four thousands, a 10457 zip code. The interest rate for 14 and a half percent, more than double what other people pay. The $64,000 question was why: were the Guzmans in bankruptcy? But if so why would Empi have made them a loan?

The other docs were smaller loans -- two thousand here, five thousand there -- each with a weird print-out list behind it. Maybe it was what the people had bought with the loan, Kurt thought. There was camping equipment, an electric typewriter -- what can that be worth, Kurt wondered -- and a $5,000 loan for a bed. When he looked closer he say that most of the finance charge was insurance.

"So is it good?" Candida asked, coming out of the kitchen with a tall glass of wine.

"Good for an exposé, but bad for the victims," Kurt said. "Gimme a second -- I need to e-mail this wacko and ask what some of this means. And how he got the documents if he doesn't work there anymore."

Here we go again, Candida thought -- another fixation, another addiction, another windmill for Kurt to waste his youth tilting at. She'd had about enough of it. She could no longer believe. She gulped at her wine and felt her smooth white walls suffocating her.

* * *

It was night and Gina was following Bernie's advice. Picture it -- hadn't he said that? She drove up the Hutch, then the New England Thruway to Greenwich, past the exits for Larchmont, Mamaroneck and Rye, strange signs for Cos Cob, the smell of money in the air. For her this was the best motivator, to cruise the private streets by the Sound. Tonight she even jotted names. When she got her Series Seven these were the people she would pitch. You couldn't see most of the houses from the street. Lush green hedges and wrought-iron fences, family names on copper signs hanging from troll-like horse trainer figures, none of them black. They had lawn jockeys in Greenwich -- Gina'd read that word, some controversy about racism, nothing she cared about. There was an overpriced diner where she liked to eat, chopped lettuce salad with no dressing and a Diet Coke -- she told herself it was not to meet a man, but only to think, without the racket and tensions of The Bronx, for visioning as Bernie said, to see it so clear you could drool and kill for it.

Today the West Farms Mall, tomorrow Cos Cob. And that was the name of the salad. Maybe tonight she'd have ranch.

* * *

Tom Bain arrived on MetroNorth at eight. He felt at a crossroads -- the train tracks helped -- and wanted to give Elizabeth one more chance, see if destiny would finally make him knock on her door, before falling headlong in pursuit of this Nour. He'd taken this ride before, and always returned on an empty train feeling lost. He could afford to live here if he wanted but it felt dead to him, these lawns and sweater shops, these new Volvo station wagons as a second car. Maybe it would make sense to live here if you had kids. That was probably Elizabeth's vision at her wedding. Tom had gotten an invitation and torn it into pieces so small his fingers hurt. It was heavy stationary of the lightest yellow and it hadn't been easy. It had been like an alarm: you are now entering the fourth quarter of your young adulthood. Your college squeeze has tied the knot with another guy. And you have exactly what? A Bloomberg terminal and a high-rise condo shackled with debt. You could buy a pet but it would be too pathetic. You had the best drugs in the world, delivered by messenger to your office or home. Death on a platter; a life wasted daily in arbitrage.

Tom Bain sucked on the cool night air, walking on the thick green grass by the side of the road. Various European luxury cars slowed as they passed. What was a man in a suit doing walking? Even for the quarter-mile to the commuter train station people bought second and third cars. Here was Elizabeth's mail box; there was Elizabeth's wind chime and her little garden, baby carrots and a small planting of thyme. He remembered when she'd cooked for him, and he for her, mostly reheated *charcuterie* from an expensive French deli he hadn't cared the cost. She'd thought he was soulless; he'd thought he could do better. Now she was right and he was wrong. The automatic sprinklers turned on and while they squeaked Tom crept to the window.

Elizabeth was home, facing her computer in her book-lined den. Tom put his cheek on the window and tried to see. Was she writing a poem? An e-mail? Trading stock? Her face looked softer, sadder somehow, more wise, impossible. She sold real estate now, that's what he'd heard. Her ex paid the mortgage but she might have to move. Maybe that would be the time to appear, the time to finally speak, to propose some spur-of-the-moment vacation to France, to show he had a soul and not just a Titanium AmEx card. He'd thought tonight would be the night but when he envisioned knocking, her answering the door dreamy-eyed from Yeats, he felt empty. He had nothing to say. He had no news, no self-knowledge, nothing but Ecstasy. He felt barren as he watched a rabbit cross the lawn. It might have been a haiku but that was too long ago. Elizabeth looked self-content and Bain was filled with self-contempt. He turned and retraced his tufty steps, condemned by the synchronized sprinklers which made this bitter heaven fertile.

* * *

He'd just missed the train and had twenty two minutes to kill. He'd have a burger rare and dripping, avoid for this night his microwave's desolate ping. In the diner there was a perfect family with their perfect kids. It was disgusting and Tom knew they smoked rock at Greenwich Country Day. There was a woman alone picking at a salad and reading a motivational book that Tom recognized from work. Maybe she was waiting for a man like him -- like him but not dead, like him but braindead, fucked and lucky -- to get off the train and drive her home. Perhaps there was a nanny taking care of their kids, though she looked a bit young to have kids you'd want to entrust to a stranger though women were hard-driving now so who knew? Bain ordered his burger -- "so rare you can see the blood," he said -- and sidled over toward the woman. The morning's near-moot Connecticut Post and the New York Times were for sale on a rack beside her table. Bain opened the Times to the Wine Section, loudly flapping the pages like a pheasant showing plumage in the wild.

Gina looked up from the fourth effective habit because this guy was rustling a newspaper and staring at her, cocky bastard it would seem but he was cute in his way, his suit fit him nicely though he looked flushed and sweating. He kept looking at his watch and then at her. She turned back to her book but couldn't concentrate. She felt his eyes on her as she drizzled a bit more ranch dressing on her salad.

"Uh, excuse me," the guy finally said. "Do you know what time it is?"

It was transparent and pathetic; there was a clock on the wall and the glint of a watch under the cuff of the guy's suit jacket. Gina looked at the thin-band watch on her thin wrist and said nine thirty-four without looking up.

"Train's in sixteen minutes," he said. "Are you going to the city?"

She closed her book 'round her finger at the page she was on. "Are you trying to pick me up?" she asked, with the glint of a smile. She was used to this. Fat ugly or old she would just ignore them. Guys like this she'd confront, just to see how they wiggled out of it.

"I read that book," the guy stammered. "So I just... wondered how you like it."

"You didn't answer my question."

"You looked lonely," Tom said. He was usually not this direct, but the waiting and panting at Elizabeth's window, the impotent feeling and the smell of his burger defrosting on the grill made him bold.

"You must think you're very perceptive." What the woman said was snotty but she was smiling, like this was a game and perhaps it was.

"You only live once," Tom said, hoping that the hundred meanings would be clear. You only live once so let's take the train to the city and fuck all night with the curtains off the windows and the planes closing in. You only live once so that's why I've taken my shot, flapping the newspaper to get your attention -- I'm a gambler not a loser. You only live once: don't eat salad alone when you could take the train with me to wherever you want to go, to the very end of the rails by the Arctic Circle.

"So I've heard," the woman said. Bain's burger was ready; he was being summoned to the counter to either eat it there or have it wrapped.

"For here," Bain said, then, "do you mind?" He sat down, gulped ice water to clear the dryness from his throat, wondered at the absurdity of being unable to speak to a women he knew yet coming on so assuredly to a stranger with a self-help book. Some blood from the burger seeped out on the bun; there were ocean-salt chips and a quarter of pickle. He could take a later train. He could take any train he wanted or no train at all.

"So what *do* you think of the book?" Bain asked after swallowing the first bite of the burger.

"I take what I want and leave the rest," Gina said. She'd driven here straight from West Farms, hadn't left a message -- let Vinny be the one to worry for once -- no one knew where she was and she felt like a college girl again, like anything in the world was possible, this guy was probably a jerk but he seemed more relaxed than her colleagues at the training today. No need to talk of consumer finance; she could pretend to be anything she wanted. "I'm married, you know," she said, just to put that on the table.

"Lucky guy," Bain said, some watered-down blood dribbling down his chin.

"*I* think so."

Bain decided to experiment with the truth. "I think those books are garbage," he said, putting the burger down and looking into her eyes. "If it was as easy as they say, everyone would be a millionaire. The only ones getting rich off those books are the authors. Or only the publishers, really."

Gina shrugged. "I like biographies more," she said. "Memoirs or whatever you call them. The guy from Virgin Airlines--"

"He's a charlatan," Bain cut in. "Sodas and airplanes and CDs -- what's the connection? He's more like a pop star than a businessman."

"Don't we all want to be pop stars?" Gina asked. She liked to hear her voice in this nowhere talk with this nowhere guy, knowing that her car with its The Club™ and alarm was right outside. This was not the type of guy who you'd meet in the West Farms Mall. This guy and Jack Bender, it was like two different species. "What's your name, anyway?" she asked.

Bain almost lied then figured what the fuck. "Tom Bain," he said, then the name of his company. It was a boutique, a recent appendage to a Germanic universal bank so he had to add, "I analyze stocks."

"What companies?"

Again, why not? Start with the largest, the pop-star loan sharks with the name recognition. "EmpiBank," he said. "And some regional banks in the South."

Gina was broken from her dream by the mention of her employer -- her mind whirled trying to figure out if this was a good or bad thing. How could he help her? Should she say where she worked? What would the world's most effective people do? Defer, she decided.

"Look I have to go," she said.

Bain was disappointed -- she'd said she was married but he'd quickly envisioned an affair, maybe some insight into Elizabeth, some surrogate Elizabeth, fucking getting back to her in some parallel universe -- so he tried to stall. "Have a coffee or something," he said.

"No, really." She was standing up now.

"Do you live around here?"

"In the city." Gina said it before thinking. She could have said yes but he might have asked where. She had a house in mind, the one that when she closed her eyes she saw, but he might know the occupants. Anyway, it was done, she'd said it. He was nodding now.

"Me too," he said. "I was going to take the train but maybe--"

She shook her head -- he might be a psycho, right? -- and he seemed to expect that because he was pulling out a business card, writing on the back, his home number. "You can check me out on the Internet," he said. "So you can know that I am, like, who I am. Summaries of my research reports are up."

"Have a nice ride," she said. The phrase would resonate with him on the lurching ride though Rye and south. Maybe that was fate, he decided. He'd gone to play peeping Tom with Elizabeth and he'd met a nice self-actualizing young woman. Nothing she'd said had impressed him too much -- it was her whole way of being, her carriage, well yes, her body, her thin salacious wrist when she checked and said nine thirty four.

14. HomeQuik

When Jack saw the Guzmans' loan docs on the 'Net he felt good. WatchCorp Kurt had used a magic marker it look like on their social security numbers and precise address on Park Avenue -- everything else was left in, including the interest rate, the credit insurance, the mandatory arbitration, the whole nine yards. But what the guy was lacking was analysis. He'd written a sidebar pointing out at most ten percent of the problems with the loan. WatchCorp didn't list a phone number, just an e-mail address. Jack switched to his Jackal screen name and typed wildly, "these people are getting fucked, I could get you their credit reports to show you they could of gotten six percent, you're sitting on a time bomb and don't even know what it is - Jackal."

This Kurt guy must never sleep -- maybe it was a committee like at SUNY they said Shakespeare was, again the floating though of the mad Dane king -- he responded right away, asking for more docs, asking to meet off the record.

Jack was nude and drinking beer and wanted more. "You got to go somewhere with this," he wrote, "I'll get more docs but you send them out, not just on your little web site but to bigger places like 60 Minutes do you know anyone there?" Jack pushed send and waited. He *had* no more docs, he'd already faxed the best stuff he had but he thought he knew where to get some more.

Candida was naked but Kurt didn't care -- this Jackal source was threatening to take his info elsewhere, it wasn't ready for 60 Minutes and they'd probably never trash EmpiBank anyway. Still he had to keep Jackal's hopes high and so he wrote, "I know a lot of people in the business press but I think we should line the whole story up before we pitch them." It was time to get more specific. "Since the files you faxed are all from the Bronx I figure that's where you worked -- true? Don't worry we never reveal our sources. But if that's where you are I could come up there and we could plan how to play the story the best way." He typed in Candida's number, it was time for that. "Call me, you don't have to give your name," he wrote and pushed Send.

"Come to bed," Candida mumbled. The pharmaceutical cocktail she'd stolen today was almost like a date rape drug. Kurt didn't like it this way; it felt like creepy necrophilia. It was too late to fight about sobriety. They were both junkies in their different ways.

The phone rang and after Candida's fake-bubbly outgoing message complete with pop music and a joke a voice came on. "It's me," it said. "The Jackal."

"Jackal!" Kurt said as he picked up the phone, as if they were friends. You had to develop your sources, it was almost like running a cult like Gino Ramos. "Was I right, about the Bronx?"

"Yeah," the Jackal said. "Where is this I'm calling, anyway? You got an office that you're there that late?"

Kurt looked at Candida dozing on the leather couch and said no. "It's just a temporary number," he said. "I'll let you know when I change it."

"You should go talk to the Guzmans," Jackal said. "Since you already put all their shit on the Web."

"I blacked out some--"

"I noticed, that was nice. But you need to hear from them what the bitch Gee-- what the loan officer told them. And she only did it 'cause her district manager said to. That's Janet Peel. That's the one you really got to get."

Kurt asked for the spelling of names; he looked at Candida's caller I.D. but it was blank. It was only seventy-five cents to block it and this Jackal wasn't stupid.

"So how do I talk to the Guzmans?" Kurt asked.

"Just call 'em up," Jackal said. This Kurt didn't know much. At EmpiFinancial they cold-called people every day. They had a quota to meet, they'd work late some nights until they roped ten suckers in apiece.

Kurt thought back to hawking copy paper for FOCO, cringed at the thought of just cold-calling these people like some telemarketer.

"Why doncha just call Janet Peel?" Jackal asked. "Just call and ask her about this fucking loan. It'd make her sweat, I'll tell you that."

Jackal gave him Peel's number, said maybe he'd reach out to the Guzmans if Kurt didn't want to. "We'll set it up," Jackal said. "They're nice people." Actually he didn't know them at all, just watched as Gina put the screws to them. He'd need a pretext. It was now or never to get revenge.

* * *

Jack was broke but he wasn't stupid. There was a place even further down the food chain from Empi, consumer finance outfit based right outside Chicago, HomeQuik. They had a second floor space on Fordham Road at the Concourse, across from the Marine Recruiting station where the finest flower of the Bronx' youth signed up with G.E.D.'s to fight the Arabs. From Subway to Saddam Hussein, it wasn't for Jack. But he went to HomeQuik and made his pitch.

"Why'd you leave Empi?" the guy asked. The guy was old-school loan shark, the only thing he lacked was a jeweler's monocle, maybe a green see-through visor and a pair of brass knuckles. It would do.

"Couldn't make enough money there," Jack said. "They had too many freakin' rules, too long a turn-around time to get the loans done. They send everything down to Baltimore for the okay. I heard that you guys--"

"You heard right. Every office is authorized to make its own decisions unless the delinquencies get too bad. We've been needing some experienced people. But you'll start on commission, you know that, right?"

Jack needed a pay check but if there was one thing he knew it was loans. "I'm ready to go," he said. "You have prospect lists, right?"

The guy -- his nameplate said Ehrenreich, he should have changed it for Bronx business but Jack didn't say anything -- shook his head. "We get data from EquiFax and send out mailers."

"What's the response rate?"

"Two percent, maybe three."

Jack laughed. "I'm gonna show you the Empi way," he said. "You go to the county clerk and look up all of last week's mortgages. The new filings. Then you call 'em up and say you can do better."

Ehrenreich considered it. This guy looked a little sleazy but he talked a good game. "How about personal loans?" Ehrenreich asked.

"There's another way to do that. But let's do mortgages first."

* * *

On St. Ann's Avenue the electricity was off. The wires that came in from the street were old and thin; they'd burned through, the super said, when two of the tenants installed air-conditioners bought on credit from the Crazy Prices discount -- meaning "stolen" -- electronics store on Melrose Avenue. Mrs. Morales bless her heart had taken Duwon and the girls to the public swimming pool in St. Mary's Park. Bertha lay on the four-poster bed, pulling the trigger on a spray bottle from time to time. The breeze from the window would evaporate the water and she'd feel cool for a moment. Then she'd spray again.

As inexorable as the heat were Bertha's thoughts of her two dead loved ones. Arthur's death had at least been foreseeable: you couldn't blame God for lung cancer, or at least it took a few more logical leaps to do so. But what kind of God kills a girl like Penny Zade with no notice, for no reason? Micah's Old Testament God like a drug kingpin gave no excuses. The evangelicals who raised their tent in St. Mary's Park every summer were another story. They claimed their God was peace and love; when tragedy happened they blamed it on free will or sometimes on the gays. Bertha hated them for that, blaming the death of her Penny Zade on people she didn't know, decisions that hadn't been hers. Bertha tried to spray and evaporate the thoughts from her mind: they did no good. She remembered a phrase from a poster in the school board's office: fight like hell for the living. She'd like to do that when the chance arose. When it wasn't so hot. The water from the spray bottle mixed with Bertha's tears, soaked into the pillows on the four-poster bed.

* * *

That night Jack took the Two Train from Pelham Parkway to One Seven Four. He was working for two masters, or four if you considered Zalie and his own needs. Even the Rent-A-Center was closed. A rent-a-cop dozed in the PhotoMat booth. Jack slipped to the back of the mall as if to take a piss. There behind EmpiFinancial's back door was his target: a five-yard rolling garbage dumpster on wheels. Jack knew when they came to empty it because he'd sent up the contract himself. Garbage went out to the dumpster every night as close of business; the BFI only came three days a week, just before dawn, its metal jaws hungry for paper.

Jack set up by the dumpster as if pissing on it and pushed up on the metal top. Gotcha! The dumb bitches! There was a space for a padlock was it wasn't in use. Inside there were three see-through plastic garbage bags of docs, none of them shredded. Idiots, Jack thought. You could give a loan shark a shredder but you couldn't make him use it. Without a car he couldn't just take the three bags; he had to go through them. There were print-outs from Monstro; there were pay-off forms and some memos from Home Office. Ehrenreich better hire some more people to refi all these bullshit Empi loans. And WatchCorp better have enough server space for all this crap. The stop, Sixty Minutes. It was dawn when Jack was done, hiding in the weeds watching the truck carry away the chaff. He had one see-though bag of wheat. Feeling rich already he took a gypsy cab to Olinville. Even the drug dealers had turned in for the light. He carried his bag and three forties of Englishe up the stairs. If this was garbage he was Albert Schweitzer. There was gold in them thar dumpsters and Janet Peel would pay and pay. He'd make her forget all about the fax, make her tell the police that she'd sent it to herself. Then he'd sue Empi for money and set up Zalie as the little princess of Rosarito Beach. Jack had a plan, a reason to get up and get outside even before jerking off -- and that was saying something.

The kicker was they'd thrown out the spare Guzman file, must have scanned the docs into Monstro and tossed the dead trees to make more space. It was all here: copies of Amado's hospital bills, his pay stubs from construction jobs, EquiFax confirming an unblemished history of servility to debt. Did the wife work? The file didn't say. Jack needed to know 'cause he'd go there today. It was time to offer the Guzmans a lower rate, and try to flip them against the company that'd first fucked them. Jack always knew that he shoulda been a lawyer. If he'd spent more time at SUNY in class and not on drugs maybe he coulda. If that bitch Diane had been more supportive, if Jack'd been more ambitious, maybe he woulda. There was the litany, unpacked. Life was what it was. Jack took the BX 12 to Fordham Plaza, then the X15 to Crotona Park and walked west.

There were furniture stores offering in-store credit -- he could get those contracts for HomeQuik, Jack thought, and maybe flip Sicilian too; there was an old bank branch become a church, a sweatshop in a vaudeville theater. There was a wide railroad cut where the MetroNorth ran. The Guzmans' house was north of Tremont. Two-and-a-half story attached with a metal gate like Mad Max. There was a separate entrance to the basement, its window dark. Perhaps it had been a candy store once, when kids played in this street instead of inside behind metal bars. Jack stood at the fence and rang the bell.

Milagros Guzman peeked out the door. Her hair was tinted purple and her brown complexion clear. "*Jes?*" she asked.

"M'name's Jack Bender. I came to talk about your loan."

"You're with EmpiFinancial, right? I saw you in the office. Look, I know we only sent half but it was just the first payment, with the hospital bill it is not easy--"

"Don't worry Mrs. Guzman," Jack said. "I'm not here to collect on the loan. I don't work for Empi anymore." He paused. "Can I come in?"

"It is almost time to take Amado to the hospital," Milagros said. "If you don't work there, why--"

"I work at another company now. I know you're paying too much and I think we can do better. I think EmpiFinancial ripped you off."

"But you were the boss, no?"

"It wasn't my loan." Jack didn't have a HomeQuik business card yet; he felt pathetic talking through this wire mesh fence. "They charged your fourteen and a half percent interest," he said. "I think I can get you six, and no insurance."

"Why did they not tell me this?"

"That's what I want to talk with you about. I think you could sue them, or go to the press."

"We just need to pay less each month," Milagros said. She wondered if this was a trick, the man from West Farms coming here talking about lawsuits.

"*Quien es?*" Amado called from in the house.

"*El tipo del Empi -- dice que ya no trabaja ahi.*"

Amado came to the door, leaning on a crutch in a muscle t-shirt, his arms well-toned. "What you sellin' now?" he asked. He did not like these gringos. He had gone for the loan since he had no choice, but he didn't want them at his house, bothering his wife.

"I'm sorry 'bout what they did to you," Jack said. "I work for a better company now and I want to make it right."

"Where you work?" Amado demanded.

"A place called HomeQuik, they have an office on the Grand Conc--"

"I have seen it. To me your companies are all the same. They bleed the poor man dry, take what he has because he has no options."

"I'm offering six percent interest," Jack said. "At least four hundred dollars less in payments each month."

"You show me in writing and maybe," Amado said. He turned to Milly. "*Dile al jodon que ya tenemos que ir.*"

"We must go now, to the hospital."

"I will bring a contract tomorrow," Jack said slowly. "I will bring another man with me who is with the press."

"*Vamos a ver,*" Amado said and slammed the door.

15. *Un Hombre* of the Left

Nicole Nour took the One Train uptown to catch of glimpse of her future. It was a graduate seminar in investigative journalism, a panel of pompous British gumshoes in a high ceilinged room at the top of Loeb Hall. Nicole had gone to Columbia J-school -- that's when she'd come to the States, over her father's objections and with him paying the bills. They sent her their monthly calendar of talks and this is the one she'd attend. If you wanted to get ahead you had to listen, how ever begrudgingly, to those who'd arrived.

A man from the Times of London played with his hair and talked about the Official Secrets Act. "You Yanks have all the freedom in the world but you don't use it," he said. He'd served jail time, for Christ's sake, for exposing a corrupt privatization under Thatcher.   "Use it or lose it," he said. Nicole wrote that down.

Afterwards she crossed Broadway to Ollie's Noodle Shop and ate dumplings alone, leafing through the Columbia Journalism Review. They tried to celebrate the written press but everyone knew that off-camera talent was increasingly cheap. Exploding tires could whip up some interest. Accounting scandals if you were the Money Honey™ were just the ticket. But the hum-drum reporting of earnings was for drones. She thought about her source -- she even thought of him that way, generically, hadn't written the name "Tom Bain" down anywhere and might never do it, he was perhaps good for only one scoop, his promises of more just a play to get laid. She'd wondered about his motive, had figured he was selling Empi short for his own account. Reporters had to take their sources as they found them, self-interested, half-stepping, moving the market then moving on. A guy at the Times had exposed a source as a pay-back for lies. It was an ugly business; now the guy worked for a P.R. firm. Protecting the source was the sine qua non. If you back-slid on that, you might as *well* be a hack. Nicole was a true believer, perhaps the only one in her graduating class. She finished her dumplings with chop sticks and grabbed her cell.

Bain was immersed in a vicious video game when his phone rang. The three CDs took up half of his hard drive but the blood look real; you moved the axe with your mouse, chopping and chopping at the gnomes of your fears.

"Bain," he said into the mouthpiece, like an astronaut or air traffic controller, not a moment or movement wasted.

"It's me Nicole from the Journal. You said you had more so I thought I'd call."

Tom hit pause, the blood still dripping on the walls, and sat up straight. You had to prioritize your lusts. Peeking in at Elizabeth had felt final; the chit-chat aborted pick-up only whet his appetite. "I'm working on it." But he had nothing to say. "In fact I'm working on it right now. I'll get back to you soon."

"You have my cell number," Nicole said, watching the ghost-like pimply students float by outside the plate glass window. "Just be sure to bring it to me first."

Oh I will, thought Tom. He stared at the gore on his frozen screen and wondered how.

* * *

In the loft over Fordham Ehrenreich shook his head. "We don't do it at six," he told Jack.

"It's worth it this time," Jack said. "The Guzmans know a lot of people, they'll talk us up and you'll have more customers than you can handle. Here--" Jack opened the accordion file into which he'd put the hottest lead from last night's forage -- "look at their fucking credit score. Seven-eighty, off the charts. These people never miss a payment."

Ehrenreich wouldn't have even thought of doing it, except for the slew of names and numbers that Jack had brought in. The pages were crumpled and Ehrenreich wondered where Jack got them. But the people were real; he'd checked a few on Fair Isaacs and in the phone book. "Just this once," Ehrenreich said. "When the referrals come in eight's the lowest we'll go."

"Yeah chief," Jack said. This guy was so slow Jack could take over this office in a month, the way he saw it. But that wasn't his goal. He needed to fuck Janet Peel and get them to drop the case. He needed to get a second slice of severance from Empi, get his daughter then clean his soul. It wasn't too late and at six he was doing God's work. His commission would be less but in context it made sense. He had to play this WatchCorp Kurt 'til Sixty Minutes came along. He'd lie on Rosarito Beach and he could always feel proud of what he'd done for the Guzmans. To be moral in a sleazy world was not easy but Jack'd caught a glimpse. Sometimes you had to destroy to create.

* * *

Jack'd arranged to meet Kurt the next day on Fordham Road. Not in HomeQuik but at a hotdog stand across the street. That Kurt didn't have a car was a bad sign. Jack needed a real journalist, not just some fucker with a web site and a dream. Kurt was fast, though, you had to give him that. He put the docs online the same night for the whole world wide web to see. Kurt was hungry and Jack liked that. Without passion the underdog could never win.

If Jack went home now he knew what he'd do and he was sick of it. It was time to conserve his chi -- you had to picture the enemy day and night, envision his downfall or in this case hers. What he needed were documents with Janet Peel's signature on them. Or proof that she'd signed off on what Gina and Maye were doing. It was barely dark but Jack headed to West Farms. No one could stop him from having a three meat taco, could they? Maybe he'd go to Rent-A-Center, see how the other half was living.

Gina's car was in the lot but so was Janet's too. Fuck yeah thought Jack, he'd catch those carpet-munching bitches screwing a new customer, get the docs from the dumpster and give 'em to Kurt. Jack ducked down behind a van, tied his postal walking shoes tighter. This was war and he was ready. He'd never written down Janet's license plate number so he did now. He had a friend at the DMV, could get her home address and whole driving record. He could make this bitch's life miserable if he wanted. And he wanted.

He should have just waited but he couldn't resist. When Janet came out in her pants suit at dusk he popped out behind the van. "The Guzman loan's gonna come in for pay-off," he told her. "Then a lawyer's gonna review everything that you did."

The balls on this cracker, stalking her in the West Farms lot. Janet was scared -- she could admit that to herself -- but more than that she was angry. "I'd stay away from here if I were you," Janet said evenly. "You might be out on bail but when you lose at trial they're going to put you away."

"It'll never get to trial," Jack cackled. "You got no proof that I did it."

Gina came out and Janet was glad. "You're a witness," Janet said. "Now he's stalking me."

"It's a free country last I checked," Jack said. Gina was looking good. Jack wished he could project a different face to each of them but it was not possible.

"Want me to call the police?" Gina asked.

"Yeah," Janet said. "Captain McBride said to call if he ever showed up." That wasn't quite true but how would Jack know?

"I got every right in the world to be here," Jack said. "Call the FBI for all I care. It's a big mall and I'm here to shop."

Gina and Janet went back inside the office. The El rumbled by and Jack's sass seeped out of him. He should have come at midnight. Or come with the Guzmans to pay off their loan with a consolidation check from HomeQuik. But he'd be damned if he'd turn tail and run now. It was public property and him being here didn't prove nothing.

Gina came out and called him over. "The police are on their way," she said. Not as abrasive as Janet but not friendly either.

"Look, I got no beef with you," Jack said.

You got no beef at all, Gina thought. Her mental genital banter was near-constant; there was no reason, however, to further incite the Cracker with double-entendres. These days she saved her word-plays for Vinny. They seemed to make him redouble his efforts which was good. You had to draw a line, between your work and private life.

"I got another job," Jack said, trying without reason to establish rapport. "They hired me one-two three. HomeQuik. It's straight commission, the more business you do the more you make. You should come check it out. She--" Jack gestured over Gina's shoulder to the office window from which Janet looked out --"she'll only let you rise so far. HomeQuik's like the wild west. Survival of the fittest." Jack paused. "And you're fit."

Gina's heard of HomeQuik but there was no future there, no Series Seven, just a lifetime of loan sharking which was not what she had in mind. "Good for you," she said sarcastically. "Especially if you're working you should get out of here."

"So how d'ya like my job?" Jack asked, trying to keep the conversation going, such as it was. But Gina went back inside. Maybe she wasn't joking, about the cops. Jack walked, slow as if he didn't care, out to 174th Street and east to Boone. Without a car you couldn't go whoring. But that was probably a blessing for now.

* * *

Kurt took the D Train from Central Park West, express under Harlem and the Concourse, to the empty echoing Fordham station. He'd borrowed a video camera from Candida. She'd used it in her divorce case with Stewart but he didn't know how. He'd like to interview these Guzmans if they let him.

Jackal was right where he'd said he'd be, eating a hotdog with onions on the counter by the street. For some reason Kurt'd thought that the Jackal was black, but that wasn't the case. This Jackal was dumpy and pink, except for the orange onion sauce that dribbled down his chin.

Jack too was surprised. This Kurt was white, like most of the Fordham students who walked this strip with trepidation. They'd be two white men in Tremont, each with his own agenda. But fine. Jack had the docs he got when he doubled back last night. "Call me this time once you've read 'em," Jack said. "Before you put 'em online let me tell you what they mean."

Kurt opened his backpack -- this was no time to read, he was eager to see The Bronx, get some footage from WatchCorp, some authentic street scenes the site could stream if he could get enough server space. Kurt took out the camera but Jackal said no. "You flash that thing around and we're gonna get mugged," he said. "And I don't want you filming me. I'm off the record, remember? At least for now."

"I thought maybe the Guzmans--"

"No way," Jack said. "It'll scare 'em off from signing the docs. C'mon, we gotta boogie. The husband goes to the hospital every day, we gotta get there first."

The bus down the Concourse moved slowly in traffic. Kurt stared out the window at the teeming streets, six story Deco buildings, fruit stands with what looked to be hairy coconuts, a standing-room only crowd on board in the air-conditioning.

"So have you reached out to TV?" Jack asked.

"Not yet. I thought if I got some footage--"

"Maybe after they sign," Jack said. "Just follow my lead."

Milagros looked out through the peephole, saw not one white man but two. "*Llegaron*," she called back to Amado before opening the door then the gate.

"Six percent, just like I told you," the guy said. Amado had convinced her last night that if the man came back they should do it. Otherwise they might lose their house, everything they'd worked for. He'd busted his back and she'd put up with shit from those rich Jews in Riverdale. Their son was with the Marines in the Philippines -- they held their breath when the watched the Univision news. When he got back he could live with them, here in this house, while he looked for a job, maybe college, found a wife. They needed a better loan or it would all fall away.

"Let me see the papers," Amado said. He put on his glasses --
they were just magnifiers, bought for two bucks in the subway but they
helped him read. It was right there, six percent.
"Who's this?" Amado asked, pointing at Kurt.
"He works with, uh, a community group," Jack said. Then, "He's
a journalist. It's like I told you, I think you can sue EmpiFinancial. You
refinance the loan with HomeQuik then you sue them -- this way you
even *make* money off the deal."
Amado didn't answer. He'd heard many promises on many jobs,
and who exactly was it who was helping him now? No one but
Milagros. They grew up across a muddy street from each other in a
colonia in Tijuana; sh e was the best thing in his life, the only thing, she
and his son Marcos. People back in TJ had a half-dozen kids; they'd had
one. It was expensive in America and you had to focus your resources.
Especially since Milagros still wired money back each month to her
mother in Maclovia Rojas, money for cinder blocks to shore up the
house, for a new tin roof when the old one blew off. Soon she might
come and live with them too, get treatment for what ever disease would
eventually kill her up at St. Barnabas Hospital.

Kurt waited until the Guzmans signed the docs before he spoke.
"I'd like to interview you," he said. "To ask what EmpiFinancial told you,
when they charged you fifteen percent."
"Fourteen and a half," Amado said. "And what's this for?"
"He's trying to get a big television show to cover it," Jack cut in.
"Like Sixty Minutes." Nothing. "Prime Time Live."
"*Occurio Asi*," Milagros said. A gotcha-ya show on Univision.
"I don't know," Amado said.
"It's for a web site," Kurt said. "It's called Watch Corp dot org
and it tries to defend the poor--"
A communist, Amado thought. And not judgmental either. As a
man who'd earned every dollar he had just by breaking his back, he had
no bone to pick with the left. The PRI, the Institutional Revolutionary
Party, now that was a joke. But so was Vinny Fox, the blow-dried
cowboy from Coca Cola. The Guzmans had WebTV although they
rarely used it.
"Show me," Amado said, walking over to their seventeen-inch
TV. There was a keyboard and Kurt typed in the URL. Amado skipped
from page to page, nodding. "It should have a part in Spanish," he said.
"If you want the people to read it, the Spanish people."

"I've been meaning to do that," Kurt said. He'd asked Candida to translate but she kept putting it off.

"Okay," Amado said. "You want to ask questions, I am ready."

16. I Love My Baby

Jack left at four to go back to Fordham Road. Actually he went to West Farms, to get the pay-off from Gina then file the loan. Kurt stayed at the Guzmans, expanding the interview to cover anything Amado wanted to say. Amado spoke of TJ, of years of shit from INS, *la migra* he called them, his pride when he got naturalized on Liberty Island where no one could go anymore. Milagros served them coffee, strong Café Pilon with heated Carnation milk and *dulce de coco*. She liked to see Amado laugh; she liked that this boy -- that's how she saw him -- was interested in what they had to say. She called St. Barnabas and rescheduled Amado's appointment for next week. There are many ways to return to health and that hospital had few if any of them.

They decided to move into the small back yard. The boy was still filming, asking
Milagros about the garden she'd planted, the *tomatillos* just coming up, the cilantro. There was probably lead paint in this dirt Kurt thought but didn't say. He felt blessed to be in this yard, with these people who didn't dissemble. He liked the wife even more than the husband but he talked more. The digital camera had almost gone dead; they plugged in his power pack to recharge the battery. That's when he saw the basement, looking in through a cobwebbed window at the clean empty space.

"That's an apartment?" Kurt asked Amado.

"It was a tailor's shop in the past. We want to put in a toilet so our son can live there when he returns from the war."

What war, Kurt thought -- the endless chasing of Muslim shadows in jungles and steppes as seen on infrared? But he had an idea. "It has a door to the street?"

"Yes. That's how the tailor got his business."

It was too soon to ask. But when would he be back here? Kurt felt like a pushy American but what could you do? "Uh, I've been needing a space, like an office, for Watch Corp... I could help put in a sink, a toilet, whatever, pay you some rent, whatever you think is fair..."

Milagros heard this, looked again at the boy, thought of Marcos, looked at Amado and nodded. He was surprised but when has Milly been wrong? "*Puede ser*," Amado said. He wanted to talk with her about it alone. It was all moving fast. But the rent would help to pay the loan.

* * *

At West Farms Gina was disconcertingly nice. The Guzmans' loan was hers; Jack couldn't figure why she wasn't more pissed it was being paid off before she even got credit. She hadn't signed the form yet; she'd made a call and now asked about HomeQuik.

"I just think we can do more for our customers," she said, "being affiliated with EmpiGroup. We have the appraisers in-house, the insurance--"

"That's a rip off and you know it," Jack said.

Gin smiled; she made herself smile. Janet had been melting down all day, went to the court in the morning, called Gina twice on her cell and now was on her way. She had to humor the cracker, keep him in one spot, it shouldn't be hard. They could of course debate credit insurance, the cracker's incongruous bugaboo.

"I think on a real estate loan it makes sense," Gina said.

"Yeah but not single premium," Jack said. "And on personal loan it's just a pure scam. When did we ever foreclose on a bedroom set? Even a four-poster bed like that Bertha--"

Janet came in to the office with a cop behind her. "That's him," Janet said to the cop. Jack stood up, glancing back at Gina's betrayal, the pay-off form still in her hand. Bitch, he thought. Bitches.

He was expecting handcuffs -- this was getting routine for him by now -- but instead the cop handed him three sheets of paper stapled together. "You've been served," the cop said. Then to Janet, "You want me to stay?"

"Yeah. Until he leaves."

Jack looked at the papers. "Order of Protection," it said at the top. "What the fuck is this?" he asked the cop.

"You can't be within five hundred feet of her," the cop answered. "If you violate it we'll pick you up."

"Hey I'm not here to see *her*," Jack said, gesturing at Janet who was standing behind the cop with her arms crossed. "I'm a mortgage broker, I'm here for a pay off." He looked back at Gina, who looked guilty he thought. "One of you got to sign that," he told her. Then to the cop: "I have to come here for my *work*"

"Five hundred feet," the cop said.

"I got a right to make a living, I'm not gonna--"

"Take your papers and get out of here," the cop cut in. Gina had signed the pay-off, held it out to him.

"The bitch is crazy," Jack told the cop as he walked past him to the door.

"You're the one with the rap sheet," the cop said to Jack before the door closed behind him.

The sunlight in the mall was too bright; the Bronx was an oppressive concrete place where he had no friends. You move around for a job, Jack thought, and you never really get to know anyone, like how they think and feel. You work with them and they plot to take your job. You make a few mistakes and you're a skel, just another loser to the cops. What did it all come to, all these pawn shop loans, these bullshit bonuses that Uncle Sam took half of, these people victimized then sweet-talked again, the empty rooms and Asian whores, actresses they were, working for peanuts, streamed in real-time to a hundred lonely cells, you car in hock your future bleak. It boiled down to a single word, fuck, a word of a hundred meaning, mean-spirited fucking and happy fucking and getting fucked up the ass by your bosses, getting set up, digging through garbage to clear your name what a joke and finally just the raw interface of consciousness and world and that word, Fuck. No car to drive no bitch to fuck, the sun too high and nothing like it was supposed to be, no character arc or heroic quest... Tacos that give heartburn, ex-wives that give heartache and smokes that give cancer. Cause and effect like an in and out in this forsaken mall: fuck.

Jack would walk home but he didn't like his mind so he took the Two Train where there were no seats, jostled by fuckers who would kill him if there was no law. On Olinville he dodged the dealers and trudged up the stairs to his hole. He needed reason and a center so he dialed the bitch Diane and lit a smoke. There was something that he'd made, something that he loved beyond any calculated reasons. She found their talks boring but he needed her now, just to hear the simple voice of youth, the freedom for which he worked and paid, the happiness that soon would fade -- Zalie.

Of course it was Diane who answered the phone. She sounded happy for a moment, fake bouncy and hot-to-trot until he said hello.

"I just wanted to talk to Zalie," he said, "but I mean, how're you doing?"

"Oh I'm fine Jack" -- she said it like a challenge, he thought -- "I'm just fine."

He wanted to ask if she was working but she'd take it wrong. He wanted to ask if she had a boyfriend but that wasn't his business anymore. Or only indirectly. "Is she there?" Jack asked. There was the sound of a TV in the background, the whiz-bang-pow of cartoons so she must be. Unless Diane had regressed again.

"Yeah we were just sitting here waiting for you to call," Diane said, sarcastic and firmly in control, impossible to talk to her outside of this dynamic, she who'd seem him drunk and seen him cry 'cause he thought he should when his momma died. "It's your father," Diane called out.

Zalie didn't come to the phone as fast as Jack would have liked. He'd wondered this often, whether the things he done with her before he left she'd even remember. Do kids remember when they're four? He didn't remember much and the thought made him sad. If it kept up this way he'd be a non-entity, just paying the money and no reason to call.

"Hi Daddy," Zalie said into the phone and Jack felt weak, to be addressed tenderly by anyone after so long a time.

"Hi baby -- I've been missing you but I've been working hard but I've been meaning to call you. How's school?"

"We paint pictures but my teacher--"

"Mrs. Robertson," Jack cut in, trying to show that he knew, trying to make a connection.

"That was *last* year," Zalie said. "Miss Craig is always gettin' mad at us and so she don't let us paint, we just sit there."

Jack was no grammarian but his daughter was off to a bad start, he thought, talking like a Bubba, her mother would never correct her 'cause she talked that way too, all headed to a bad end, the absentee father now with a rap sheet.

"Doesn't," Jack said softly but Zalie ignored him. "I'm trying to come down and see you," Jack continued. No way she could understand Judge Birnbaum and the bail and all this bullshit. "I'm going to talk to your mom about it. Maybe we'll go on a trip."

"To Disney World?" Zalie asked. "Jenny Byers in my class went there at Christmas, almost everybody's gone but me."

"We'll go somewhere nice, honey, I promise." Jack wondered if she'd like Mexico, or if she'd think it too dirty and no Mickey Mouse.™ They had some bush league Disneyland out there, so low-tech now they might soon close it. They could just disappear into the crowd and never come back. "What have you been doing?" Zalie didn't answer. "What sports are you playing in school?"

"Like dodge ball but the boys throw too hard, they try to hurt you."

If Jack still lived in Bubba-land maybe he'd have done something, gone drunk to talk to the bully's father, or taught Zalie how to kick and aim for the balls -- did it even hurt when you were six, Jack wondered -- but he wasn't there and he hadn't done anything like that while he was.

"Look Daddy my favorite show's coming on."

Jack felt lost but shouldn't show it, there was no reason to be mad at her, that's just how kids were. "Okay baby I just wanted to talk to you, to let you know I'll be coming down this summer."

"Here Mommy," Zalie said and then she was gone. Jack woulda liked to hang up, the sickness in his stomach a mix of longing and hatred for Judge Birnbaum and Empi -- this wasn't the time to pitch Diane on the trip anyway but here she was.

"Don't go promising her Disney World when you can't even pay-_"

"I didn't say nothing bout Disney World," Jack cut in. "I just told her I'm going to come down this summer."

"Oh are you now," Diane said. "It'd be nice to ask me before you go promisin' things to your daughter you might or might not be able ta do."

Jack lit another smoke, ran his tongue over his teeth. Like he needed the bitch's permission to go to Charlotte. The only person's permission he needed was Judge Birnbaum's, and even that was a joke. "She my kid too, ya know," he finally said. "I mean I'm paying--"

"Not this month you ain't--"

"Look I had a little problem but don't worry 'bout me, I'm solving it and like I said I'm coming down--"

"When?"

"Don't know yet. That's why I didn't tell you. Soon as I know I'll tell you the days. I want to take Zalie on a little trip."

"Yeah we'll see about that," Diane said.

There was no reason to argue now. The way Jack saw it she should be happy that he wanted to do something with Zalie. If she had a boyfriend she could probably go on a trip at that time too. He'd like to ask but how to do it? "Ya working?" he asked, wincing before even finishing the words.

"Yeah part time at Shoney's," Diane said. "And this month I'm sure glad. Otherwise we'd be starving, if we counted on you."

He let that one go by. She'd worked at the Shoney's before, he'd never liked how the manager looked at her but now he didn't care.

"Eric was asking about you," Diane said.

"Yeah I'm probably gonna call him. He still work for Empi?"

"How should I know? He came in to Shoney's with some skank, him and Maggie are like separated, she found him in some titty bar and threw his bony ass out, served him right."

If gossip were news Diane could be Dan Rather. Jack knew the strip joint Eric liked, he'd gone there himself sometimes after Blitz Night to unwind. Diane never knew but what the fuck. She watched soap operas, fruity Italian men prancing around in just a towel and how was that different? "D'ya know where he's living?"

"Like I said, I don't know and I don't care. I saw him in Shoney's is all. He asked about you then he left a stinking dollar tip on a ten dollar check. Whoever the skank was, she'd givin' it cheap."

At first Jack'd liked it when Diane talked dirty. She was younger than him but had probably had more partners -- when he was drunk he'd asked and liked to hear, he'd make picture in his mind that made him angry and hard at the same time, Diane with the guy who now worked at Midas, Diane fighting off the advances of that chemistry teacher who everyone said smelled like death. It wasn't really that he got sick of Diane, but she of him. Further and further apart 'til drunk and impotent he'd lost control. He didn't like to think of it and so didn't.

"I'll let you know," he said.

"If you don't send the check don't bother coming." Then the dial tone.

17. Death Row / The Vague Basement

Kurt had a theory that corporations were killing the world. Tonight Candida'd had to listen for at least the dozenth time. Perhaps it was therapeutic for him, she thought, to replace one grandiose theory of life, FOCO's, with another. They were at the Saigon Palace on Broadway and 98th and Kurt wouldn't stop talking.

"You ask yourself," he said between bites of a spring roll, "I mean, I ask myself, why do the people at EmpiFinancial do what they do? How does the company beat them down so they think nothing of fucking over a couple like the Guzmans, charge them the highest rate possible and lock them in with a prepayment penalty--"

"There's just doing their job," Candida said. "You talk like every company is just a bunch of crooks. How would stuff get made? Maybe you think it's boring and dirty. But it has to be done."

"I'll tell you how they do it," Kurt said, ignoring her. "They tell them it's not them fucking the customer, it's the Monstro system. Monstro analyzes each applicant down to the level of what insurance coverage can be sold, every last opportunity to gouge. If you don't do what the system says they keep track. You don't get a bonus. Maybe you get fired, like this guy the Jackal."

Candida was tired of this, the half-eaten spring roll in Kurt's right hand, the way he looked around the restaurant, talked loud like he was trying to impress someone when nobody cared. "You should finish that," she said.

Kurt put the spring roll down then thought the better of it, popped it in his mouth. The pastry was crisp; there was mint or something in it. Amazing, Kurt thought, how America had napalmed the Vietnamese but expropriated their cuisine, which itself was a product of French colonialism. Maybe WatchCorp should run restaurant reviews, a set of anti-imperialistic recipes, a hundred and one way for tofu and ginger to fuck on your plate.

Candida had taken the bait, despite herself. "It's not like you say. Most people are not always getting screwed. They live their lives, they try to be happy, they accept the backdrop of systems and things, airline schedules for example, get a mortgage when they need it, change companies if they don't like it. These people you think you're helping, this noble Mexican couple that you describe, why don't they just go to another place for the loan?"

Kurt was surprised. Maybe it was a good sign that she'd spoken at length. She usually only argued when what he said implicated her; sometimes he did it on purpose but often not, just out of control, just locked in his own head, just trying to end the thing or make her different than she was, make her what he wanted her to be, what he'd thought she was, when they got together... Kurt was still thinking of Milagros Guzman, the elemental way she walked, the aura of integrity, her hair pulled tightly back, like a painting he'd seen of the Mexican revolution a voluptuous woman leading the *braceros* into battle. And that was probably based off the French symbol. And he shouldn't be thinking of a happily married woman, a heroically married woman, *una mujer recta y directa* -- such was not for him, the self-hating spawn of the bebop middle class. But back to Candida's question. Kurt had a theory and he rose to the challenge while the baby corn got cold.

"Government's given up," he said. "They don't regulate these fucking companies anymore. The corporations have only one goal -- profit, as much profit as possible. The only thing that keeps them from killing people is competition, and worries about their reputation... The middle class people you're talking about? They're lucky. They have things easy. If they don't like T. Rowe Price, they just to go Charles Schwab. People *care* what they think, so their tastes are catered to. But in the ghetto it doesn't work. People need the money desperately, right now -- the company knows it and they fuck them as hard as they can. The middle class doesn't care that the poor are being fucked, no one will report it, and so reputation doesn't work either."

"You're talking about a *mortgage*," Candida said dismissively. "Not torture."

"Sure it's worse in other countries," Kurt said, tipping his hat to her Peruvian back-story, which she rarely talked about, the vague basement in Queens making all that came before a topic to avoid. "But the structure is the same -- no competition, no ability to effect the corporation's reputation with anyone they care about. And so just the old in-out, bloodsucking, business...".

"I guess Gene Ramos was right, then," Candida said. "Power to the people." She wanted to go home and change clothes; then she wanted to hit the nightclubs with her friends from work if not with Kurt. Kurt was a downer. He'd never be the man for her. It was too late. She gestured to the waiter for the bill.

Kurt could have played the victim -- how can you joke about the cult I barely escaped? -- but he had big thoughts, he had a theory and three Sing Tao beers, he had something to say whether Candida cared or not.

"So communism failed," he said. "I'm not like a defender of Stalin or anything. But even if you didn't like it, it least it kept the U.S. in check. It's the same structure -- competition. As long as there was another ideology in the world, America had to pretend to be concerned, to also care about the poor. Do you think it's a coincidence that it was only after the Berlin Wall fell that Clinton did so-called welfare reform?"

"Don't *talk* to me about welfare," Candida said. Kurt missed it and kept right on going.

"It's like each system kept the other on its toes. Now America rules the world. It's not even just America, it's consumerism, a mindless worship of corporations, of bigger is better, blander is better--"

"It's called progress," Candida said, having paid the bill. "I'm leaving now but don't mind me. You can stay here and keep on talking."

Touché, Kurt thought. Touché but you're outta here. A few more ass-fucks and we're done. *Vaya con Dios.* No one's hands are clean.

* * *

The bitch Diane would never agree but so what. Jack wanted out, he wanted his daughter and a brand new life. He'd rather not be looking over his shoulder for the cops so getting Peel to drop the case was key. From five hundred feet out the best he could do was tele-harass her. From payphones 'cause of fucking Caller I.D.. Bastards charged seventy five cents for Star Sixty-Seven and who knew if the shit worked anyway. Putting the squeeze on Empi was his only way out. If they told Peel to drop the case she would. So though he didn't like it, Jack Bender found the full-page ad in the Bronx Yellow Pages and called Micah Levine.

"Have you been hurt in some way?" the secretary asked.

Lemme count 'em for you bitch, Jack thought. "I used to work at EmpiFinancial," he said. "Levine knows me -- tell him it's about Bertha Watkins' loan."

"Just a moment."

Jack stared at the ad's cartoons of wounds -- a throbbing thumb, a toddler eating what looked like potato chips but was probably lead -- then Levine came on the line.

"You say you work at EmpiFinancial?" Levine asked. This might be his lucky day. A whistle-blowing employee, a confidential source; he could kick him some of the money back and still make a profit. Winning a case for Bertha would come first -- he'd make sure she *saw* him win it then take things from there.

"*Worked*," Jack said. "I left about a week ago. But I know where the bodies are buried." Jack'd heard this phrase in a few movies; it sounded dramatic and like it would get this shyster's attention. He had to fuck Empi and have them know that it was him, behind Levine, who was fucking them. Dole out some information and keep some for later. You want my silence? Then let me know, with a nice severance and a fucking letter of reference.

"Don't tell me -- you're the guy in the parking lot?"
"Three meat taco, that's me."

Micah laughed. The guy's looked so pathetic it was hard to imagine how much info he'd have. But it was worth pursuing, this turncoat cracker. "We should meet," Micah said. "Can you come to my office?"

"Yeah," Jack said. "I'm gonna bring somebody with me."

This, Levine didn't like. "A borrower?" he asked.

Jack had meant Kurt, but why not the Guzmans? Their HomeQuik loan had closed. But maybe that's the one he'd hold back. Give the Jew the dirt on Bertha, promise a Mexican victim too if all went well. "A guy I trust," Jack finally said. Though whether he trusted Kurt he wasn't sure.

* * *

This kid Kurt was a get-over, Jack thought. He'd brought him to the Guzmans' to film and somehow the kid had now rented their basement. He had a dust mask on and was sweeping the walls with a broom.

"You movin' in?" Jack asked.

"I need an office for WatchCorp," the kid said through the mask. "But yeah I might move in."

Jack shook his head. Olinville might be bad, but this was the real South Bronx. The block was quiet, sure. But at night they'd kill you for a five dollar bill, a loose cigarette, maybe even your shoes. It wasn't Jack's problem. "I talked with a lawyer," Jack said.

"For the Guzmans?"

"Yeah probably, down the line. First about that other loan I sent ya, the lady with the five thousand dollar bed."

Kurt remembered the one. He hadn't put it on the Web site since it wasn't a house. But selling insurance on a bed was almost funny.

"I'm gonna meet him," Jack continued. "I want you to come."

Kurt wondered why, but what the fuck. He'd play it as he had here, pulling out the camera only later, documenting the whole process: the predatory loan and attempts to fight back. "When?" Kurt asked.

"Tomorrow. You need some help?"

Kurt nodded, thinking of the table he needed to move downstairs.

"I'm gonna go get us a six-pack," Jack said. "Then we can really get busy."

* * *

The basement was pretty much in order -- a desk in the front, some half-ass bookshelves made of milk cartons, the plywood off the windows in the front and a rotating fan -- and now Jack and Kurt were drinking the beer, the third of Jack's six-packs, the cans lined up like a firing squad on the window sill.

"They tryin' a sue me," Jack slurred. It was time to tell the kid what they had on him, make him promise he wouldn't turn the camera on the Jackal himself.

"For using the loan files you took?" Kurt asked.

The kid knew nothing of the dumpsters -- and why should he? "Nah. For death threats," Jack said. Might as well cut to the case.

Kurt laughed. "Who'd you threaten?"

"They got no proof at all. Somebody sent 'em a fax, saying that Janet Peel should die. She got her panties in a twist and went to the cops. But they got no proof so it's bullshit."

"They charged you with it, though?"

Jack nodded. "They're scared I'm gonna refi all their loans now that I'm at HomeQuik. Like I did with the Guzmans." That couldn't have been it, Jack knew, since they'd been fucking him even before he took the job on the Concourse. But it was better this way. Let the kid think he was a hero, fighting Empi for the same reason he did: for nothing.

"What'd they say when they charged you?"

"They said it came from a Kinkos, they got some sleepy-eyed Negro" -- Jack used the word when drunk, learned it from his momma and had heard Colin Powell use it so it must be okay -- "to say it was me, showed him my picture. But I talked to him an' he said he wasn't sure."

Kurt was loose with the beer but the word Kinkos gave it away. That's where Jackal'd faxed him the first documents from. So the Jackal was wacko -- who cared? Docs were docs. And Kurt kinda liked the poor fuck anyway. "You got a lawyer?" Kurt asked.

Jack thought of Lorraine Thompson; it was hard to say yes. "Yeah kinda," he said. "Maybe I'll ask this shyster tomorrow to represent me. They say I can't leave--" Jack stopped. No reason to spill his beans to this kid. If he left the state why leave a trace.

"You were in jail?" Kurt asked.

"Just a few hours waiting to see the judge," Jack said.

How this all fit together Kurt didn't know. He cracked another beer and put his feet up on his new desk.

* * *

"I used to know a guy on death row," Kurt was saying. "He was in jail in Huntsville, Texas, filing appeals that were denied one after the other."

"How'dya get to know him?" Jack asked. He'd heard of women who went looking for husbands on death row. It made him mad since he was out here free and available but the bitches wanted the idea of a man rather than a real man. Why Kurt would be trolling death row he did not know. The kid was a voyeur.

Kurt hadn't told Jack anything about FOCO, about the theories of the wheezing Gene Ramos and didn't want to. "I worked with a group in Brooklyn," Kurt said. "They published a newsletter and I was an editor. The guy from death row -- Bobby West was his name -- he sent in an article."

"Sayin' he was innocent?" That's what the skels always did, Jack thought. It was one thing to play games with the truth about stalking a bitch like Janet Peel, a bitch who deserved it. But if you killed somebody you better stand behind it.

"No. That's why I liked the article. He said he did it, even said he understood why he should never be free again. But he didn't think that he should die."

"Who does," Jack said. That was the bargain, those were the loan documents God or whoever was in charge put on the table. Though maybe it was different, knowing the day and time and all that, and that the government would do it, not cancer or ciggies or AIDS from some bitch.

"I went down to see him," Kurt continued. "Drove down to Huntsville. The jail was like a castle in the middle of rice fields, stone walls thirty feet high. They lowered down a basket for you to put your driver's license in, then swung open these big steel doors."

"I betcha they were mostly black," Jack said. He didn't really mean that Negros did more crime -- maybe they did but you weren't supposed to say it, that's why he tried to use the word "black" with this kid -- they were poorer, anyway, most of them. Jack'd seen a movie about death row, maybe it was news -- it was drama, all of it, the world through the funhouse mirror of TV -- and the skels had all been Negros.

"Mostly African Americans or Latinos," Kurt said.

Jack noticed the fancy words, the double-talk that changed every year -- what the hell was a "Latino" anyway, Julius Caesar with a pina colada? He wondered at the gulf between him and Kurt, wondered what this kid wanted in life if not an ex-wife and a buncha bills, where he thought his laptop would take him. Somehow the kid must have money, Jack thought. Otherwise it made no sense, the shit he was doing for free.

"Bobby was white," Kurt continued. "But there on death row he got along with everyone. Not the guards. But he helped the other prisoners right their appeal, once they'd run out of free lawyers or before they got one for the final step."

"What's the guy do?"

Kurt lit another smoke and wondered how to put it. Brutally, just like the act. "He beat a gay john to death with a baseball bat in Houston."

"He was a faggot, this Bobby?"

Kurt shook his head. "He'd been in and out of reform school as a kid, said he got beaten with a hose full of sand. When he got out he snorted angel dust, he needed money so he became a gay whore."

Jack thought about that, another guy fucking you up the ass. Not for all the money in the world. He'd asked a lot of women for it and never gotten it. Diane turned him down flat but she probably gave it to others now, while he paid the bills and jerked off until his shit was raw. Fuck, Jack thought. He didn't give a shit about Kurt's death row friend. Kurt was just looking for sickness and freaks. "Why'd he kill the guy?"

"He didn't say. Probably the guy asked for something Bobby didn't want to give. Maybe it was to rob him."

Jack wondered how to ask. "This Bobby, did he pitch or catch?"

Kurt caught the euphemism. "I'm pretty sure he pitched. He said what the hell difference did it make what you stuck it in."

That, Jack could understand better. If you wanted to cornhole a woman, then why not a man? Get drunk, close your eyes -- people did it in jail, did it in the army too he'd heard. Romans had done it. That Latino motif again.

"Anyway he killed the guy. He got caught, tried and convicted, sentenced to death."

"Live by the--" Jack paused. Live by the dick. Maybe they shoulda just castrated this Bobby West then put him in a dress to service the other skels, work off his karma 'til the walls of his rectum gave way.

"When I visited him he was down to his last appeal," Kurt said. "They bought him into the cage in shackles. Two guards stood behind him the whole time we talked." Kurt paused, thinking back to that airless feel, to the way his mind wandered as he drove back north, not stopping through the night straight through DC and to New York. "When the time was up Bobby refused to leave, he made the guards drag him by the chains. He was spitting and kicking and that's the first and last time I saw him."

"Fucking animal," Jack commented. A kid he'd gone to high school with in Charlotte now worked there in the jail. It paid okay but it was a job for a sadist. The kid had been a bully and it wasn't surprising. "He said a lot of guys did that. They'd wait in their cells for the guards to come in. They'd shit in their own hands, stand their holding it, just waiting to throw it at the guard when he came in."

Jack tried to picture that: a guy shitting standing up then holding the turds in his hands. He pictured flies and a warm wet ooze. Mother fucker, he thought. The lock-up at arraignment was nothing. He had to get to Peel or head down south to Mexico.

"I almost understand it," Kurt said. "The way Bobby put it was that the guys had to express themselves. Once you give in you're already dead, he said. If all you can do is throw shit at the guards then you do it."

From flies Jack's mind returned to the dumpster. Was that what he was doing? Throwing shit at Empi while waiting to die? Is that what Kurt meant?

"They killed him," Kurt said. "I heard the news on NPR. TV didn't bother to cover it because they kill so many people in Texas, what the hell."

"I gotta go," Jack said. He was tired of Kurt and his bullshit stories. "Meet me in fronta Lincoln Hospital tomorrow. That's where the shyster's office is."

18. Swanker's Subpoena

Ernest Swanker didn't like to be played for a putz. The way he saw it Rudehart had him on ice. The promise of dinner and political schmoozing held out to keep him in check -- "don't do anything while I'm gone," Rudehart had said -- but when was it going to end? Swanker'd seen on Bloomberg some speech Rudehart had given in Mexico City, how markets had to be open, how money wanted to be free just like people, just like goods and services and three out of four wasn't bad. A real fucking statesman, Swanker thought. That day he'd sent a civil subpoena to EmpiFinancial, putting in writing and broadening his earlier request for all record reflecting training and compensation related to credit insurance practices. Fuck 'em. Let 'em dig up every print-out in Baltimore and cart the crates to 120 Broad -- he hadn't disobeyed Rudehart, hadn't even mentioned credit insurance to him yet. Micah Levine had given Swanker a fresh piece of meat, an interim dog treat, and Swanker'd use it to raise the stakes. News would reach Rudehart on his Mexican junket. I'm not a man to be trifled with, Swanker thought with some pride. I'm not going to languish with this tin shield for long. It's DC or Wall Street and you're either with me or you're not.

But the ripples caused by Swanker's subpoena did not reach Mexico. Empi in Baltimore was like a bunker: they liked to solve their problems without bothering Sandy and his circle of stuffed shirts. They were used to beating questions with a blizzard of paper. In response to Swanker's first call they'd sent Keith Mudnick to The Bronx. They could document that a branch manager had been fired; they could say the problem if there was one had been quarantined then eliminated. Now he wanted training manuals. They could send him a truckload. They were covered with dust but they had them.

Mudnick looked out over St. Paul's Place while he dialed Janet Peel. She'd said her life had been threatened so he'd better show concern and ask about that first.

"Any more threats?"

"The guy was stalking me in the West Farms Mall... But don't worry, I got an order of protection. If he does it again he's back in jail."

I wasn't worried, Mudnick thought. "Look, your state A.G.'s on our ass again. It's just a fishing expedition but I think for now we wanna watch our p's and q's. Why he's so interested in The Bronx we don't know--"

"He's from here," Peel cut in. "Little rich kid from Riverdale."

"Maybe that's it," Mudnick said. He'd never heard of Riverdale, couldn't give a shit one way or the other, really. "The point is, we think you should be hands-on in West Farms for now. You should manage the branch."

"But Gina--"

"She hasn't been with us long enough."

"She's been going to trainings." Telling Gina wouldn't be fun. And Janet was a *District* Manager -- she was supposed to oversee a half-dozen branches, not run just one. She wanted to go the whole tri-state region.

"Look, when the pot is hot we send our best people in. Hold down the fort for a few weeks, just until Swanker backs off. We're very impressed with you down here."

That, Janet liked. She was becoming a troubleshooter, the best person man or woman for the job. "As long as it's temporary," she said. "You know these politicians -- they see a hotter angle and then forget all about the first one."

Janet knew of Gina's dreams -- the Series Seven, private banking one day, asset management. Half of Janet's job was managing people. Jack was unmanageable but Gina could be stroked. Janet drove to West Farms to deliver the news, almost *hoping* she'd see Jack there so she could call the cops. Janet'd given a copy of the order of protection to the rookie D.A. Wing Tsai. He'd put it in a file but said there wasn't anything he could do right now, he'd raise it at trial. Meanwhile the Cracker was running wild, picking off loans to refinance and drive her numbers down. She pulled into the mall but there was no sign of Jack.

Gina'd moved the coffee machine to the front of the office; she'd put some stupid poster of Lorraine Robinson and a black opera singer on the wall. "It makes 'em feel more comfortable," Gina said as Janet poured a cup.

"You need Hispanics," Janet said. "If you're gonna do it right. Look, I got a call from Home Office..."

Gina didn't like the sound of this. That's the phrase Janet's used in her first move on Jack. Maybe it was the cocaine making her paranoid. Gina smiled, smoothed down her blouse and waited.

"They said there's some investigation, the state A.G.'s asking for all kinds of docs and they want to be safe."

"Everything's in order," Gina said. And everything that wasn't had been thrown away.

"They want me to run the office for a few weeks," Janet said flatly. "Don't take it wrong. I told them you've been going to the trainings, they think very highly of you down at Home Office"-- here Janet lied, but that was half of managing people, wasn't it? -- "they just want me to say I'm in charge for the next few weeks."

Those stupid fucks, Gina thought. Here she was busting it out at night, turning down Vinny for sex so she could read the self-help books, and they wanted to demote her. "I understand," Gina said with a fake smile. There was no reason to argue with Janet. Janet was a good Nazi, carried out the orders while dispensing her stupid advice of putting spic posters on the wall. Nuremberg redux.

"It's only a few weeks," Janet said again. Gina's reaction wasn't what she expected. You had to know your people. Janet wondered if she did.

* * *

A building had burned in the Melrose flats; there were three ambulances and a television truck in front of Lincoln when Kurt arrived. He had the camera with him so he filmed, the gurneys rolling by, a kid with all the skin burned off of his hands, even the drug dealers stopping to look. There was a tap on his shoulder and Kurt turned with his fist clenched.

"Easy, boy," Jack said. The kid was gonna get himself killed, flashing this thousand dollar camera in the South Bronx streets.

"There was a fire," Kurt said.

Jack shrugged. "The whole area's a fire trap. C'mon, the shyster's waiting for us."

Micah was watching the ambulances through his venetian blinds. He'd seen the guy filming, then the three meat taco guy go over to talk. Micah didn't like to be recorded -- you couldn't talk honest that way. He went into his outer office to greet them.

"Who's this?" he asked Jack.

"Kurt Wheelock. He's been filming some of the borrowers, putting it up on his web site, trying to...".

"Hold EmpiFinancial accountable," Kurt finished Jack's sentence.

Micah preferred things being solved in the court, in closed-door talks where money was paid without admission of guilt. Companies wouldn't change -- the fucked you will always have with you -- but Micah could get good money for some of them, braindead babies' parents winning big downpayments for houses in the Hamptons. "Don't film in here," Micah said. "I'm eager to hear anything about EmpiFinancial, especially Bertha Watkins' loan. But nothing on tape."

Jack nodded, then Kurt did. Micah'd thought of inviting Bertha to this meeting, but he wanted to hear it first for himself. If he won for her, he wanted her to think it had been just him, and that he wasn't just a flunky using some dirt from this whistle-blowing cracker.

"So whatd'ya got?" Micah asked, taking out a yellow pad, all business.

"The insurance they sold to that lady--"

"Bertha--"

"It was just a scam. I know 'cause I worked there. They only ask what the loan is for so they can jam insurance into the loan."

"Do they ever foreclose?"

"Are you kidding? What would EmpiGroup do with a used bed?"

"I'm just asking because they're sure to have a defense. In the whole time you worked there -- how long did you work there, by the way?"

"Almost a year, up here. Before that I worked for them in Charlotte."

Micah and Kurt both noted this, the origin of Bender's drawl. The NASCAR Jackal, Kurt thought. The holy grail of consumer litigation, Micah thought: the South with its pre-compute loans and asbestos-ridden illiterates. Neither knew they had Starbucks in Charlotte now, well-staffed offices of indicted accountants, software programmers from India eating corndogs at Shoney's.

"In that whole time, what's the cheapest thing you ever saw them take?"

Jack thought about it. "Sometimes down in Charlotte we'd go out and pick up a car. Not 'cause we'd resell it, but just to put the pressure on. When it's your only way to get to work, you pay the loan."

Micah nodded. "Okay, cars. How about furniture?"

"Never. The only exception was TVs and stereos. We took a few of those. Mostly the loan officers took 'em home and used 'em."

"Ever repo-ed a bed?"

"Like I told you, never."

Micah looked over at Kurt. It might be good to tape this, so he could take it to Swanker and get him off his ass, get the ball rolling on a class action that could be settled, it now appeared, for *mucho dinero*, as Micah's Univision ad put it. But how to get a tape from this hair-shirt?

"If you record what we're saying, can you get me a copy?"

Kurt nodded. Candida had two VCRs. He reached for the camera.

"But don't put it on the Internet," Micah said. "If we're going to use it in court, or even to prepare a case, we don't want the other side to see it and pick it apart."

Then what was the point, Kurt thought. And what was the point of trying to use it in court, if Jackal's credibility could be shat all over with the death threat charge. Kurt had assumed Levine knew about that, but maybe not. Kurt didn't owe this ambulance-chaser anything anyway. He'd give him a copy but after that all bets were off. He didn't nod one way or the other. He just pointed the camera at Jack and hit Record.

"So in your many years at EmpiFinancial, you never saw or heard of foreclosure on a bed, is that correct?"

"That's what I *told* you," Jack said. He wanted to get at Empi, sure -- but a tape, that never went away. Down in Charlotte some guy'd taped his girlfriend sucking dick; he showed it at a bachelor party and they put his ass in jail. Jack never even got a copy. Didn't they have some way to jumble the screen, make his voice like a robot, the spy who came in from the cold?

"Say it again for the camera," Micah said. The shit about beds was true enough. Jack repeated it, getting into it now, wheeling out his Bubba-jokes.

"I've seen people who sign with an X," Jack said. "Most people didn't even know what interest rate they were payin', or that they had insurance. We'd jack 'em at the table, change the docs, sign 'em later, whatever we had to do. It made you sick, sometimes, what you were doing. They took the staff to this theme park just over the South Carolina border, Six Flags over Jesus, they called it. Holy rollers sucking the equity of out of people's homes, sendin' the money to Baltimore and getting ten cents back on the dollar, if that. I thought it'd be better up here but it ain't. It isn't."

This poor dumb fuck, Kurt and Micah thought at once. It was like watching a car crash. Outside the ambulances screamed. They stopped when Kurt was out of tape, out of memory, down Charlotte's memory lane with this confessional cracker. They learned of his Three Tooth Rule; they heard of primer-covered TransAms and mobile homes on cinder blocks. Kurt thought of FOCO -- Gene Ramos should go recruit down in the Carolinas. Micah thought of the p.i. lawyer from Durham who was now in the U.S. Congress. It was a gold mine Jack described -- a steaming drawling gold mine for corporate sleaze and class action suits. The Jackal was almost like Faulkner, Kurt thought. He painted a picture of strip malls so bleak you could taste them. This was the way of life that Al Qaeda had hit. Jack described a bank tower's prong standing alone in the center of town, a football stadium named for a Swedish cell phone company; he mentioned an ex-wife and daughter and once again Kurt and Micah thought, the poor fuck. Then Micah thought of Bertha and Kurt pictured Milly under Amado on a bed. They'd both lost their chances. The poor you will always have with you.

19. Calamari

Gina had a cell phone, Gina had a friend on Wall Street who lusted for her and she used it. The guy who'd come on to her in that diner in Greenwich -- Bain, his business card said -- he or his bosses would love to know the trouble brewing in this company they covered. The key was, how to make the trade, how to get some assurance, that she could have a job at the i-bank now or if her career at Empi led nowhere as it seemed to be. To make this call she went to Manhattan. It was a Manhattan kind of call, nothing Vinny had to know about, a line thrown out into the future, a rope she could use to climb the mountain, right over Janet Peel and that lifeless auditor from Baltimore, the one who'd looked her up and down then gave her the kiss of death. Fuck him; fuck them and fuck their trainings, she was calling the future because the future wanted her, had asked for a ride from the diner into town, would have done anything, over that burger, to have the things that Gina had. Not just her body but her mind. She was two steps ahead and she dialed the phone.

Tom Bain had a new video game. It came from some sadistic software genius on the Philippines, by way of Steve the Sleaze. You didn't feel like a kid, some fairy tale swinging the axe. In this one you had guns and knives, nylons to tie the cyber-babes down. There was even a hijack sequence if you could just get through to Level Three.

The phone rang and Tom Bain let it ring, on the Caller I.D. it was neither of Nicole Nour's numbers so it could wait. The machine beeped and then a woman's voice came on.

"Uh, this is for Thomas Bain, it's the woman he spoke to at the diner by the Greenwich station, I have information that I think--"

Bain picked up the phone without pushing pause. His alter-ego with his guard down was blown away by the cops. That was okay. Bain remembered the diner babe, he hadn't thought about her since but this just proved the point: cast your seeds upon the waters. You had to be in it to win it. Bain turned on the charm, such as he could.

"I'm glad you called... Of *course* I remember you... I've been thinking about you...".

She was still playing that this was about information, that she had some dirt on EmpiFinancial that he would be interested in.

"You didn't say you worked there."

"You were being very pushy. I mean there's a lot I didn't tell you. I was surprised that I talked to you at all."

Yeah I'm grateful, Tom thought. Maybe she was a whore, this was her little game, camp out in a diner in a rich suburb, let a guy come on to her, call him and pretend it was normal. Or maybe she was just horny and in the hunt. What different did it make? He couldn't spend half of the bonus he made. Paid or free what was the difference?

"Yeah well I'd love to see you, you name the time and place--"

"It's not for free," Gina said. Ah ha, thought Tom, just as he'd pegged it.

"I have money," he said.

This struck Gina as strange. Should she just sell some files to Bain, let him figure out just how badly Empi'd cooked the books? That was looking too low. She wanted Wall Street not a little pay-off. She wanted Bain's job is what she wanted.

"Not enough," she said. "It's that I've been preparing to take the Series Seven, I mean, I've always wanted to work on Wall Street, I majored in finance..."

Now Bain was confused. Maybe these were some code words; maybe she thought the phones were bugged, investigation into Wall Street call girls. He played along. "You seemed really driven. I thought you already worked on the Street."

Gina liked that. It was the look she cultivated. Dress for the job you want, not the job you have -- that was just one of the helpful squiblets of information she'd gleamed from the management books. It made the men drool, too, some fantasy of S and M, Margaret Thatcher with nubile tits, Mary Magdalene with an MBA.

"So I need a deal," she said. "That if I give you this information, there'll be a job for me."

Bain had no authority for this, none at all. But let her dream. "Hey if it checks out, we're always looking for hard-charging people. Especially women." He wondered how that would go over, the reference to Wall Street's dodging of employment discrimination by gender lawsuits. There was a case still pending against Empi, brokers on Long Island called strippers in, and drank their Bloody Mary's from garbage cans in the Zoom-Zoom Room.

Affirmative action by sex was no problem with Gina. "I'm qualified," she said. "I just need a chance. I'll give you the info for that chance then take it from there." She wondered if she should get it in writing -- she'd prefer it that way but didn't want to show how green she was. The SEC must look for just that kind of memo. They had their ways to do business on Wall Street and she'd play along. She had another trump card anyway: the horny way the guy'd looked at her in Greenwich. Though that only paid off half the time if that.

"I'm sure you will," Bain said. "Let's get the process started." He suggested they meet as his apartment; she resisted. Fine, Bain thought. A fancy place on West Broadway. It used to be jammed but since Nine-Eleven sat half empty. "Nine o'clock," he said. "We can sit outside if you want."

* * *

It was time to take the Jackal to the Great White Way. Kurt had branched the Guzmans' cable down to the basement and now had the 'Net at near T-1 speeds. He ran searches on different words: EmpiFinancial and scandal; Sandy Vyle and predatory lending. At the cusp of the two he found the Heard on the Street. The Journal's site was for-pay only, but other places put the stuff up free. The byline was a hyper-link, nnour@wsj.com. He should call her, Kurt thought. It was too easy for an e-mail to fall through the cracks.

"You've reached Nicole Nour at the Wall Street Journal," her message said -- a bit cocky, Kurt thought, a bit too proud of this three-word newspaper name. "I'm either on the other line or away from my desk. Leave me a detailed message and I'll call you straight back."

Kurt focused his mind and made his pitch. "My name is Kurt Wheelock. I work with a non-profit group, WatchCorp dot org. We've been looking into EmpiFinancial, trying to fight predatory lending, and we've come across stuff you might want to cover. I saw your article. Check out the Web site -- what we've published there is only the half of it." Kurt left Candida's number. He'd ordered a phone line from Verizon but who knew when they'd come. He hung up and wondered what he'd say if Nour took the bait. She could interview the Guzmans, maybe this client of Levine's that Jack kept talking about. It was time to take the cracker Jackal to the Wall Street Journal. He was glad he didn't have any Gene Ramos breathing down his neck. He felt free. There was freedom of the press and, how ever marginal, he had his own press. The Journal was the big time. The Journal could make Empi scream.

* * *

Bain worked out with weights between seven and eight -- he liked the way they made his veins stick out, made his hands look like a medical model, made him feel like an animal again, stalking the plains of Lower Manhattan. They treated the stock analysts well, he had to admit it. They had a gym in the building, a shower room, sauna -- you could get your laundry picked up, daycare if you had a kid, even program your secretary to buy and send birthday presents to your mom or wife if you had one. All so the focus on numbers would be pure, or if distorted not by distraction but by self-conscious sell-out to build the boutique's other business: M&A advisory, co-underwriting of stocks, fairness opinions and the like. What a joke: fairness opinions. Two page letters for which CEOs paid over a million dollars, covering their ass with some intern's opinion that the price they were selling at was fair. Comparable transactions; reasons for differences -- you could justify just about anything as fair, especially when you had the wild card of post-Nine Eleven fluctuations. Maybe this Gina whoever she really was could write fairness opinions. It wasn't Tom Bain's job to give but his word carried some weight -- about as much as this two-pound fruitcake's barbell.

Tom showered, moussed his hair, put on his best striped shirt, his hunting shirt he called it, the one he'd worn to meet Nicole in the coffee shop's loft. He hadn't called her because he didn't have information. Maybe he'd get some tonight.

Gina took the subway to City Hall Park; she walked north to Duane Street to avoid the tourist gawkers at the corner of Vesey and Church. The ins and outs of the Towers' fall were beyond her. She had her own towers to climb. If they could kill all the terrorists, fine. She didn't like to wonder if she'd die on the way to work. That was her link to the War on Terrorism. What more could she do?

She'd heard of this place Odeon. It had a faux-Art Deco sign and the air of the insiders' lair. It was mentioned in the Post's Page Six, which Gina read like so many others. The bold-type people, their peccadilloes and flaws, their sex and money, the way they were chronicled while the rest of the drones just read. Gina was not a drone, she'd known that since high school or even before. She had girlfriends that gave hand jobs like hand bills, just to pass the time, just to fit in the crowd -- not for her. Everything had a purpose: either to move forward or for her own pleasure. She was not like those dowdy ghosts in Afghanistan on TV, floating through the rubble of Kabul in their light blue bags. You've come a long way, baby -- Gina remembered those ads. She didn't usually smoke but she stopped at an Arab's newsstand on Church Street and bought a pack of low-tar 100s, she remembered the divas in black and white movies with their cigarette holders, the way they held a man's eyes, the way they had their own world. She do it on Wall Street and she'd start right here.

The horny guy'd taken a table outside and was eating calamari.

"It's such a nice night," Bain said, standing up to pull her chair out for her. She looked like a little doll in her knee-length dress, better than she had in the diner. He wanted to play this right, maybe not even deceive her. Maybe it would all work out.

"Did you talk with your bosses?" she asked.

This was the knock-out question; this was a landmine that had to be defused. "Yes," he said. "They're very excited."

Gina wondered; Gina ordered a Campari and soda since she'd seen it on a show and it looked debonair. Dubonet, too, that was a name that stuck in her head. Odeon's menu was short and the prices too high. She was glad there was English by the French in italics. Seared fish with some kind of Latino chutney. Bain got a steak as he always did. The night of the hunter. The calamari was greasy when cold.

At Gina's request Bain described the work of an analyst. She nodded as if she knew; much of it she'd read about, her autodictat Vinny-less nights, all bearing fruit now. The moon as low over New Jersey and the moment was now.

"It's the way we refi loans," Gina said, dabbing her fish in the mild spicy mango. "A lot of loans, we *know* the people can't pay. But we refi them before they go thirty days late. Sometimes we just extend the due date."

This left Bain cold. Flipping was a fact of life in the loan shark world. He pretended to be rapt. He had a hard-on or near so. His apartment was near. "Go on," he said. "This is fascinating."

"The other part's the insurance. We're supposed to put it in every loan, whether or not it makes sense, whether or not the customer asked for it, or wants it... We've written unemployment insurance on people that never had a job; we've written life insurance for people with no relatives."

Bain faked outrage though he'd heard all this before. It only mattered if the suckers sued, and they never did. But then Gina said, "Now the state attorney general is asking for documents, my supervisor's all worried about it, she's a District Manager--" Gina stopped. She didn't want to say she'd been demoted. No one on Wall Street wanted damaged goods.

"Swanker?" Bain asked.

Gina nodded. That was his name, stupid as it was. Bain whistled through his teeth. "This is big," he said. "This could cost Empi a bundle." It was bound to happen, he thought. A press-hungry A.G. and a predatory lender. But Swanker usually went after the small fry. If he took on Empi it would move the stock. If Bain's firm traded on it before it was public they could make a bundle. Maybe he even could get this Gina a job.

"Don't get me wrong," Bain said, "but how do you know this?" Gina put down her fork. Was this the time to hold back? To make sure an offer was on the table? The waiter came over -- some kind of Mexican, probably illegal, Gina thought -- and she nodded, waited while the plates disappeared.

"I'm thinking of changing jobs," she said.

"You were saying."

"So I just need to know what kind of offer your boss will make."

Bain's boss was skiing in Chile, the bastard. There was a hiring freeze in place but exceptions were made from time to time. Bain's focus was on the here and now. The night was so nice that if it slipped away he'd feel even emptier than usual. "They pay well," Bain said. "More than any of us have a right to." There was her previous lie -- "Any of us without kids," he added.

He was looking at her ring finger; his meaning was clear. Gina wasn't like her slutty girlfriends. She held out the promise like a check and never cashed it. She'd mastered her desires. Vinny was her safety net for now.

"Let them make me an offer," she said. She gave him her cell number. "Don't use any of this until the offer's made."

Hah, Bain thought. He could confirm this Swanker business on his own. Was time to play that card? If it failed he'd never get a taste of Gina. There was a topless bar on Murray Street anyway. He could afford to be classy. He charged the dinner to the firm and flagged a cab for Gina.

She rode in the cab to 14th Street only, then switched to the Four Train the rest of the way. Waste not want not. She had the horny guy in the palm of her hand. She smelled Series Seven. When she got it she'd leave The Bronx forever.

20. *Tamarindo*

Nicole sipped her chai from the Starbucks downstairs while she played back her voicemail. Various flacks pitching various spins: these flurries always happened in the wake of a Heard, when they saw your byline, your power to move the markets with some reheated rumors.

One message stood out because it was so amateurish: some guy from a community group saying he had the goods on Empi. It wasn't Hill & Knowlton; the number when she called was a private apartment, some Spanish name, a woman's voice -- she almost hung up. But what was the down side? "This is Nicole Nour from the Journal, returning a call to"-- she looked at her notes -- "Kurt Wheelock. I'll be in most of the day but on deadline from about three o'clock on. If you have documents you can fax them--"

There was a click then a male voice, the same one from the message. "Yeah Miss Nour," he stuttered, "I'm glad you called, wait a minute." The machine was still recording. She heard a beep. A community group that didn't even have an office. This was probably a waste of time. While she waited she opened her browser, typed the U.R.L. in, WatchCorp.org. It wasn't fancy but there sure were a lot of words. It seemed like every other one was "predatory." This guy needed an editor. The amateurs were stinking up the world with their rumors. He came back on.

"I read your article, it was right on target. I think if you talk with some EmpiFinancial borrowers you'll see there's even more to the story."

"What will they tell me?" Nicole asked.

"How they got their loans, what was said to them and what wasn't said. How they got ripped off, basically."

"You're in Manhattan?"

"Uh, yeah, right now. But the borrowers I have in mind are in The Bronx."

Nicole pictured abandoned buildings and junkies. At Columbia J-school they'd done a project about The Bronx, a sort of fake newspaper that no one there read. She'd traipsed around some hell hole called Melrose, wrote a profile of a toothless Dominican man who ran a restaurant out of an old yellow school bus. She'd gotten an award. She'd made up some quotes since her Spanish was far from perfect, but nobody'd been the wiser.

"Where in the Bronx, Melrose?"

Kurt was surprised. "Some of them," he lied. "But the ones I have in mind are in Tremont. They got a home equity loan from EmpiFinancial at fourteen and a half percent -- then another lender made the same loan at six percent."

"Meaning--"

"That Empi wildly overcharged them, yes."

"They're willing to talk?"

"I'm pretty sure," Kurt said.

Nicole looked down at the phone like, why have you been wasting my time? Kurt heard the silence and rushed to fill it. "I'm going there later today," Kurt said. "I'll ask them to make sure. I can have them call you or you could just come up."

"It's better in person," Nicole said. She remembered the school bus restaurant. "Do they speak English?"

"Pretty much. And I could translate the rest."

She should get a real translator, Nicole thought, but she wanted to work this on spec. If it was going to be a Page One Feature she wanted the whole credit. She'd like to do the pencil drawing herself if she could. Goodbye earnings round-up; hello GQ or even Esquire. "This will be exclusive, right?"

Kurt hadn't thought but said yes. "I'm the one who called you," he said. "But it'd have to be fast." The Jackal was a time bomb. If he could get Chris Bury or even Jerry Springer all bets were off. "Did you check out the web site?"

"I'm reading it now." Nicole reopened it by hitting Back. She didn't like to read the 'Net, thought it corrupted her style. But she'd better bone up before heading to The Bronx. The race goes to the quick, and anyone could read the crap this guy had posted. "Their names aren't on here, are they?"

They were but not their address. "No," Kurt lied. "I'll call you from The Bronx."

Candida watched Kurt on the phone: the way he bobbed and wove, the way his eyes were wide, the way he lit one cigarette after another and hardly took a puff while they burned down in the ashtray. Kurt used to tip his hat to her desire for clear air, only smoke at the window looking down on the Hudson. Now he didn't care anymore. Neither did she, in a way. But she'd wasted time with him, precious time while her ovaries grew harder and more sporadic, bothered her. Sometimes either getting high or coming down she had a plan: she'd get pregnant by Kurt whether he stayed with her or not; she'd raise the kid alone, she and her girlfriend, teach it to be either the smoothest gigolo man or a sharp 21st century woman. Either way it would do better than they had, it would give her a reason, she would have no regrets.

"Where're you going in such a hurry?" she asked, as Kurt zipped up his ridiculously big backpack, as if he was going camping.

"Gotta go up to the Bronx. There's a journalist interested and you know how they are, when they say jump you say how high."

Candida thought that was just for Gene Ramos. "Lemme come with you," Candida said. Maybe if she tried harder to get interested in the things he did, they could keep it together at least 'til conception occurred. After that the shit was fated.

Kurt paused. He'd rather go alone, for more reasons than he wanted to articulate. He wanted Milagros to think he was single; he didn't really want Candida to know where his office was, in case it all broke down and he left her, without even a note, or something short and poetic, "We've taught each other a lot." But each thought was heartless, even he could see that. And Candida was Latina; he'd stand out less that as the solo white man. Maybe they'd think he was her pimp. "Okay," he said. "But hurry up. I said I'd call the reporter back this afternoon."

Candida got dressed as if for safari: her two hundred dollar inflatable aerobic sneakers -- made in Myanmar, Kurt always pointed out, the fucking kill-joy; her baggy khaki shorts, a nice push-up bra and a pink belly shirt. She sprayed perfume on both sides of her neck and she was ready, a real killer, a succulent playmate for a Bronx afternoon.

Kurt noticed the get-up and felt a rise inside his Y-fronts. Ol' Candida could still do that. Too bad there wasn't time--

"You got a Metrocard?" Kurt asked. He had one, the unlimited weekly for seventeen bucks. To buy one for Candida would slow him down.

"I've got a FunPass™ that I never used," Candida said. It was still in the plastic. Four dollars to any corner of Gomorrah. She put on a hundred-dollar pair of RayBans and her fanny pack. "*Vamos p'al Bronx,*" she said. He loved it when she spoke Spanish. *Papito*'d been his favorite word.

After 96th Street all the white people'd left the train. Two tall Puerto Ricans, one with a thin line of beard along his jaw, were staring at her. Kurt pretended not to notice, or didn't notice. He was looking though a file of papers. Candida felt the look, liked it but also wished Kurt would do something. He was a wanna-be Latin with none of the kick. A macho manqué, a workaholic with his head in the clouds. "So are the Guzmans nice?" Candida asked. He'd talked to her about them but she hadn't paid attention.

"They're all right," Kurt said. Candida and Milly was a combo he wanted to avoid. Maybe Milly would be at her job in Riverdale, playing nanny and housecleaner for some rich fucks whose names Kurt didn't know. Amado could talk on the phone to Nicole, then Kurt could take Candida somewhere and fuck her. In the basement? No. Amado's tell Milly. He'd tell her anyway. The lady was married and Kurt should forget all about her.

They got off on Tremont. To Candida it looked like Queens, the graffitied parts like Jackson Heights, maybe Jamaica. There was a wide street; the little Incas selling coco cherry rainbow, water ices in white paper cups, the older 'Ricans shaving blocks of ice to pour *tamarindo* on. "C'mon let's get one," Candida said. "I haven't had one for so long."

The cheapest *piragua* cost a dollar. Kurt got a fifty-cent *cocito* and they set off down the hill, mangos and *verduras* out on counters on the too-narrow sidewalk, the smell of piss from a doorway, a check cashing place with a line of people out the door. "Park Avenue, eh?" Candida said. "I didn't know it came all the way up here."

"It stops at Fordham Road," Kurt said. There were drunks on the stoop of Bronx Lebanon's A.A.; they whistled at Candida. "*Deje este blancito*," one of them slurred. "*Vente con un verdadero hombre.*"

"Don't mind them," Candida said.

"I'm not."

Webster was wide, the gypsy cabs flying by, a run-down hotel with a crowd out in front. "That's a real hotel?" Candida asked. "I mean, people can stay there?"

Maybe she meant her and him, Kurt thought. It was a fleabag used to house homeless people with AIDS, the settlement of some class action lawsuit, a room of your own in the months before you died. "The City's rented all the rooms," Kurt said, not wanting to mention AIDS, not wanting to bring on bad luck. He'd offered to use condoms but Candida always said no. It felt better that way, but still.

East of Webster is was quieter or more desolate, glass half-empty or full. There was a soul food restaurant on the corner of Park. They turned north, long blocks of two-family houses attached, metal fences covering their front, sad somehow, this last stand, this need to live as in jail even as homeowners.

"It's here," Kurt said. It was a house like all the others, except that it had a driveway along one side -- semi-attached, then -- and a rolling gate on a door to the basement. Candida saw the sign and laughed: "WatchCorp, by appointment only."

"You didn't say--"

"I'm just starting," Kurt cut in. He climbed the stoop and rang the bell. A man came to the door and Candida's stomach dropped. He looked like her father. The same swagger, the same dark eyes with their hint of sodomy, the same fake-gentlemanly question, "*Quien es tu amiga?*"

Kurt made the introductions; Candida shook his hand but looked away.

"*Milagros esta?*"

"*No, esta trabajando,*" Amado answered. He was alone in the house, watching the rebroadcast of a Mexican soccer game, Cruz Azul against Oaxaca. Kurt explained about the reporter, how the pot was hot to kick Empi in the balls.

"But what about a lawyer?" Amado asked. "Newspaper is nice but it is not court."

Kurt had wondered why all Jack'd pitched to Levine was the bed, the Bertha Watkins loan. "We're getting a lawyer ready," he said. "But let's call the reporter, it'll help." Maybe they could get someone better than Levine. That guy's neon ticker-tape sign did not inspire confidence.

"In a bit," Amado said, pointing at the TV. It was the thirty-seventh minute of the second half, Oaxaca up two to one.

"We'll be downstairs," Kurt said. "When the game's over just give us a shout."

Back outside Candida was glad to be far from the man. It stirred things up in her: hatred and pain and surprise, her strongest feelings, Stewart always said she should go to a shrink and she did, but not about that. Kurt opened the padlock and pulled up the gate. It was dark inside, just a rickety desk and some half-ass bookshelves.

"This is where you've been working?" Candida asked. He'd been gone in the mornings when she'd gotten up, coming home late at night babbling about The Bronx this, The Bronx that. She didn't like basements either, on principle.

Kurt ignored her question. He plugged in his laptop. "Let me clean up a bit while we wait," Candida said. He'd be bringing this dust home into her bed. Anyway she didn't want to sit, didn't want to think, didn't want to feel. Those eyes and this basement. Now she knew why she hated the outer boroughs.

Kurt watched her sweep, the curve of her ass in her khaki shorts. Why didn't he love her, he wondered. She was bouncy, she was pert; there was something desperate about her but in bed that sure didn't hurt. He approached her from behind, while she swept at the walls with the rag-tag straw broom. "*Luego hacemos el amor aqui,*" he said in his stilted Spanish. Candida thought to correct him then didn't. She put his hands on her breasts and closed her eyes. These twists in her brain, the bad hand she'd been dealt in that Queens boiler room, they could all be changed. If he were only different than he was. They kissed and rubbed and then Amado shouted down.

"*Estos jodones de Oaxaca,*" he was saying, as the broadcasters did *Minuto Noventa,* named the *Jugador Mas Valioso, patrocinado por* Wendy's *y* Coca-Cola and some Mexican telephone service that Kurt had never heard of. "This reporter, what should I tell him?"

"Her," Kurt said. "Just say what they charged you on the loan, what they told you, and then the price that HomeQuik gave."

"Mister Jack?"

"Yeah, Mister Jack. He works for HomeQuik." Kurt dialed, made the introduction then watched while Amado explained and re-explained, in Spanish and broken English, his view of Empi's sins.

"*Ella quiere hablar con tigo,*" Amado finally said, handing Kurt the phone.

"So what do you think?"

"It's a good story. I'm going to need to see the documents then talk to my editor. I'm gonna need to call EmpiGroup, too."

"Of course," said Kurt. "He said, she said."

"It's called balance. When can you fax me the documents?"

"Tonight," Kurt said. "They're in Manhattan."

"I'm going to call EmpiGroup's spokeswoman now, just to get the ball rolling."

Kurt looked at Amado, wondered what the down-side might be then said goodbye.

21. The Cajun Wings (of Penny Zade)

Micah had good news for Bertha: the cracker's tale made clear that she'd been fucked, that it was a pattern and practice of fucking and might even give rise to punitive damages if they pushed it. Micah sat in the half-light across from Lincoln Hospital and felt what he knew was a conflict. The serpent in him -- call it The Cunning Advocate -- knew that the matter was larger than Bertha. What the cracker'd said applied to all of Empi's loans. At least personal loans where the property list was stuff that Empi'd never repo. Bertha could be lead plaintiff, the named plaintiff, but she'd get no more than any other member of the class. The insurance might be cancelled and the premium returned, plus maybe a piece of the punies if they got them for the time she spent in litigation. But another part of Micah wanted something faster, a quick win for

Bertha, the congratulations maybe consummation. Micah's snake was strong and said, perhaps you can have both. If Bertha could see the bigger picture, perhaps she'd thank Micah for that, right then. They could work on the case and all the attendant time together. Micah picked up his wheels from the municipal lot and drove east on 149.

The bed was hardly the largest of Bertha's problems. Duwon was due in summer school but refused to go. He spent his days with his video games; at night he asked for money to take the train to Times Square with his friends, attending movie premiers and returning at midnight or later, once with a leather coat he said he found but still -- if Arthur were around he mighta beaten some sense into him. Bertha tried with a broom once but then felt sick. She lay on the bed then, hugging Shaniqua against her, while Starquasia asked Duwon about the lump on his head. It was a long hot summer and it wasn't yet July.

Micah brought plums from the Koreans on Brook. Micah tapped fists with Duwon -- that wasn't helping, Bertha thought -- and asked him how he liked the Yanks chances.

"They gonna win again," Duwon said. "Ain't no team can buy playaz like the New York Yankees do."

"*Isn't*," Bertha said. "Isn't no team like the Yankees."

Duwon rolled his eyes and returned to his game with a plum. "I have news," Micah said. "But more importantly how are you doing?"

Bertha motioned with her head at Duwon. "It's not easy," she said. "I *need* some good news. What's up?"

"Remember the guy we confronted in the parking lot?"

Bertha did. "That sorry-ass white trash flunky who said that everything was legal?"

"Yeah well he quit, or got fired, who cares which -- and he came to my office."

"He came to confess?" To Bertha this seemed unlikely. Maybe the guy needed a lawyer for his own self, for his own reasons.

"Sort of. I got it all on tape, him saying how they *know* the insurance is useless, but they sell it anyway. It's very damning."

Duwon's ears perked up: the Jew boy was using swear words.

"So what'd we do with it?"

"That's what I wanted to ask you. If this weren't such a good case, if what they'd done to you wasn't so outrageous"-- Micah's snake was laying it on thick here, but all for a good cause -- "then I'd just call

EmpiGroup's legal department, let 'em know we have 'em dead to rights, and get your insurance cancelled."

"But you're not gonna do that." Bertha could tell.

"There's another way to approach it. We could file a class *action* lawsuit, suing on behalf of other people like you who got the insurance."

"Then what happens?"

This was the crossroads for the snake. "We could get insurance cancelled for a whole lot of people. We could also get punitive damages, the kind I was talking about after Pen--" Micah stopped, don't say that name, don't ring that bell, it was an intimacy they shared but it didn't lead where he wanted to go -- "well you remember. We could sue for more money."

Bertha noticed his stutter, wanted to say go right ahead, say her name, her Penny Zade, keep her alive in that way -- to pretend it had never happened was like pretending that she'd never lived. But Micah was weak. Or sensitive. A white man. Pussyfooting around the cold black facts. "And you'd get a fee," she said.

Micah's face turned red. He nodded.

"I'm not judgin' that, I mean it's fine with me. And the punitive damages too. If you think the class action is better, let's do that. The bed ain't goin' nowhere."

"Isn't," Duwon muttered, just to fuck with her.

"Have a plum," Micah said, glad that the snake had won out. His next stop was Swanker and he was taking Bertha with him and the tape of the cracker's tale.

* * *

Swanker was driving his interns crazy, reading EmpiFinancial training manuals until their eyes glazed over. He had better things to read: this morning's Wall Street Journal had a Page One profile of some victims in The Bronx, a Mexican man whose drawing made him look like Pancho Villa, ripped off by Empi and not taking it lying down. God bless the press. They did so much of his work for him. He needed to talk with these Mexicans -- there was a wife mentioned in the article but not quoted, typical Taliban sexist shit -- so he put in a call to the Journal's reporter, an Arab herself it appeared. She'd probably run a follow-up that his office was looking into it, newspapers loved to promote themselves that way, keep a story going but that was fine. Any mention of his name in the Journal was gravy.

That bottom-feeder Micah Levine was in his Planner: his secretary had asked and he'd said yes. That was about EmpiFinancial too, but something different, some bullshit about a bed, nothing high profile like a house and these Mexicans. Swanker thought of canceling it but decided no. Then he'd only have Levine barking around his heels for another chance. And he wasn't like Rudehart, tangling the promise of face-time than pulling it back. Fifteen minutes, no more, he told his secretary. She knew the drill: come in and say some pressing business called, some drug-bust in a state prison, some antitrust case against TicketMaster or the cigarette makers. He was an important man. Levine should be happy with fifteen minutes.

There was parking galore in the lot on Fulton Street. Even Micah had used to take the train down here, before Nine Eleven,™ before some many Wall Street firms quietly shifted their shit to New Jersey. They all waved the flag while they jumped the ship like pin-striped rats. They'd tried to blow up the Towers from the garage underneath in '93; one of the planners of that had said "we'll do it again and with planes" and no one paid attention. Twenty-twenty hindsight Micah thought as he clicked to make sure the doors were locked.

Bertha loved the Seaport - Arthur had taken the five of them down, Penny Zade with her pink thingees on, on a day he got paid. They'd sampled the food court -- Cajun wings and pork fried rice, cornbread and ribs and some Indian things -- and sat out on a wooden deck looking at the Jehovah's Witness Brooklyn Bridge. There was the honking of tug boats and the sense that they lived at the center of the world. Then two deaths, two falling towers; sullen Duwon and the crackheads downstairs. How fast it slipped away.

When Swanker saw the black woman he glared at Levine. I don't have time for sob stories, he tried to convey. He needed those Mexicans since he knew what they could say. "Sit down," Swanker said. "Ms..."

"Watkins," the lady said. "You can call me Bertha."

I don't think I will, Swanker thought. Even saying the name felt racist, like Aunt Jemima -- not good for election.

"Did'ja see the Journal?" Swanker asked Micah.

"Yeah. It's interesting but that's a one-off. Ms. Watkins has a case that is more systematic. I brought a tape--"

Here we go, Swanker thought. A fucking movie screening, while Empi was probably chasing those Mexicans to pay them off to shut their mouths. Micah walked to the VCR on top of Swanker's wet bar, popped in the tape and hit Play. "It speaks for itself," Micah said.

On the screen a dumpy white man spoke of credit insurance. He used loan shark slang -- ripped, packed, flipped and one he really seemed to like, jacked -- and Swanker was drawn in, he had to admit. "Is this guy stupid or what," he muttered.

"He quit," Micah said. The guy's probably been fired but why muddle the story?

"I know all about the Bertha Watkins loan," the guy was saying. "The insurance was bogus. We'd never repo a bed. In all my years with Empi, here and in Charlotte, we never took back no furniture but a TV set or stereo."

Micah pushed Pause. "Predatory *per se*," Micah said -- the Latin made Bertha think ever so briefly of her Penny Zade -- and Swanker had to agree.

"Unless the guy's lying," Swanker said. "Or unless there's some dirt in his past that Empi could use. Often these whistle-blowers are not what they seem. Have you checked him out?"

"Yes," Micah lied. "You heard where he talked about Charlotte? I think we better sue, both of us, before he goes. You do the enforcement action and I'll do a class action."

No reason to tell Levine about the training manuals, Swanker thought. But he could use this bottom-feeder's passion. Rudehart thought Swanker was bluffing, just angling for a contribution without the cards to back it up. "I've got a meeting with Empi," Swanker said. "I'll let you come if you follow my lead."

Micah'd rather sue then talk. "With who?" Whom was correct but it sounded stilted.

"Rudehart. You know, the--"

"I know. Sure I'd love to come."

"After we make the pitch I'll need to talk to him alone."

Micah nodded. Swanker could try to cut his own deal, but he couldn't sell Micah's case out. And what could Rudehart say about the tape anyway? He'd make Swanker mad and they'd be off to the races.

Bertha watched the white men joust and was nonplussed. Micah was licking this other Jew's ass. Maybe for a purpose but Arthur didn't do it. Arthur was dead. He and Penny Zade were in heaven she hoped. And here she was with vipers.

Over the intercom a woman's voice cut in. "There's a problem you have to attend to," the voice said. Swanker shook his head and apologized. Micah knew the game and Bertha didn't care.

"As soon as Rudehart gets back from Mexico," Swanker said. "I'll call you."

* * *

"What'daya think?" Micah asked as they walked up Nassau to Fulton. There were no cars allowed on this street; there were cheap shoes in the window that Bertha stopped to see.

"I don't trust him," she said. "And who's the guy you're gonna have dinner with?"

"A big shot," Micah said. He bowed down to no man but he knew the flow chart. "Used to be secretary of the treasury under Clinton--"

"The thin guy? Grey hair?"

"That's him."

Fruit, Bertha thought. Big shot fruit. "Let's stop at the Seaport," she said. "The kids love the wings they make there."

The Fulton Fish Market was abandoned; now in the Bronx and bad-mouthing it too. There was an old wooden boat parked next to the Seaport. Arthur'd taken Duwon on it that day, told him about black pirates who once ruled the seas off Jamaica and Haiti. Arthur knew shit like that, or made it up if he didn't.

Bertha filled a Polystyrene clam shell with chicken wings. "Let me pay," Micah said. He felt grandiose, ready to cross swords with this Rudehart, ready to play the hero for his damsel in distress. Thirty-three and a third of the punies. If all went well he could open franchises like Jacoby & Meyers.™ Bertha let him pay; she thought of Penny Zade, toddling around on the wooden deck outside. Neither thought of Al Qaeda. Neither thought of any towers but their own. And that was fine.

22. Roshomon on the Intercom

They met in the basement -- Milly, Amado, Jack and Kurt -- reading and rereading Nicole's article. Milly said the drawing wasn't her. Jack said fuck, inside, his trump card gone, Micah'd be here any second and then what would Jack have to trade? Kurt wondered if he'd shot his load too fast, passed off his best lead to the right-wing Journal. But there's be more, wouldn't there? The Jackal had all kinds of files. Amado said, "Isn't it time for a lawyer?"

Kurt agreed. Verizon had finally installed the phone line. He could start calling around tomorrow, or maybe just fax the article to the biggest plaintiffs' firms in town. You had to hit a beast like Empi fast, before they could regroup.

* * *

Vile was going apeshit in his second-floor lair over 48th and Park -- he called in one flunky after another without satisfaction. His flack Lena Jones had given him a heads-up, otherwise her head would have rolled -- it still might, because her quote was too defensive, "we review all irregularities and act on them." Fuck that! She should have said, we are a market leader with best-practices, blah blah blah. This loan as best as Vyle could make out, there was nothing wrong with it. Caveat fucking emptor, that was Vyle's motto. These wetbacks had needed a loan and they'd got one. They found a cheaper deal later, fine. Where's the sin? Where's the crime? Lena said the Muslim bitch called with a follow-up question, whether Empi was aware of A.G. Swanker's inquiry. Fucking vultures all trying to stop a good business in its tracks. A settlement would be like a tax, like bread to the masses, Marie Antoinette. Vyle was Louie, fourteenth and no later. Vyle was Napoleon: he'd go to the island that he'd bought if all broke down. It was just off Anguilla but it was sovereign in its own right. Like Nauru in the Pacific, a perfect place to run a bank. Fuck these vultures. And where was Rudehart anyway? Hadn't he said he had Swanker in hand, that he knew his type -- Vyle loved that, these knowing looks from the flunkies he hired.

Vile jammed down the intercom button for Lena Jones. She'd pay for her weak quote with extra work. "Tell that Nelson fucking Mandela Rudehart to get his ass back up here. This is what we pay him for, not stroking those wetbacks when we already bought their bank."

Lena Jones cringed. Two ethnic slurs in a single sentence. She often wondered when she'd see Vyle quoted verbatim in the press and have to deny that was what he said. Empi paid better than Burston Marsteller, the p.r. firm she'd worked at after the Post and her government days. She'd worked for Swanker once though he wouldn't remember -- she'd been number three on the quote chain, the upstate papers her domain, the Rochester Democrat & Chronicle and the Buffalo News, strictly *verboten* from the Times much less the national press which Swanker craved. The loan Nicole'd described was indefensible: she could see it through Swanker's eyes, through the eyes of the readers of the Amsterdam News. Vyle didn't get it: you couldn't just no comment that one, you had to show caring. It was like the Red Cross lady who went down in flames after Nine Eleven -- the first words out of your mouth had to be, "it's a tragedy." *Then* you'd start the spin, hangdog and sneaky. These were the fine points but Sandy Vyle didn't care.

If she didn't watch out he's just *hire* Nicole Nour as his number one flack. Since that would just motivate more reporters to break their chains and go after Empi, he'd probably call the Journal and get Nicole sent on assignment to Brasilia or Mexico City, some Third World dog house like the sweat box in Papillon.

"Right away, Mister Vyle," she told the intercom. She liked Robert Rudehart better. He was slick and knew the press. He could slip a knife in Sandy's back without breaking a sweat. But he wouldn't: forty-five million a year before options to be minister without portfolio for Empi, to never dirty his hands or his legacy with loans like this, it was Rudehart's dream-job, his payoff for serving his country -- and Empi -- so well under the Arkansas horndog. These Democrats were slick -- she was one of them -- Al Gore'd had a sista as his chief of staff and his melt-down hadn't been her fault, she'd made the race proud. Lena hoped to, too. Not in this job but in her next. As soon as my options vest, she thought.

The Mexican version of the Wall Street Journal didn't carry the Guzmans' tale. There was clearly a local angle but it wasn't the bolsa or NAFTA, not Pemex or Cemex or even Coca-Cola. Rudehart had his laptop though and read it, had already scheduled the EmpiGroup jet to take him to White Plains. He wouldn't talk to the press -- that was beneath him, might tie him to the vicious roots of Sandy's empire -- but he'd go have that dinner with Swanker. That bastard should have called. He was a two-bit A.G. who took the short view. He'd have to remember to undercut Swanker's fundraisers unless he backed down soon.

* * *

Gina was one of the Journal's few home deliveries in The Bronx. She'd believed their advertisements, that if you read it your future was assured -- in the alternative since all your competitors read it, laziness would leave you in the dust. Gina listened to Bloomberg Radio; she watched CNBC and MoneyLine. This was the first time she'd ever been mentioned and it made her high and sick. Her name, Gina Sunday, in the paper of record. But tied to a bed loan gone bad. She'd wanted to remain anonymous while she climbed the lower rungs of the finance world. Later erase her West Farms days. Now it was immortalized, it was archived and searchable, she could never pretend she'd come straight outta Wharton and taken The Street by storm.

Vinny stumbled out of bed, his penis jangling against his thighs but Gina didn't care. She was on his level now, pegged as a loan shark.

She might even get fired. That Bain has surely read it. If they hired her now it wouldn't look right.

"Whatza matter baby?" Vinny asked. "Some stock you own went down?"
Vinny liked having a money-makin' bitch. Some of his friends were already tied down with three brats and a cow, busting their hump to move to Yonkers where the schools still sucked. Gina paid half his rent, the whole thing if he needed her too. Sure he got some pieces on the side, he'd always had a way with cooze and it was a damn shame to waste it -- but Gina was a bitch worth riding while it lasted. An uppity climber but in bed that was just the ticket.

Vinny wouldn't understand, he wouldn't even know why it was bad, this mention, he might brag about it to his friends, those idiots he played softball with like they were still in fifth grade. "I gotta go," she said.
He didn't ask but she knew the request: leave money on the kitchen table. Most of the time she liked it like this. She wore the pants, she had the balls, she paid and so didn't have to answer his questions. He was handsome but lazy. He ate her out but was a deadbeat. You've come a long way baby, she thought. She left two twenties on the table and left without a word.

Downstairs in the downscale Bronx streets Gina grieved for her lost virginity. Her name had been in print; she'd been pegged as a lowly loan officer for EmpiFinancial. This catty Nicole Nour whoever she was hadn't even called for her side of the story. Gina'd seen Lena Jones' name before but what did Jones know? She'd made it sound like the loan was bad. And now the info about Swanker looking into it, her ticket to a job at Tom Bain's firm, was public knowledge. Its value had shrunk to zero, like Vinny when he was too drunk to even perform.
Gina wanted some trinket to make her feel better, some accessory of the fast-lane life. Not a Starbucks in sight, buncha Spanish restaurants and a Burger King with rats. She'd been to Odeon, she'd had fish -- she should have closed the deal right there. Now the deal if there'd been one was probably off. Bain could have called to say don't worry, your spot's still ready but he hadn't. It was desperate to call him but she did.

"I'm sorry," a secretary said, "Mister Bain is in a meeting. Is there anything I can help you with?" The bastard was probably right there pantomiming that he wasn't, writing her off as some cheap outer borough floozy. "Tell him it's Gina Sunday. Tell him it's important." "He's not here like I told you. Does he know how to reach you?" "Yes," Gina answered and heard the crack in her own voice. She was going to cry, for God's sake. This was not what a powerful woman would do. Scented baths were fine but this was business. There was an angle to be found but all Gina saw were the sodden Bronx streets.

* * *

Bain had read the article nude and alone and glad for air-conditioning. Nicole mother-fucking Nour --she'd found sources beyond him, nailed a detailed mortgage loan and landed on the front page. And she hadn't even called him, to see what he had to add. The bit about Swanker was still worth money. He put on yesterday's suit and tie and flagged a livery downstairs.

Sitting in the back in the traffic it suddenly hit him: the loan officer mentioned in the B section was Greenwich diner Gina. He'd been lying that a job was on tap and now it didn't matter. Her name was mud -- the Street didn't hire from the gutter, not that gutter anyway. His lie was erased: the job had been there, you understand, but after this we'll have to wait. She kept her legs crossed and now must regret it. Could he get a fuck of desperation? Only if desperate himself. He had trades to execute, shorting the little extra juice of the Swanker bit. He should get credit for this. Let the firm profit and know it was him; trade a bit for himself and call it a day. Maybe try to reach Nicole and congratulate her. If it depressed him enough he'd call the loan shark skank with this new balance of power. It was dog eat dog and Tom Bain this day felt the hunger surge.

He fired his orders off to Datek Online then took the internal stairway down to the Equity Desk. These were the glassy-eyed cowboys who took their meth before the opening bell. Bain went to the glassed-in box of the boss. "I got a tip," he said. "The Empi story is worse than it seems. Short the fucker 'til the next news comes out. It shouldn't be long."

The Equities chief knew better than to ask why -- it was only insider trading for the one who could answer that question. Bain jogged back upstairs to check Datek again. His trades had gone through, intricate shorting until Empi fell into the net. Then he'd unwind and be one step closer to telling them to take this job and shove it. He might start his own hedge fund; he might start a militia. He was Timothy McVeigh with an MBA. He was king without a queen. Nour was a name of Egyptian aristocracy -- he'd checked it out on Google, that's how love struck he was -- he dialed her now and agreed to be put on hold. He started Level One of the kidnap game again to kill the time. Finally she came on.

"Hat's off," Bain said fake jocular. "That's the kind of story I've been trying to get for you but you obviously have other sources."

Nicole wanted to cut to the chase -- do you have anything solid for me? -- but was innately polite. "Just luck," she said. "A guy in The Bronx called me and gave it on a platter."

"The Mexican? I mean--" Bain looked at the article again -- "Amay-dough Guzman?"

"Ah-mah-do," Nicole said. "No it was some guy from a community group--" She stopped. You should never name your sources, even to another source. It made them wonder whether you'd sell *them* out, to someone else. "There's going to be more," Nicole said to change the topic.

Bain knew better than to ask. So he offered instead. "Swanker's looking into it."

This Nicole knew, from Swanker's office's call for the Guzman's number. But how did Bain? "Where'd you hear that?"

"Got a source inside Empi," Bain said. "I've been working on them to get you some more."

This guy was all talk and no action, at least since the first and only lead he'd given her. "Who else knows about Swanker?" Nicole asked. She thought she had an exclusive follow up for tomorrow. But if the Street already knew...

"Just the people in Empi and me," Bain said.

"Thanks," Nicole said. "Be in touch." She put down the phone without waiting for his goodbye. On Wall Street this was not considered rude. He must have sources in the executive office at Empi, Nicole thought. She'd called Lena Jones and already Tom Bain knew. She filed that away and set to typing. They could get the Swanker news in the afternoon edition, put it on WSJ.com, stay ahead of the pack.

23. The Cracker Jackal's Play

"Hello *Lena*. The old man hasn't been driving you too crazy, has he?"

Rudehart asked as if he and Lena were old friends, as if this were in confidence, as if she could say what she really thought. "No worse than you'd expect," Lena said.

"I just wanted to check if there've been any more fireworks from our honorable Attorney General before I call him, anything I should know."

"No. He seems to be leaking everything through the Journal."

"What do we know about this Nicole Nour? Did she just stumble on this? Or has she made us into her great white whale?"

Rudehart loved literary allusions -- illusions Lena called them, because Rudehart talked down to what he supposed was in his interlocutor's library. Moby Dick was presumed to be in the collective unconscious -- or unconscience if you wanted to peg Empi and its peer group with a noun. To Kill a Mockingbird, Tom Sawyer: there were only a few that Rudehart used with the workaday drones. When alone he read Harold Robbins or some harder stuff. But he had the Ivy League pedigree, kept it up with the Capsule Summaries for Executives,™ an almost parody of itself by which busy machers kept au courant. Lena almost liked Sandy better. He was just who he was, a hard lender from Brooklyn.

"It's from Moby Dick, I'm sorry," Rudehart said. Lena left him out on a limb, standing lithely and lightly in his thousand dollar Italian suits worried about racism, the off-change of an employment discrimination case.

"It was the 'white' that threw me," Lena said. "It's more like the guy with the windmills. They'll never stop trying."

"Touché," Rudehart said, fruity and relieved. "So I'll call Swanker. Tell Sandy I'll be down to see him in a moment."

I am a public-relations professional, Lena thought, not some note-taking functionary. But her quote had put her in the shit house and she had to crawl out.

Rudehart's suite was on the third floor over Sandy's. His was better decorated, the cream from Empi's art vault in Queens. Chinese vases looted in the days of Chang Kai Chek, a few nudes by Picasso that left Rudehart cold, a miniature Diego Rivera that he loved to study, laughing at that leftist's naiveté. Rivera worked for Rockefeller, and he for Sandy Vyle. Who was more effective? He'd leave that to his biographer. He often wondered in which graduate school his Boswell now toiled. Harvard it should be; perhaps Yale or Princeton, no lower. It's not that he was an elitist, he told himself. But a man is known by the company he keeps. He'd toured the South Bronx, in his days of public service, held an AIDS baby in Lincoln Hospital and read to some immigrant kids in Hunts Point. He wanted his story told *right*, damn it. Why the head of Goldman Sachs would give six years to Uncle Sam. He wanted a legacy. A good story well told.

Swanker'd be lucky if one of the SUNYs made him a case study. His Republican predecessor, where was he now? Flacking for Waste Management, dodging ethical bullets if he was mentioned at all. Many are called but few are chosen. Rudehart had his secretary place the call, my-people will call your-people, the whole rigmarole of one-upsmanship. Swanker came on as he knew he would.

"Bob," Swanker said, "I hope you had fun in Mexico."

"*Muy boo-eh-no*, Ernie," Rudehart replied. He told people to call him Bob but then liked to make them second-guess themselves. There was an order of rank -- that's what Nietzsche said -- and Swanker'd better learn it. "So I hope I haven't missed my chance to taste your lovely wife's cooking."

Had he said loveless? Swanker wonder. "We've been looking forward to it," he said.

"That's not all you've been looking at," Rudehart turned the screw. "I understand that you'd have to follow up on the Journal's little tale. But why the subpoena?"

"There's a guy I know--" Swanker wondered how to put this -- "a friend of mine from the Bronx, a trial lawyer--"

"Oh, no," Rudehart joked.

"He's been jawing my ear off about credit insurance at EmpiFinancial, I thought I'd take a look. Actually, he'll be at the dinner too if that's okay."

"I love to know how our friends at the bar think." Rudehart was a lawyer too, as he managed to get mentioned in every profile, he was public policy on steroids, woulda been a doctor too if he had time. "What's his name?" Rudehart wanted to prepare.

"Micah Levine. He's just a grassroots storefront lawyer. But he has his ear to the street--" in the gutter, Rudehart thought -- "and gets a lot of walk-in traffic at his office in The Bronx."

Rudehart wondered what Swanker's angle was. Did he want to forego the political rabbi talk to let some ambulance-chaser have his precious face-time? Rudehart needed to make Swanker an offer he couldn't refuse, a carrot or stick both supplied by Sandy whose J. Edgar Hoover research operation hummed away in Queens like a server farm. "Let's get some time alone too, though."

"He'll leave after dinner," Swanker said. "I have some Calvados I think you'll like."

Then I'll sodomize you, Rudehart thought -- figuratively, of course. Politically. He'd stick a pear up Swanker's ass like a *Poire William*. Like a model ship in place of hemorrhoids. "Why not tonight?"

So he was desperate. "Uh, Carolyn has symphony tickets for us tonight. Tomorrow at seven."

"Seven thirty," Rudehart said. Sandy wouldn't like the delay but what could happen in a day?

* * *

Jack was closing loans for HomeQuik, cherry-picking Empi's biggest dupes. From the dumpster docs he compared credit score to interest rate, factored for the equity left in the house then made his calls. "I can do better" was his opening line. How he knew what they were paying he never answered. "What's it to you?" he'd ask rhetorically if they pushed it. "I can save you two hundred a month minimum. Take it or leave it."

The ones who took, Jack kept their names for later use. That fucking Kurt had wasted the Guzman case. But there were more, many more. Some he'd tell the kid about and some not. Sure fucking Empi was fun. He'd clipped 'em for a mil in real estate loans already. But he had to keep his eye on the ball: the upcoming trial, some cards to swap for Janet to back down. Horse-trading, wasn't that what they called it? Or whore-trading. Speaking of which -- that fucking Gina Sunday was now the poster-girl for Empi's sin tickled him to no end. He knew about her bathroom snorts, the way she thought her pussy was too good for The Bronx, too good for him at least. He'd seen the beefcake in the car at the end of Blitz Night. Some Wop who ordered anabolic steroids from that Men's Health rag -- they shrunk your dick, Jack'd heard -- and squired Gina around like she was some porno star. Two-bit loan shark gliterati, now brought low by Wall Street's Bible. That was the upside of losing the Guzmans as a trading card. Gina'd be desperate if he knew her and open to a play.

He was hiding in the weeds by the West Farm mall when Gina dramatic walked out toward her car. She had on dark sunglasses like she was in mourning, a strip mall Lorraine O, carrying the weight of her dead husband or her dead career on her milky white shoulders. Jack hissed from the weeds -- he couldn't be seen, not with Janet inside as he knew she was by her car -- and Gina looked over.

The ghost of bed posts past, thought Gina. The irrepressible cracker who shoulda been the one slammed in the Journal.

"Meet me around the corner," he whispered madly. "We need to talk."

Even as she turned the engine Gina thought she'd drive on by. But the cracker's lust could be used: it was axiomatic that in crisis no asset could be overlooked. She pulled under the elevated train and rolled the passenger's side window down.

"You shouldn't be here," she said.

"Fuck Janet," Jack said. "C'mon, let me in. I don't want her to see me."

Gina wondered then clicked. She had a gun that Vinny'd gave her in the glove compartment, behind her Effective People™ books-on-tape. If the cracker got fresh he'd regret it.

They drove down the hill of Boston Road. She smelled his sweat -- the cracker took the cake when it came to personal hygiene -- and wondered why she'd ever though there was a path from here to there, from gut-bucket subprime to the Wall Street heights.

"That wasn't fair," Jack said, and for a moment she thought he was reading her thoughts. "The article," he said. "You do what you're told and the next thing you're the scapegoat." He paused -- he had a whole plan here, she saw, then asked, "What's Janet doing there anyway?"

"Just making her rounds," Gina said. But why not tell the truth? She was ashamed in front of some people, but Jack wasn't one of them. "They put her in charge for now. Something about the attorney general."

Jack whistled and shook his head. "So they fucked us both," he said. "First they set me up, then they demote you."

"It's only temporary."

"Yeah right. Let me tell you, the time I've been with Empi, I never saw anyone go down to go up." Jack smiled at his double-entendre: there had been a branch manager in Rock Hill who'd sucked her way to the top, they had a good laugh at Six Flags Over Jesus, but that was another story.

"Get to the point," Gina said. She'd parked by the zoo, watched pathetic cows with their screaming brats pour through the metal turnstile, the smell of urine everywhere, the world bleak.

"You should come over to the dark side," he said. She thought of the gun, wondered just how crazy the Cracker might be. "To HomeQuik I mean. You gonna be *called* a predatory lender you might as well let it all hang out. The money's better, I'll tell you that. Straight commission. Front end and back." The image in his head was of double scuttling but the reference was to yield spread premiums and Gina knew it. She was trying to go up and not down. She'd shoot herself before she went to HomeQuik. It was just a phrase but she didn't like to think it. Not with Vinny's gun with the self-help tapes.

"That's not the future I en*vis*ion," she said precisely, thinking of the tapes.

"You didn't en-*viz*-jun they'd be screwing you neither, did you." Jack said it flat, a statement not a question. "Lemme get to the point like you asked. The way I see it, Empi's going down. They're throwin' sacrifices to the wolves. First me, then you -- Janet thinks she's safe but she's livin' in a dream world."

"EmpiBank has stood the test of time," Gina said by rote.

"Times are different. You saw Enron -- the shit can explode in a minute. That's what's gonna happen with Empi. I just wanna speed it up a bit, give 'em a push."

"You're out on bail," Gina said. "I can't see what you could do to them."

Jack wasn't going to tell her about the dumpster. The bitch could rat to Janet then that gig'd be up. But give her a change to help the cause. Test her integrity, the way the cop shows put it. "I need access to Monstro," Jack said. "Just a few minutes on the system is all I'm askin'."

"Get out," Gina said. She might sell out Empi -- she'd tried, right there at Odeon -- but not to Jack. To cast her lot with the Cracker was unimaginable.

"Take it easy," Jack said. "I was just *askin'*."

"I'm serious, get out of the car right now or I'll call the cops."

Jack wondered why this always happened to him. Diane had done it, then Janet and now Gina lousy Sunday. She'd be a lousy lay anyway, he now realized. Too high strung. The only cock she sucked was Empi's. "Think about it," he said with the door still open. Gina squealed away from the curb and burned the light on Vyse Avenue. Jack could walk home from here. On the 'Net he knew bitches who could put Gina Sunday to shame.

24. The Buffalo Motz

Finally the night of the sun-dried tomatoes; finally the show of Riverdale's own Jackie O. Carolyn Swanker ordered Milly to and fro, the final drizzle of virgin olive oil on her buffalo mozzarella, the white wine glasses next to the puffy red, two racks of veal sizzling with thyme in the oven. Carolyn watched *Cucina Italiana* on PBS, she knew her Umbria from her Calabrese, could recite each of Rudehart's alma maters if the chance came up. They were Riverdale royalty bound for the big time. This little soirée with the Treasury Secretary was the proof of *that* pudding. Ex-Treasury Secretary, what was the difference. It was the kind of dinner you'd see mentioned in the salmon-pink New York Observer. In Talk Magazine before it folded. She'd sent the kids to sleep-over with their friends from Horace Mann. She was ready but wished this Micah wasn't here. She'd set the extra place begrudgingly, leaving one fewer fork since Ernie said that Micah Levine would be leaving early. She had sorbet on ice, impossible Chilean fruits and the Calvados Ernie or probably his secretary had rushed to buy. Who knew what else she did for him? Ernie never caused a scandal. He knew that much, her Ernie did.

Micah had driven around Riverdale to Steely Dan to kill time. The Hebrew Home for the Aged with its Alzheimer's cattle call on its verdant pasture; the Wave Hill Mansion with its tasteful plaque to Mark Twain. Rudehart was a get-over who'd try to blow him off. The thing was to stick in his craw, so Rudehart in turn would piss Swanker off. Then the double-whammy of a cease-and-desist and a class action lawsuit. He missed Bertha but this was not her kind of scene.

Swanker had a government car and even a driver, the fuck. Micah watched it pull into the driveway; Swanker rushed inside with two bags of groceries. It was like that movie The Sting: setting up a fake bookie joint on the spur of the moment. Each with their own motives. Let the games begin.

Micah parked on the lawn on the side of the house. No need to lock the car up here. He rang the bell. A vision in pearls with a Plastisene smile appeared, "Oh I've heard so much about you," she said -- what would she do for Rudehart, Micah wondered: drop to her knees on the marble floor and blow him? He'd brought flowers, he was nothing if not smooth, and Mrs. Swanker handed them to a good-looking Puerto

Rican woman with insulting instructions. "Cut them diagonally so the water can get in," she said. The maid was in black with a white doily apron, a blast from the past, slimmer than Bertha but from a world incomprehensibly far away -- Micah cut off the thought.

"So you know the game plan," Swanker said, stirring them gin and tonics on the sidebar. "Chit chat over the cheese, credit insurance over veal then you're outta here."

"I'll say I have to meet a client."

"Whatever. The sherbet's your cue."

"Sor-*bet*," Swanker's wife said. The Spanish chick should kill her. The world wasn't fair.

Rudehart had a driver too: Chuck Stewart. Chuck had a gun. Twenty years on the FBI strike force and now a nine-to-five at EmpiGroup. Every once in a while he had to do a job at night. The psycho branch manager with her brow-beat in Kinkos, hadn't that been a pisser. As the deputy chief of security he usually didn't drive, but the runt in the back seat they called precious cargo. Maybe he was like that scientist on Channel 13 with his head lolling over.

They pulled into the driveway. "Here we are, Mister Rudehart."

"Thank you Chuck," the runt said. Like Jeeves, like he was some butler. If the guy'd been elected to something it'd be different. Chuck stayed in the car, watched a white lady in pearls throw herself on the runt like he was Mick Jagger or something. Like a Barry White without the heft. Fake fucks these people were. He had some nice R&B and two hours to kill. He'd hit White Castle when it was over, after he dropped the runt on Park Avenue. He could taste those greasy Sliders™ now.

Rudehart cased the joint like a cat burglar. Swanker had family money, from a slumlord the tabloids said. The white couches stunk of it, the view of the Hudson and the Palisades, the trophy wife -- she had some crow's feet, okay -- the dark-skinned French maid, Martinique perhaps, or a rare mulatta from Senegal. Rudehart didn't like to drink. He was a man of SlimFast and the StairMaster, power was his drug, the only one he'd ever needed. "Just water with lime," he told the maid, smiling, he'd like to know her name. But that wasn't the point. Listen to this Micah Levine then get him the hell out of here so he could make his pitch. It'd been Sandy's idea but he'd improved it as he always did.

Micah played with his sun-dried tomatoes while Swanker and Rudehart shot the shit about the HMOs. Prescriptions for seniors: supposedly elections turned on this but Micah couldn't tell why. Neither party offered to cover the shit like they did in Sweden. The national debate, at least down in Washington, had been shrunken so much it could fit in a pill jar, with a child-proof cap. What about the Tobin Tax? What about the corporate death penalty? The more he knew Bertha, the lefter he got.

"We'll paint the Republicans as in bed with Pfizer," Rudehart said knowingly.

"Aren't we all?" Swanker countered. Carolyn Swanker tittered, quiet pleased with this repartee. She wanted to make a joke about Viagra but it might be a sour joke, at least with her husband.

"I read your speech at Harvard," she said to Rudehart in a lull. "It was wonderful."

"Did you go there?"

Of course. That was the reason she'd asked. "Milly!" she called out. "I think these carnivores are ready for their veal."

At last, Micah thought. He'd had it up to here with the DNC humor.

Milagros carried Rudehart's half-eaten mozzarella through the swinging doors. These people were haughty, *come mierdas* as they put it in Tremont. It meant "shit eaters" literally, but "full of shit" was the better translation. Mistress Carolyn -- she called her that sometimes, to Amado or even here without the stuck-up brat even noticing -- giving her lessons in preserving cut flowers as if she knew. Back in Tijuana Milly'd grow food and spices in their *casita*'s back yard. Her mother taught her how to do it; her mother did it still as her house fell down around her. Even here on Park Avenue, Milly grew peppers and could keep the flowers Amado bought her on *el dia de las madres* alive for two weeks, changing the water daily, adding powder from the *botanica* on Fordham Road. She'd have quit this job if not for Amado's injury. Maybe the lawsuit would solve that problem. She'd give them two days notice, maybe less.

The platter of the veal was hot, but Mistress Carolyn didn't like her to use the puffy oven mittens. *'Ta bien*, she thought, let them eat their cow fetus and speak of the poor as an issue, a slogan for every four years then *no más*. Amado was more into unions and their coalition politics but she had a gut sense for fakers and she felt it now. This dinner guest who drove the Mistress so crazy -- who was he? She laid the veal platter down, stood meekly to the side while Master Swanker pretended that the carving was difficult and heroic. Juice squirted on the table; she would have to wipe it up. These people were full of illusions. She wouldn't eat their food if she were starving.

"This is *won*derful, Carolyn," Rudehart said, nibbling on a small bite of the still-pink meat. Micah had hardly spoken but now he stirred.

"I'm sure you wonder why I'm here," he began. Carolyn Swanker flinched. These sixty dollar racks of veal, and Ernie's gauche guest was going to ruin them with business. There was always the Calvados and sorbet.

"Ernie's told me a bit," Rudehart said, glad for an excuse to put down his fork. "Something about credit insurance. It's not my area of expertise, but I'm always interested in what our company is doing. So tell me."

"I have a client," Micah said. God he wished Bertha were here with him, and Duwon and the girls, just to see the sorority sister squirm a bit more, at a woman of color she couldn't order around. "She took out a loan from your finance company--"

"That's Sandy's baby," Rudehart commented, trying to disarm with honesty and distance himself at the same time.

"I've seen the documents and half of the charge is insurance."

"I've heard we sell it," Rudehart said. "It's not illegal."

Micah put down his fork, let the suspense such as it was build. "What caught my eye is *what* they'd written the insurance on."

"Go on," Rudehart said. This Levine had a real stage presence. He probably winked at female jurors, smiled and implied that he'd split his fee with them.

"It's a bed," Micah said. "A bed and she's paying twenty five hundred dollar in insurance."

"Queen-sized, I hope," Rudehart said. Carolyn laughed, too loud, fake. Swanker shot her the look. Micah kept his gaze on Rudehart. Bertha could wipe the floor with his type in a minute.

"Look," Rudehart said, "I don't mean to be callous. As far as I know, the products we sell are all voluntary. Do customers sometimes have second thoughts? Who doesn't? But I'm sure this insurance can be canceled."

Micah thought of the cracker: the first day he'd seen him in the mall, then the embarrassing confession in his office. "That's what I tried first," Micah said. This really wasn't a bad story, he thought. Not a bad case at all.

Rudehart looked at his watch. Time was a'wasting and still this bed. "Don't tell me -- they wouldn't cancel it."

"Correct. And I'm sure that's what most customers hear if they try."

Caveat emptor was Sandy's phrase. Rudehart was more elaborate. "These loans get securitized. We can't go changing the terms at the drop of a hat. But in the appropriate case it shouldn't be hard. Your client's lucky to have such a persistent advocate. Just--"

"There's more. The man who'd refused to cancel the insurance, he came to my office later with a story to tell."

Spare me, Rudehart thought. Could this shyster be any more heavy-handed? He designed a come-back. "You know that as a lawyer you shouldn't talk to a target corporation's employees. It's black letter law."

"He'd already quit. So he's not an employee--"

"He's a whistle-blower," Rudehart mockingly completed his sentence.

Micah nodded. "He says that at least half of the insurance EmpiFinancial sells is on personal property they'd never foreclose on."

"Never is a big word," Rudehart said. "Peace of mind in itself is a benefit. No judge would second-guess a customer's desire for it. To do so would be--" he smiled -- "patronizing."

"But if we can show that EmpiFinancial routinely sells insurance that has no conceivable value -- worthless insurance with no benefit to the borrower at all -- it's a set up for massive punitive damages," Micah said. "It wouldn't help your stock price either."

"Are you suing?" Rudehart asked, turning to Carolyn and smiling.

Swanker'd had enough. "Okay, you've made your pitch, Bob's heard it," he said to Micah.

"We have a tape," Micah added. "The stuff in the Journal's just the tip of the iceberg."

"These things have a way of working themselves out," Rudehart said. Soon it'd be his turn to pitch. Why was this shyster still here?

"Milly!" Carolyn called out. "I think we're done. I don't want to rush you Bob--"

"Oh, it was delicious. My stomach's just a bit tender from my time south of the border."

Milagros pushed open the swinging doors she'd been standing behind. Her mind was swinging, too. She'd heard "EmpiFinancial," heard the *pato* defend it. So this was Mistress and Master Swanker's dinner guest: *un prededor rapaz.* She'd have to tell Amado. She'd have to listen more. It would be the sweetest revenge. She owed these people nothing.

As she cleared first the platter, then Rudehart's still-full plate, the other man -- the man of the people it seemed -- continued to jibe at the *pato.*

"It's an indefensible practice," he said. "It's systemic fraud."

"It's the business," Rudehart said. "It's not my favorite part of Empi but it has stood the test of time. People sue and they lose. Most people don't sue so they must like it."

"Bob you don't have to--" It was Carolyn.

"Oh don't worry. I'm not ashamed of our business at all. We give the people what they want. If some lawyer doesn't like it, too bad." He turned to Micah who was biting his lip. "The beauty of America," Rudehart continued, "the beauty of markets, is that they're constrained by competition and brand equity. If things were as you say, Empi simply wouldn't be in that business. And your client, this poor little victim with her queen sized bed -- why did she take the loan? If there was a better deal out there why did she come to us?"

Rudehart didn't like to lose his cool and was only half-playing at doing so now. His dander was up but he took the long view. Once Swanker was back on the reservation, once this Nicole Nour was exiled to some dysentery bureau, it would all blow over. Then there'd be only this putz and his bed. The clean-up squad from Baltimore could handle him and his type. They always had. Money talked and bullshit walked. On that, he and Sandy agreed.

"Blaming the victim doesn't work in the courts," Micah said. "What you do here you do worse in the south, say in Charlotte--" he was thinking of Jack, of the Pandora's box opened up by that tape, I-95 with full-throttle Steely Dan -- "and you're planning to do it in Mexico too, from what I hear. You're on notice."

"Duly noted," Rudehart said. "Really, your etiquette could use some work." Cocksucking trial lawyer, a moderately big fish in a the puny pond of Bronx slip-and-fall. It took all kinds. Now to put the screws to Swanker.

"I'm sorry Bob, I had no idea," Carolyn said while Milly went to close the door behind Micah. Swanker begged pardon and followed, confronted Micah on the porch.

"Good work," he hissed. "Now they'll never settle."

"He's a pompous prick," Micah said. "I don't *care* if he worked for Clinton. He's a smug bastard... We're going to sue, right?"

"You'll be the first to know," Swanker sneered. "You should go to a gym or something, work out your frustrations. Or to a shrink."

"Don't get too soft," Micah said over his shoulder. "Empi's got the money but you don't have to beg for it. Sue 'em and you'll be famous."

I already am, Swanker thought. Micah was a putz. Carolyn would go back to sleeping in her own private bedroom but that was okay.

Chuck saw them argue on the porch, wondered whether the runt might be in danger back inside. Getting his salami shaved by Miss Pearly Whites, more likely. The runt had a beeper he could press to summon muscle. Chuck watched the one who'd left squeal out the gravel driveway. It was a real soap opera up here. Like Dynasty or Dallas, or the crap they showed at 2 p.m.. "The way you touch me," the back-up singers crooned. Oh yeah, thought Chuck. The way you touch me baby.

Inside Carolyn had her hand on Rudehart's arm. "You must apologize to Bob," she scolded her husband. "We invite him to dinner and he gets ambushed by a Communist with a law degree."

"Micah's no Commie," Swanker said. "He's a capitalist in his own way."

"I know his type," Rudehart said, out loud before he realized. Carolyn waited for more but there was none. Already the sorbet was melting. She'd told Milly to serve one course after the other -- she was like a robot, Carolyn thought, no improvisation, no sense of the gastronomic moment.

"Passion fruit," Carolyn announced. "And sorbet of a pear found only in Tierra del Fuego."

Swanker got the calva and the Cuban cigars. The U.S. Senate was the lowest he'd land. Micah hadn't been a bad warm-up act, really. Micah was the Talking Head, but Swanker was MegaDeath, deaf-making heavy metal, Ozzy Osborne about to hold this pigeon's head between his teeth and ask how much? How much support can I count on not to turn your corporation inside-out in the public view? Rudehart was old school and he was the new.

"Give us a moment," Swanker told his wife, escorting Rudehart out to the terrace, some tanker ship inching north up the river with toxins.

They lit their cigars with dramatic puffs. There was no reason to speak of Micah: they both knew he'd just been the opening act. The maid stood by the door, mopping something up on the tablecloth. It was time to deal.

"It's taken a while but let's cut to the chase," Rudehart said. He didn't like to smoke either. But there was something Godfather-like about it, something necessary. He didn't draw the fumes into his mouth: it was the doorway to his smokeless soul.

"My thought exactly," Swanker said.

Milagros inched closer to the door. Mistress Carolyn was schizing out with biscotti, all to the good.

Rudehart blew out on his cigar and looked at the river. "EmpiGroup can make or break a political career -- you know that, don't you?"

"I trust in the voters," Swanker said. "But go on."

"I've told Sandy that you're one of us -- a man of the Street, a believer in markets, globalization with a human face, the whole Blue Dog catechism."

Swanker waited. Talk was cheap.

"Who knows when we'll have a Democrat president again," Rudehart said. "If Gore runs again it'll be a fiasco. But you could move to the House, no problem -- with Empi's support. *Comprende?*"

Milly stifled a laugh at the Spanish word. She wanted to memorize what she overheard, to tell Amado and maybe the kid downstairs. This was like the final days of the PRI, the bastards who sucked Tijuana dry and left her mother without sewage lines or even a paved street. It was naked corruption. Blue dog she did not understand. But Amado would know, or the kid.

"I could win a House seat on my own," Swanker said. "Winning a case against EmpiGroup would probably help my chances, not hurt them."

"We'd fund your opponent."

"Some tinhorn councilman? I've got name recognition."

For now, Rudehart thought. Next year you could be at Waste Management paying bribes to make ground water violations go away.

"I'm looking at the Senate," Swanker continued.

"Those seat are filled," Rudehart said. "We both know that."

"That's what primaries are for. I'd just need enough money to break through."

The balls on this guy, Rudehart thought. It was time for the stick. "Let's not get ahead of ourselves. You think it's all upside but there's a downside too. No job is forever. There's a good D.A. in Rochester--"

"Basso?" Swanker asked. "You can't be serious."

"Sandy likes him very much, Basso's pitched him about what a truly pro-business Democratic attorney general could do for us."

Sandy'd never heard of Basso -- why would he have? Lena'd found the guy, some quotes in the upstate press screaming between the lines of Basso's ambitions for higher office. They could offer him the Faustian bargain tomorrow and he'd take it. Swanker'd be beaten or at least damaged goods and he knew it. Rudehart liked having another man's testicles in his hand.

"Basso's a nobody," Swanker insisted.

"With Empi behind him, a nobody becomes a somebody so fast it makes you head spin. Keep your feet on the ground, Ernie. You play ball with us, we'll play with you. Take the long view."

This Basso threat made Swanker sick. If he caved right now he'd just be a Basso one rung up the food chain.

"I'll see what the documents tell me," Swanker said.

"You do that. Lay off the subpoenas, think about it a little. Take your wife on a vacation, for God's sake. When you get back we can talk about the House seat. You might have to move-- " he gestured at the house, saw that delicious maid still standing at the door and wondered why -- "but only for like a week or so, some rented place in the district before you move to D.C.."

"I like my job," Swanker said more uncertainly than he'd have liked.

"And that's another reason. C'mon, let's have another Calvados. I want to tell your wife how delicious this has been. Even that Micah stuffed his face."

Swanker's thoughts were dark with Basso. Rudehart felt sweaty balls in the palm of his hand. And Milly wrote the whole thing down in the kitchen bathroom, Senate and House and this name Baso. Like *vaso* the glass, or *ah-so* the Japanese phrase of enlightenment. In a flash by the door she saw the breadth of corruption, as if illuminated by lightening. She knew which side her heart was on. Mistress Carolyn was the pampered wife of *un coruptido*. A man in the bag of *un prededor rapaz*. She thanked God again for the man He had given her. *Humilde pero recto*. She said the prayer again when Master Swanker dropped her off at the One Train on Broadway. Once he'd put his hand in her crotch and she'd slapped his face. It had not happened again. This time he did not even speak. Did he care how long it took her to get home? He did not. She splurged on a gypsy cab. Amado'd be awake and they could plan what to do.

25. The Morning After

On his way from the train Swanker did something he was not proud of. He pulled to the side of the road and unzipped his fly. It was a reflex, to make sure it was there. It was a pretext, to stretch it long and make it hard, thinking of Milly or any number of hotties from law school, anything for release, so that this reflexive hunger couldn't be used by Carolyn. She'd want him to apologize for Micah's hard-line, as if that made any difference now. She'd want to know the blow-by-blow of what was said on the terrace. She was a political wife, a good counsel perhaps -- but who'd cop to emasculation? If he told her the deal she'd file it away, use it if they got divorced, use it in arguments, perhaps tell a biographer when the time came. *If* that time came. She'd say: take the deal, of course: lay off of Empi and take the House seat. She had the brownstone in Georgetown already picked out. He couldn't get hard, worried about his State of New York plates. How pathetic was it when you couldn't even get yourself off? He cursed Rudehart and that bastard Basso in Rochester. His dilemma was shameful, he felt. He had no one to turn to.

* * *

Rudehart had no such conflicts. After the StairMaster, after the Power Shake, he plugged Micah Levine into the J. Edgar Hoover machine. The first check is simple: was this joker even an attorney licensed in the State of New York? He was. He'd listed his office address, 149th Street and Morris Avenue. Getting his home address shouldn't be hard. He'd been a night student at Brooklyn Law School; he'd been a co-editor of some second-tier journal on Ghetto Law. This made Rudehart laugh. American academia, even the law schools, was going to the dogs. They had Chic-eh-no studies -- what chicanery, Rudehart thought -- they had post-imperial studies, even the newest defeatist flavor, "Post-Development." What the hell did that mean? That the maquiladora drones he saw down in TJ didn't want a fridge that poured ice cubes from the door, didn't want buffalo mozzarella and sorbet like last night, and even a maid? Post development? More like psycho nay-sayers, Rudehart thought. He was on several committees of the International Monetary Fund and the Wolfsberg Group. Since '99 they'd had to play lip service to something called civil society. As if there were some society somehow more moral than Empi, more vibrant and pure, just because they ran interminable meetings and never made decisions at all except to break windows in one city after another. He'd been in Seattle for the WTO; he'd been in Prague and even Doha, saw some Commie Italian rightly shot down by the *caribinieri* in the streets of Genoa. Now *they* had mozzarella. Rudehart hardly ate but the Italians for all of their failures in business, they had a taste for the finer things in life. Sophia Loren, a fascist stripper in the parliament, a Dolce Vita Rupert Murdock running the country while his cameras rolled.

He ran a web search now on Micah Levine. There wasn't much -- a marginal loser, just as Rudehart'd pegged him. Here though was something of interest. A web site called WatchCorp, with a pseudo-journalistic write up of EmpiFinancial's supposed sins, mentioning Micah Levine and something about a bed. It had the bed-owner's address: Bertha Watkins of East 149th Street. Rudehart wrote it down. When he'd left the Treasury Department he hadn't expected to get this low in the gutter. But this was the case that Micah Levine deluded himself would bring Empi down. The way to cut the shyster off at the knees would be to go around his back, cancel the insurance on the bed, hell give her a new one, cut this bottom-feeder off from his chum and watch him starve. Lena could invite the press. He'd have to ask Sandy.

Something about this WatchCorp.org bothered him, though. Its tone was in-the-know; it ended every write-up with the breathless word "developing." It promised more dirt, unfolding stories, "stay tuned," it said. Rudehard clicked through to the contact page but not surprisingly there was no name listed. Cowardly bastards spewing anonymous libel, that's what the 'Net had fallen to. He did a WhoIs search, half expecting a limited liability company, some inscrutable offshore partnership like Empi would have done -- but no. Kurt Wheelock, it said. With an address on Riverside Drive. Some pinko Upper Left Sider stirring up trouble north in The Bronx. This too could be taken care of.

* * *

Amado'd been asleep when Milagros got home. He grunted, rolled over and kissed her. She had much to tell but this wasn't the time. The gate to the basement was locked. The kid had said he might move in but hadn't yet. Milagros took off her ridiculous white apron, the too-tight black skirt and turned on the tube. They rebroadcast *novelas* on TeleFutura at this time, one from a few years ago, "Traviesa." A girl who dresses up as a boy and works as a clerk for the rich. The rich man's son, a lawyer, falls for Traviesa and pursues her through supposedly Mexican streets in a convertible. The streets looked like none Milagros had seen in Azatlan. Dream on. These shows like fairy tales always had the poor girl saved by a prince. Milagros wasn't buying. The rich were corrupt, as she'd seen tonight. She was grateful for Amado while she listened to him snore.

In the morning as she boiled water for coffee the kid arrived. She heard the gate being pulled up and went to the door.

"*Que tal Milagros,*" the kid said in his ridiculous Spanish. Well at least he tried.

"*Quieres café?*" she asked.

"*Como no.*" He came up into the kitchen. Milagros switched unilaterally to English. She wanted him to understand this.

"Last night I see something I want you to know. I work as a maid -- I told you this, no?" He nodded. Somewhere in Riverdale. He wished she didn't have to. "My boss, he is big lawyer in New York State."

Kurt perked up. Some corporate pig? "Do you know where?" he asked.

"For the State of New York. He is, how you say, general attorney."

"Attorney general? You work for Ernie Swanker?"

"Yes. Him and his wife Carolina. I call her Mistress Caroline." Milagros laughed. "I never think my work may be connected to my house."

Kurt remembered Nicole Nour's update: Swanker was looking into the Guzmans' loan. "Did he ask you about it?"

Milagros shook her head. "No. He does not ask me anything." She thought about it, pouring the steaming water through the filter. "He does not know where I live." She thought of him putting his little pink hand in her crotch. The coffee overflowed. "Last night they have big party. Not big but very important. Two men come to the house in separate cars." Kurt mopped up with a paper towel. If Swanker didn't ask, what was the connection to the Guzmans' home? He waited.

"One man, he gets loud. He is a lawyer, his name is something like Miguel but that's not it. Russian name maybe. Mikhail... No. His name is Mee-cah."

Kurt stopped wiping the counter. "Micah Levine?"

"Yes. They call him that."

Mother *fucker*, Kurt thought. The shyster was selling them out. Or maybe not -- maybe he was planning a case with A.G. Swanker. "The other man--"

"This is best part. He has strange name, I cannot forget it. Rudehart. *Como corazon.*" Milagros pointed at her chest. Her breast, Kurt thought. Why did he always fall for women whom he shouldn't pursue? "Rudehart work for this Empi, the ones who make our loan."

"I know."

"Mee-cah yell at Rudehart, but Rudehart only laugh. Then Mee-cah leave."

Maybe a settlement talk, Kurt thought. But it couldn't be about the Guzmans' loan, since Micah had never met them. Maybe that bed. A big pow-wow in Riverdale about a bed? Hard to believe.

"Rudehart take Master Swanker outside. I stand by the door -- I am cleaning up the table, I am not spy -- but I can hear them."

"*Y que dijieron?*"

"Rudehart tells Swanker he must, how you say, back up. No sub-peony." Actually it had sounded like a bad word to Milagros, the worm in a man's pants. She did not want to say this, and so a flower.

"Subpoena. What did Swanker say?"

"He talk crazy -- he talk about Senate, about Washington, mention this company I see in the news last year. En-ron. 'It can slip away so fast,' Master Swanker say. But Rudehart is not scared. At least he does not act it."

He should be, Kurt thought. Unless they have something on Swanker.

"Rudehart say House -- like *casa* -- then Senate. Rudehart say if Swanker make subpoena he will lose his job."

"But he's elected," Kurt cut in, thinking out loud.

"I know this," Milagros said. "Rudehart mention some man from Rock-chester, Basso he is called, Bossa Nova, they will give him *mucho dinero* to try for Swanker's job."

Kurt'd never heard of Basso but it was all too perfect. No reason for Milagros to make this up. Empi was playing hard ball. "And what did Swanker say?"

"No answer. Rudehart say, take a vacation, take Mistress Caroline away, come back and talk of the House."

The offer itself was newsworthy, Kurt thought. He could make a sworn statement for Milly, but no. How could Swanker have missed this? Kurt took his battered copy of the Wall Street Journal out of his backpack. The drawing of Amado; Amado's quotes about this woman Gina Sunday. No mention of the Jackal, no mention of WatchCorp -- and no mention of Milagros by name. Just, "Mr. Guzman's wife." Very enlightened.

Milagros continued. "Master Swanker drive me to Broadway -- he never drive me home and this is okay, one time he try--" She stopped. No reason to say this.

"He try what?"

"He try to drive me home but I say no."

Kurt sensed some sleaze, wondered if this "drive me home" was a euphemism in Spanish. The horse in the stable he'd heard of. That bastard.

"He look sad. No -- he look scared. He drop me on Broadway and not say good night."

"He   didn't   know   that   you   heard."

"No. But in my mind I am sure -- he is scared, he not fight EmpiBank no more. He must talk to Mistress Caroline." Milagros laughed and stirred in the milk she'd heated. "That is his punishment."

"Milagros this is amazing. We need to use it but I don't know how." How to ask? "Look, I'd like to report this on WatchCorp but I don't want--"

"Do not worry. This job with Swankers, I am near the end. *Son come mierdas.*"

"I won't say it was you that heard."

"Okay. But if they know I do not care. It is corrupt. It is often the servants, *los trabajadores*, who can expose these things. In *Mehico* they will try to kill you. I do not think that happen here."

Kurt wasn't sure. Gene Ramos always said there were threats on his life. He may have been crazy. But how about the Black Panthers? There'd been a tenant organizer dumped headless in Hunts Point. Kurt wasn't so sure. And even genteel there were other ways they had. "Did they make you a sign a contract, when you went to work for the Swankers?" He was thinking of the suits the British royals brought against gigolo horse trainers, butlers who collected pubic hairs, the life-long gag orders rock stars tried to get.

"There are no papers," Milagros said. "Nothing to sign." She thought again. "They do not pay taxes on me."

"No W-2?"

"No. No forms, no taxes. No social security. This is why I cannot list what I make when we apply for a loan." She thought back to that day at Empi, the fast-talking *blancita* and Mister Jack in the corner watching her.

Kurt shook his head. This was the so-called nanny problem: it knocked out some corporate ice queen from Greenwich from Janet Reno's job; it knocked out a judge named Kimba Wood or so the paper's said. The Swankers had a nanny problem. Empi had leverage on Ernie, whoever this Basso was -- but now so did Kurt. He wanted to kiss Milagros but it wouldn't be right. He'd fuck Candida with abandon tonight, maybe order a maid's uniform if they stayed together that long.

"You're amazing," he told Milagros, the double meaning as thick as his coffee.

"There is something I like about this Mee-cah," she said. "He was not scared of Rudehart. Since Amado wants a lawyer, not that he's in papers, I think that maybe Mister Mee-cah is right one."

"I'll call him," Kurt said. If the Guzmans could win a case, Milagros could quit before the Swankers fired her.

26. Poisonous Hormones

"Get the bitch a new bed -- I like that."

Sandy was again bright pink in the steaming water at Armonk. It was just him and Rudehart today. Blowman wouldn't bring anything to the table. What he sold he called strategic thinking. But this was a matter of tactics, pure Clausewitz. Chuck had driven them up --˙ you couldn't be too careful -- and he could be deployed for the first advance. The bed bitch then the WatchCorp guy on Riverside Drive. There was just one missing piece.

"You think he's really got a source? Or he's just blowing smoke up your ass?" Sandy farted and it bubbled to the surface. Rudehart cringed.

"He said it was the guy who refused to cancel the bed insurance. I've got his name already. Jack Bender."

"Never heard of him."

"He worked for you -- for us -- in Charlotte. His numbers weren't bad, but they wrote him up for going too light on insurance."

"Why'd we fucking promote him?"

"He'd put in a request for a transfer. We needed to staff-up fast to open the branch in The Bronx--"

"Fucking moonscape," Sandy commented. Rudehart paused in case Sandy had more to say. He did: "But there's money there for the taking. Ya know we own that mall, right? And the land under it. If this shit keeps happening, we should close it down. Or maybe blow the whole place up."

Rudehart nodded. If he were still in government this might be controversial. "So for whatever reason Bender was the guy. He'd never flunked an audit 'til he got to The Bronx."

"Audit-shmawdit. There's two keys to this business, Bob -- hitting the bonus numbers and *believing* in what you do. The moment you waver you're fucked. That's what I told Lena."

This reminded Rudehart: "If the bed woman is willing, we'll bring the press up there."

"Too defensive. Just pay the cunt and move on. You wanna do press, go up to Rochester and put your arm around Basso. That'll make Swanker's sphincter pucker, I guarantee." Sandy went underwater. He looked like a bloated corpse, Rudehart thought, his few remaining strands of hair floating up like seaweed, his eyes open like an octopus or a squid. He resurfaced and sneered. "We need to break this Bender's balls," Sandy said poetically. "What'daya got on that?"

"He's doing it himself. Just before the audit -- during it actually -- he got arrested for whoring."

Sandy snorted. This didn't make Bender alright. Sandy liked cheese fries and so did a million other schmucks. It didn't make them brothers.

"Then, get this: he got arrested again for faxing death threats to the district manager."

"You talked to him?"

"Her. It's a woman, covers lower Westchester and this one in the Bronx. There's more. This guy Bender, he's been stalking the D.M.. She took out an order of protection. The legal department's got a whole file on this guy."

"And we're the last to know."

"Typical low rent bullshit."

"Until now." Sandy got out of the water and Rudehart turned away. Sandy noticed and didn't give a fuck. When you were rich enough you could eat what you wanted. Rudehart was a fairy like the little boy who ran England for now. "So Bender's ass is grass," Sandy said flatly, not a question but a statement, a schoolyard couplet he'd carried from Brooklyn.

"Yeah we'll make sure that his trial's done right. I'm putting out some feelers down in Charlotte too. See why he requested the transfer."

"Sounds like a plan." Sandy paused over the cold water, considering going straight for the rub-down without this shock. "One more thing Bob -- only tell me what I need to know. You're the one who let Swanker roam too long. So it's on you to clean it up."

Mother *fucker*, Rudehart thought. In his days of public service he'd drawn up a few plays about the horndog's midnight blow jobs. It was dirty but the stakes were high. This low rent soap opera was beneath him. But a couple of spins of the wheel and it'd all be clean. Sandy would owe him. He could smell the options now.

* * *

In the air-conditioned half-light Jack sensed that the shit was all slipping away. He'd been closing loans for HomeQuik like crazy, almost enough to get his Taurus out of hock. But Gina's blown him off and he couldn't hack Monstro. Janet Peel had her five hundred foot force field -- as if anyone would want to fuck that glassy-eyed robot anyway. The Guzmans were stars. Kurt was gonna hook them up with Are-You-Hurt Micah without him even being involved. He had a list of the Empi victims he'd flipped but what good would it do him? The Kinkos gazelle had said what he'd said. Everybody was having a fucking party but him.

The last call with Zalie had left him depressed. He wanted to see her in-person next time, with a tank full of gas and his rap sheet clean. Lorraine Thompson was a joker, plea bargaining for a pack of crack smokers. He needed F. Lee Fucking Bailey, or the bald headed guy who'd represented Ozone Park's John Gotti, may he rest in two-bit tabloid peace. He'd settle for Micah Levine. The fucker owed him for that tape, didn't he?

Levine made him wait, with a lady whose baby had shat out his pampers, an Indian guy with a turban made of bandages. It was like a Goddamn deli in here: take a number, wait your turn. You gave 'em information and they ran. They squeezed and used you then moved on. The kid hadn't fucked him yet, that was true. But yet was the operative word. He wanted to see his name on WatchCorp at least -- he had nothing to lose, no reason to play the Jackal anymore. But the kid thought the fax shit was petty. "It's a tangent," he'd called it. A *tangent*? It was Jack's fucking life in the balance. The last thing Lorraine'd told him was that they were adding charges under some new anti-terrorism law. She'd said it was "interesting" but he could think of other words.

"Jack!" Levine came out of his office, beckoning his in like they were strip-club pals in Charlotte. "How goes it?"

"How do you *think*?" Jack answered. He assumed that the kid had told Micah the real story, that he hadn't quit but been fired and why. But Micah played dumb.

The guy was unstable, Micah'd concluded. But why had he come to his office today? He'd been careful at Swanker's not to name his whistle-blowing source. He'd just told Rudehart he had a tape -- oh fuck. He'd said that it was the guy who'd refused to cancel Bertha's insurance. Could he be sued for this? Better play nice. "What's on your mind?"

"Kurt told you, right?"

"Told me what?"

"The frame-up that Empi is putting on me."

Micah shook his head. It could still be about the tape, could still be the echo of Rudehart's wrath. "There are whistle-blower protection laws, you know--"

"I need a lawyer."

The magic words. How mad could this cracker be at him if he sought his counsel? "I'm all ears," Micah said. "And just so you know, everything you tell me from this moment on is privileged." He made a note of Bender's nod. There. He'd tacitly agreed that nothing before had been covered. It could muddy the waters; it was better than nothing. Still he should have gotten a release that first day with the tape.

Micah relaxed more and more as Bender told his tale. It wasn't about him, about his slip-up with Rudehart. This poor fuck had faxed a death threat to Empi -- real smart, Micah thought, right after being fired -- and his trial was coming up.

"Who covered the arraignment?"

"Free lawyer called Thompson. Lorraine Thompson. She's, uh, black."

"That probably helps," Micah said. Especially a white defendant in The Bronx, if you were going to have a jury trial that was the best way.

Jack didn't follow. But that wasn't the point. "This law you was talking about, protecting whistle blowhards, whatever, you think it can help me?"

The timing was off. He'd sent the fax and gotten charged with it before he blew any whistle, hard or soft. Unless--

"Did you ever complain? Like officially file a complaint about the work conditions at Empi? Anything they made you do?"

Jack thought about it. He'd been written up in Charlotte, he remembered that. "I complained about the insurance," he said. "They wrote it up and everything. The only reason they didn't fire me then is my production was so good. I made more real estate loans than Raleigh and Durham put together."

"That's good," Micah said. "If they wrote it up you can get it in discovery. Tell Ms. Thompson--"

"I want you to represent me."

Micah shook his head. "I don't make it a practice to take cases from other lawyers. You need friends in this business and that's not the way to go. I'd be willing to confer with her, maybe second-chair the case--" here he was lying: he'd never take a back seat on some mundane crap in the criminal court --"but I can't just take it from her."

"I could fire her. I mean, she said I was over-income."

So she was an 18-B. Most accuseds got Legal Aid. Article 18-B of the judicial law let private attorneys -- losers, most of them -- represent some indigent defendants for forty dollars an hour. It was the bottom of the barrel since the pay was so low. Yep, Jack might need another lawyer. But Micah could dodge and he did.

"Tell her you talked with another lawyer. Give her my card. Together we can come up with something."

"They're callin' me a terrorist."

"What?"

"Some law they passed after those crazies blew up the World Trade Center. Use of the wires to induce fear, some shit like that."

Micah shook his head. The blast on civil liberties might be deeper than Ground Zero, more permanent. The memorial would be trumped-up charges for decades, the government getting people's library records without their consent, holding immigrants incommunicado and taping the few lawyers with the balls to defend them. The legal press loved this kind of thing. "That's more interesting." "That's what Lorraine called it." "Let's call *her*," Micah said. Even if the cracker had sent that fax -- and Micah felt sure that he had -- they could challenge this law, the add-on terrorism charge, make a big case out of it. The press would be all over it and maybe, just maybe, Micah Levine could leave these braindead babies behind.

* * *

Kurt sat smoking in Candida's kitchen, writing a draft of Milagros' tale. The nanny problem could be kept for later -- he could probably reach out to Swanker, penetrate his secretarial defenses using nanny as code-word. What he wanted to expose was Empi's hardball offer. Their use of campaign money, even after McCain-Feingold,™ to bend the people's purported protectors to their will. He had to confirm that this Basso existed. He found the Democrat & Chronicle and yeah there he was: locking up vaguely Arabic immigrants, shoulder to shoulder with Ashcroft out in the sticks. Swanker was sleaze but at least independent.

"When will this *end*?" Candida said from behind him. The way he talked about this *Mehicana* was beginning to bother her. The wife of the rapist who she'd not met that day; the wife of her father -- so her mother, that made her. Her dead mother returned to steal her man away before an egg caught hold. Candida had been drinking; on top of the pills it made her grasp of her family tree even looser than usual.

"I gotta do this," Kurt said. "The things Milagros heard have to be reported, before Swanker packs it in and it's all just a footnote."

"Do you think you're going to change *any* of it?" Candida demanded. "Do you think some obscure fucking web site is gonna stop anything that's bound to happen?"

"I do the best I can," Kurt said. A line from some movie, Clint Eastwood clenching his jaw. A man's gotta etcetera. Sublimating his ardor for Milly onto this shrew was not happening.

"You're wasting your time and you know it. It's like you *want* to fail, to throw yourself in front of a train and then cry." Candida gulped another slug of her Bacardi 151. It was like grain alcohol, like the fruit-flavored vodkas she kept frosted in the freezer. A girl's gotta do what a girl's gotta do. But she was not a girl anymore. "You know what I think?"

"What?" Kurt said without looking up. He'd had a few drinks too, but cut it with orange juice so he could still get hard. "Go ahead and tell me what you really think, rather'n being so polite like you usually are."

Sarcastic ungrateful prick.   "You think you're fucking Jesus, some white savior come to save all the stupid Spics who don't know any better."

Jibes about racism were more than Kurt could take. If the choice had been his he would have *been* a Hispanic. Didn't he lie about Wheelock? Didn't he give years to Gene Ramos -- who turned out to be a fraud -- and now to The Bronx? Kurt stood up, knocking his drink on the floor.

"You're *drunk*," he spat. "Why don't you go throw up all the fucking pills you've been taking and then start over. Maybe we could actually have a conversation--" he paused, decided it was time -- "about why we're breaking up, why we don't work. Like people, not animals. Go on now, go get your stomach pumped and get ready."

He felt insane; he felt like a god. His hatred for this white-walled asylum spewed up like semen, like puss from a boil. Candida looked stunned, crazier than he perhaps, throwing back her tumbler, throwing the glass at the wall.

"You *bastard*!" she yelled. "You arrogant junkie bastard!"

"Look who's talking," Kurt shot back. "Maybe I was in a cult -- but you're the one stealing pills and then wondering why you never get pregnant."

This was a low blow and he knew it. Maybe it was because she was too old; maybe it was because he pulled himself out and came on her stomach. Her ovaries were her Achilles' heel and he'd cut at the sinew. Maybe it was time to go. He snapped his laptop shut, pulled out the plug and began to wrap the wire between his elbow and palm.

"Put that shit down!" Candida raged, knocking the laptop on the floor with a crash, the screen probably broken, Kurt's mind under fire and now on fire, like his nerves were in the circuit board, like the 'Net was being taken away, the web site frozen with Milly's tale untold--

"You've gone too far this time," Kurt said, walking toward Candida with murder one on his mind. "You're gonna fucking pay for that--"

"Cheap bastard--"

"Not with money but with this--" Before he thought much about it Kurt had slapped Candida in the face. His palm was open, it was not a punch but a wake-up slap -- he was spinning it in his mind, he was not an abuser, he had never done this before, not ever, the Spanish psycho'd made him do it and now he felt sick.

"*Cobarde!*" Candida screamed, her Spanish roots bubbling out 'round her slurry mascara. "You don't know what it is to be a man!" Kurt was transfixed, he was sick. He would take it back if he could. That it was now time to leave was clear. He picked up the shattered laptop without opening it, could hear the glass of the screen crunching around inside. "This isn't working," he said stupidly, like they would on a sit-com, like this justified the slap, the raising welt on Candida's cheek.

"You think you can just leave? You think you can hit me and then go to the Bronx and try to steal that cheap Mexican whore?"

My plan exactly, Kurt thought in the chaos, minus the cheap and maybe half of the whore. No but that wasn't it, he'd never get Milagros, never even go after her. That wasn't the reason he'd hit Candida's face.

Candida was dialing the phone while Kurt filled his backpack. The rest he could get later, or maybe never. Was she calling the cops? They should give her a blood test. But that'd be no defense. It was a crime, it was taken increasingly seriously, Kurt didn't disagree -- he could think about this for years with horror but for now the Guzmans' basement called.

"I'm sorry," he said as he opened the door. Candida threw another glass, his, and it shattered in the hall. Eyes in the peepholes, a service stairway that smelled of old laundry. The doorman looked at him strangely as he passed. Some shards of glass had cut his chin. Did that make it equal? Even Kurt didn't think so. Rich fucks walked their poodles on West End and Kurt wanted to drop kick them. Testosterone is poison he thought. Blame your balls and not your cowardice. He stood on the narrow platform under Broadway and Ninety Sixth and wiped his chin. When the Two Train came it was cold metal like a spaceship. In the future these perversities will be cured, he thought. No lust no sex no violence. But this was now. He entered The Bronx with the blood on his hands.

27. The Story on Numbers

Tom Bain was an arb. Tom Bain needed to know if the Swanker shit was true, or at least if it had legs. When Nicole's update ran he'd cashed in most of his stake, as had the equity chief downstairs. But where was this going? If Swanker filed charges the stock would take another hit. Bain wanted to arbitrage that shit, surf that wave as well but he needed to know. Lunch with Nicole if she'd do it might be just the ticket. He rolled his roll-on on the pits of his shirt and made the call.

Page One made you high. You were Dow Jones' baby, a brand-name pundit of finance with all that it entailed. Nicole'd had her moment on CNBC; she'd taken a limo at dawn to Secaucus and heard Insana's tripe piped into the aerosol green room. If you weren't rising you were falling. The newsroom was full of one-hit wonders, kept around out of loyalty for re-write work. Loyalty was the buzz word now. The reporter they'd shot on video in Pakistan made them one happy family. "We're all in it together," the rat-faced head man said. Her Arabic roots were of no moment. They trotted her out just to show how open minded they were. Prejudice had no place in a market-based world. If Wacky Kadafi would just privatize the phones he'd win man of the year.

"You're a star," Bain began. "I'm honored you even take my call."

This goofball had a mole quite near Sandy. No lower than Lena Jones. He was worth listening to even though he'd provided nothing since the story on numbers.

"Let's do lunch," he said. "My treat. There's a Yemeni place in the   Village--"

"I prefer Chinese. And it's closer to my office too. One-thirty? Fine. I'll meet you downstairs to save you the security check. If you have documents please bring them."

Bain flexed under this shirt. What documents did the hell he have? He was trying to feel *her* out, or feel her up, both would be best. The meaningless sex of the jet set crowd -- why wasn't it true? Why did the ones who put out always turn out to be climbers like Gina and not the ones who'd arrived?

Pondering this, Bain took the One Train to Canal. He could have charged a livery to the firm but he felt frugal today. Frugal and fragrant. Davidoff Cool Water™ with some add-on musk. What did Nichole want, saffron? She wanted documents. And Bain's sacks were empty.

He'd checked that wacko site WatchCorp dot org. Nothing for the last few days. Maybe Sandy'd shut 'em down and this was just a ghost, a dead site walking, a memorial to entrepreneurial rumor-mongering gone wrong. Gina Sunday's name was on the site, and had been before Nicole had it. So they must know something. Maybe they'd have the skinny on Swanker. Bain had sent 'em an e-mail and got no response. Slow fucks who ignored the rhythm of the Street.

Sixth and Canal is hardly Chinese: class-B office buildings of the plasterer's union and other anachronisms. There was a boutique hotel with the New York *pied a terre* of the songstress of the moment -- the Post called her a "pop tart," zingy and tangy Bain loved that rag. One block north he saw Nicole. As prissy and slutty as always, he hoped, the promise of Casbah in the air, the scent of myrrh and of the S&P 500.

"You look smashing," he said in his best Eddy George -- Boy George, George Michael, mousse with the promise of leather, arb with the echo of freak.

She didn't respond to that. She was a brain not a broad. She was not eye candy like the Money Honey. She was hungry, sure, for the taste of Hunan fire. But lay off the slobbering. It was a decade early for that.

They walked past Church to Lafayette. Here the carps were wide-eyed and fated. Here the vibrancy of the Asian Century made itself known in winter cabbage. Nicole chose the place, full of jurors and sweatshop owners. They ordered by number then got down to business. At least she hoped.

"I saw you went short on Empi," she began.

"How do you know that?" This was a reverse feel-up, and not the kind he liked.

She shook her head. "Sources," she said. "Like you have in Empi. Who was it that told you I'd called them for a quote on Swanker?"

Bain fiddled with his chopsticks and wished for a fortune. "The mother of your children is close at hand," he imagined. He didn't really want them but it was the thing to do, at a certain point. Your legacy and all. She thought he had sources. The bimbo from Odeon and the diner before.

"You know some things, I know others. In my line of work you trade, not give." It sounded trite even to him but it had a certain rhythm. "You go first," he said. "Is Swanker in it to win it or what?"

Why not. "I put in a call but they didn't call back. It's weird, because they usually have a sound byte ready in ten minutes or less." She paused. "If I were a trader -- which I'm not -- I'd bet it's going nowhere."

"Why?"

"Who knows? Some easier pickings came along. Some analyst who forgot to demagnetize his hard drive."

That had been a field day for Swanker: stock touts who told the public to buy while admitting in e-mail that the stock was a dog. It was the paper trail that killed them. A word to the wise. Nothing had changed but Swanker'd declared victory. Even Empi'd tipped its hat to his New Code of Conduct.™ Don't ask don't tell. If it worked for the gay G.I. Joes why not here.

"Your turn," Nicole said quick, her lips pleasantly on fire.

It was the moment of truth, put up or shut up. Put out or be shut out. He'd give up the whore to the virgin and see where it got him. "I have a source in The Bronx."

"At EmpiFinancial?"

"Yeah. I think s--" he stopped himself, perhaps in time -- "the person is leaving. But for now she'd got info. I could put you in touch."

Nicole doubted it would be that simple. This horny fratboy would want to remain the middle man. She'd left her desk for this? "Where do you see Empi's stock price in a month?" she asked. "And this is on the record."

"Not for attribution."

"Fine."

Bain tried to douse the fire with a clump of white rice. I'll suck your chiles, mama -- there should be a song with that line. She was waiting.

"Down twenty percent," Bain said. "And probably another ten or more after that. People thought Sandy Vyle was the perpetual motion machine. With the new focus on numbers his days themselves are numbered." He smiled.

"You should copyright that."

"I already have."

* * *

In the basement Kurt felt sick. He'd slept on the desk, not wanting to bother Milly for a pillow or blanket. He'd gone out early for coffee, three sweet ones from the *cuchifritos* on Tremont near Park. This was a batterers' social club, he felt. The greasy meat in the window said clearly that in this life shit just plain happened. Plantains split open for *carne molida*. Chubette waitresses doting on masons with tattoos. Had Amado ever hit Milly? For some reason he'd like to know. But that wasn't the point. The game was different south of 96th. They fucked you for shit like this and perhaps you deserved it. He had lard bread with garlic and almost threw up.

Now he considered his shattered laptop and sense of self. He was an abuser, and his link to the world had been lost as payback. The internal modem must have felt Candida's pain 'cause it sure wasn't working. He fucked with the wire but no dice. There were terminals connected to the 'Net in some libraries but none of them had his Web

Publishing software. WatchCorp was drifting out of his reach and he still saw the welt, smelt Candida's victimized lunacy with a heavy dose of rum. He'd have to lie low. He was like the Jackal now, a cracker skel on the lam from love and the law. Were there men's rights™ lawyers? If so was Micah one?

* * *

Chuck did Riverside first. He was sick of The Bronx, from Riverdale to Kinkos. This Internet nerd should be easy. A veiled threat under the Cyber-Squatting Act, a well-placed bulge in the pocket, a kick in the groin -- whatever it took. He'd bring the bastard's promise to quit back to Rudehart and leave the bed sister for another day.

He flashed his old badge, fast and out of date, at the doorman and went in. There were armchairs and reading lamps on every landing, as if people'd sit and read their books right here, forgetting the elevator for Farewell My Lovely. He found the apartment, noticed glass shards on the ground. The janitor was down on the job. One cut yuppie and it'd be termination for cause hearing at Local 32 B-J.

He knocked. In the stillness afterwards he listened close and heard a woman cry. Maybe it was the Internet nerd with his voice as high-pitched as his prose. He knocked again, adding this time, "Wheelock. I'm here to see Kurt Wheelock."

There were footsteps. The crying getting closer. "That bastard is gone," a voice slobbered from behind the door. Drunk in the daytime? Some bastards have all the luck.

"I have something for him," Chuck said. He pictured Ed MacMahon, the big cardboard checks in the now-debunked sweepstakes.

"He doesn't live here, I told you." The woman sounded on the edge of losing it. Then she did: "The fucking bastard should be in jail for all I care."

On good days the word did itself. "I could help with that," Chuck said. "C'mon now, open up. Sounds like maybe we got a common enemy."

The woman opened the door. A Spanish lady, not half bad looking. Strung out and with a shiner. "I'm Chuck Stewart," he said, closing the door behind him.

The name Candida didn't like: was she dreaming? The guy was black and fifty at least. Stewart was limp and gay -- the first and only frigid man she'd ever met -- but at least he'd never hit her. Kurt thought he was her father but the bastard would pay.

"You want I should call a doctor?" Chuck asked. The lady didn't need it, ice or a raw steak would do it like in the movies. But they liked to be worried over. Instant intimacy. Baby lemme kiss your booboo and make it go away.

"No," Candida said. "I need a cop if anything."

"He hit you? This Wheelock?"

She nodded.

"Cowardly bastard," Chuck said. He'd done it himself but that's wasn't the point. They liked to hear this, outrage, it emboldened them. I can play Gloria Steinem, Chuck thought. Domestic violence is my business. There was a woman killed every eight seconds. Or was it raped? A shamus for the new century needed statistics. "You really want a cop?"

"They'd lock him up, right?"

"If that's what you want. Sure they'd do it."

Candida thought about it, as much as the pills and the hangover allowed. "I know where he is," she said.

"We tell the cops and that's it."

Now Candida remembered. "You said you had something for him."

Not half dumb either this broad. Chuck assessed the lay of the land, the nipples through the leotard. "It's a lawsuit," was his gambit. "For the freaky things he's been doing on the 'Net." He left it open that way -- let her think child porn, let her think chatroom tryst, whatever she wanted. Maybe the guy was taking boxing lessons for all he knew. He sure needed them. This shiner was strictly bush. Like a girl's slap but in just the right place.

"WatchCorp?"

He nodded. So that was the play. "I'm with EmpiBank -- let's just say I represent some people there. He's infringing on their trademark. Reducing the value of their corporate brand. I'm here to put a stop to it."

"Let's go," she said. "I know where he is."

28. The Muscle

Ernest Swanker looked out the window of his corner office in 120 Broadway, generally in the direction of where the World Trade Towers once stood, and thought about his future. He did not think about patriotism; he did not think about terrorism; he did not think about the delicate balance between civil liberties and national defense. He thought about Joe Basso, the stalking horse EmpiGroup had chosen to use to keep him in line. After his flaccid parking in neutral, Swanker'd come up with a plan as he always did. He'd bring an enforcement action in Rochester, on something Basso could have done but didn't. Leaking underground storage tanks? Public corruption by some about-to-retire city councilman? Maybe even predatory lending, against some company too small to be able to project its power by campaign contributions. He'd let the local and statewide press know that he only stepped in when he saw a break-down in vigilance, a good-old-boy culture that he and only he could shake up, since he was independent due to his family money. If Basso asked to be let in to the prosecution, Swanker would refuse. Maybe he could even indict the bastard. Self-preservation was the law of politics as well as the jungle. Swanker would K.O. Basso right on his bush-league launching pad, show him what happened when the big boys came to town.

He'd show Empi, too, in an abstract way. He'd gotten an e-mail from Rudehart, reminding him gently that he'd want to return the documents he'd collected with his subpoena. Why leave them in government files where they might become public. Rudehart's presumption enraged him. Just for that he'd keep the docs, for now; he'd let them watch as he outfoxed Basso. Let 'em sweat a bit the bastards.

But Empi, of course, could recruit another stalking horse. There was no good way and no good reason to oppose them. He'd crush Basso just to make clear his point: he was no one's sycophant. He might bend over but don't stick it in. He might give in to Empi but it was *his* choice, Goddamn it, not theirs. With that clear, at least in his own mind, he'd probably be able to get hard again. A House seat wasn't so bad. Look what Schmuck Schumer had done with it. One day he'd have his shot at Schmuck and he'd take it. But that day had not arrived.

Swanker hadn't told Carolyn. Sweet not-so innocent Carolyn -- let her enjoy decorating the Georgetown place, let her keep her illusions about her man's incorruptibility while she relished the fruits of his sell-out. If a man can't feel pride in his own fucking house, where could he? Swanker'd be happy to move. That terrace for him was a place now of trauma. He could never go out there again.

* * *

Kurt sat in the half-light typing up Rudehart's offer, adding a sidebar on nannies and taxes. He could type on the laptop though it froze from time to time. But the modem was dead and so he typed in a vacuum, an exposé he had no way to get up on the 'Net. The futility of the whole endeavor was highlighted. He was a nay-sayer only, preening

only for himself. He was a batterer without the authenticity of Jack.
Most of his thoughts he would jot but not these. Sometimes carrying on
was all you could do.

He heard voices at the door -- a woman's voice, "He's in there;" a
deeper voice, "Let me." Then a loud knocking, the door jerking in its
frame. Candida and the cops, he thought. There was a window in the
back but it was covered with bars.

"Come face the music," Candida said through the door. It
flashed through Kurt's mind to deny what he'd done. To rat her out on
drugs, maybe, or to show the broken laptop. It was almost self-defense:
the extension of his brain had been thrown on the floor; he'd flipped out,
he'd lashed out, he was sorry and a first time offender.

"Open the fucking door," the gruff voice said. Kurt thought of
Milly upstairs and the scandal he was bringing. "All right, all right," he
said, opened the door and stepped back.

The man in front of Candida was middle-aged and black -- no
uniform, no cuffs; no Miranda just yet so what the fuck. A vigilante,
then. It occurred to Kurt that this was Candida's father, the one she'd
referred to, her ace in the hole. This was better than arrest. He'd take a
beating or give one. Either way the issue could die right here.

"She'd fucking crazy," Kurt said to the man. "She broke my
computer" -- he pointed at it -- "and I just lost it for a moment." In the
half-light the welt wasn't as bad he he'd feared. "Look, I'm sorry," he
said to Candida. "We should have just known that it wasn't going to
work."

"He's a *punk*," Candida told the man. The man moved slowly
toward him, hand in his pocket, now coming out -- a gun. Mother fuck,
Kurt thought. Perhaps in Peru this was how it was done.

The man pointed the gun and smiled. "You like to hit women?"
he asked. No Spanish accent, Kurt noticed. Perhaps not her father.
Hired muscle, hospital security guard, who knew.

"I never did it before," Kurt said, hearing his voice crack. The
statement was true but didn't sound it.

"You won't never do it again," the man said. The gun was in
Kurt's face, his eyes fixed on it -- then some motion and a spark in his
head, staggering backwards, tripping over a milk carton, a throbbing.
The guy'd punched him with his left, just over his eye. There was blood
on his hand when he pulled it back, a loss of depth perception. A
cackling Candida and still the man with the gun.

"So now it's even," Kurt rasped. Shiner for shiner; an eye for an
eye. This still might end without death or arrest.

"He stole from me," Candida said, egging the gunman on.

Chuck's left fist hurt but he liked the dynamic. The Internet nerd was holding his head; there's no way that he'd complain to the cops. He'd hit a broad and this was just. But he had to make the message clear. "D'ya know who I am?" Chuck asked the kid, not expecting an answer.

"Her father?"

Chuck laughed at this. Great relationship these yuppies had. "No you stupid fuck. I'm here for EmpiGroup. Your little fan-zine Web site don't sit well with them." He stood over the kid, and now kicked him in time with his diction. "You're infringing--" kick -- "their fucking--" kick -- "trademark. You dig? Take the shit down or you'll be seeing this--" gun to temple -- "again. Just one more time."

Kurt's ribs hurt and the garlic was in his throat. It felt like a dream, crazy Candida and an Empi goon. Had Candida been ratting to Empi all along? Somehow this had to be used, corporation as thugs -- but how? Would the guy kill him? He breathed deep and it hurt.

"First Amendment," he said in a whisper, looking back and forth between the gun and the guy's foot.

The guy sneered and kicked out again. Kurt rolled back, still got it in the hip, like an electric shock. If he could make the guy shoot there's be proof. He might also be dead, though. The door opened wider: Milly's silhouette with the afternoon behind.

"*Quienes son esa--*" she began, stopped when she saw the gun.

"*Vienen de Empi,*" Kurt said.

This Chuck didn't like. The Internet punk was effectively gagged -- if he beefed it'd come out that he slapped his girl around. He'd get locked up and Chuck had his ways to make the Empi angle go away. But now there was a witness, lady jabbering in Spanish. Fuck it the messages was delivered. Chuck lowered the gun, moved to stow it away.

Kurt saw this and made his move. He charged low at Chuck, aiming at the knee to snap it back. Chuck kicked but too late. The kid hit his shin and the gun went off. The sound filled the basement, the smell of cordite, the kid behind him, not charging this time, yelling at the Spanish lady, "*Sal te,*" like salty, like salt peanuts, mother fuck this wasn't the way it was supposed to go down. Chuck pocketed the gun and moved toward the now empty doorway. "C'mon," he said to Candida.

"Fucker won't bother you again." Candida stood there until he pulled her out the door.

They got in Chuck's car and didn't speak 'til Fordham Road. "You need to remember what happened," he told her. "The fucker hit you then he lunged for me, before I pulled the gun." He thought. "Don't worry it's licensed." That was one upside. He'd have to ditch the piece and get ready to call the kid a conspiracy theorist if it came to that. "Someone from Empi" is all the kid could say. He didn't have Chuck's name and this Spanish mama wouldn't give it to him either. She was the wronged party, right? He pulled in to park in a bus stop on Jerome under the el train, leaned over and opened the glove compartment. A man's gotta be prepared. He took out the Polaroid and clicked up the flash bulb, heard it hum.

"What the--"

Chuck snapped the picture before the flash was ready. The plastic square spat out the front of the camera; Chuck put it on the dashboard in front of him to dry. "You might want this later," he said. He shifted the car into drive and continued down Fordham. He turned south on the Deegan and wondered if Rudehart had to know that the gun went off.

* * *

Kurt lay in the half-light, smelled the piss in his pants. It hurt to breathe but the bullet had missed him. He had the story of his life but his modem was dead and his hands were hardly clean. There was Milly again coming in through the door.

"*Voy a llamar la policia*," she said.

"*Espera.*" He switched to English. "I need to think what we'll tell them."

"They beat you up. They shot a gun... Who was the woman?"

Kurt didn't answer that. "Did you hear the guy say he was with EmpiGroup?"

"I heard it when *you* told me--"

"But when he said it?"

Milly shook her head and then stopped. "Maybe," she said.

Kurt struggled to his feet, leaning over to reduce the pain in his ribs. "Let's try to find the bullet," he said. The floor board was splintered. Kurt pulled it back. It was dark underneath, just dirt. He dug with his hands.

"*Tiene que estar ahi*," Milly said from behind him. "*Vuelvo.*" She went upstairs while Kurt continued to dig. When she came down she had one of Amado's trowels. Kurt used it, sifting the dirt to the side of the hole.

"Here it is," he said. A slightly mis-shaped slug. Could it be matched to a gun? He didn't know. "I'm going to call Micah," he said. The shyster probably knew ballistics.

* * *

"You're sure he said Empi?"

The kid nodded but Micah did not believe. A bank sending a gunslinger to shoot a little web site down?

"There's another part of it I need to tell you," Kurt said. Milly'd gone upstairs to make coffee; now was the time. "He came with my girlfriend -- my ex-girlfriend. I'd, uh, hit her last night. I don't know why I did it, I never did that before, I was even gonna call you in case she called the cops on me--"

Micah's doubts grew. The kid was paranoid: his girlfriend and Empi ganging up on him. But there was the bullet.

"The more time goes by, the harder it is to call the cops," Micah said.

"The part of hitting Candida, do you think..." The kid's voice trailed off.

Micah nodded. "Yeah it could all come out. But this other part is bigger, if it's true."

"What I can't figure out is why they came together. Was she in touch with them the whole time?"

Milly came in and Kurt shut up. He slurped at his coffee, wincing as he swallowed. "I think the best way," he said, "is if Milly is the one to complain. Empi sent a guy to her house and fired a gun."

Micah turned to Milly. "You saw the whole thing?"

"Jes," Milly said. "Almost all of it. But I have to ask Amado."

"You can forget about the cops then," Micah said.

"There are other ways," said Kurt.

29. Blowing BusinessWeek

Money-makin' Jack was the toast of HomeQuik. His dumpster diving -- he'd taken to calling it document retrieval -- yielded more leads than he had time to follow-up. Ehrenreich brought in loan officers from slower HomeQuik offices in Fort Lee, New Jersey and Elmsford, New York to help cold-call the names on the lists in Jack's goodie-bags.

Jack's Boys, Ehrenreich called them.　　Jack wasn't getting all the commissions he was owed but so what.　　He was making up his arrears to Diane.　　He was still looking for dirt to get leverage on Empi -- literal dirt as the documents were mixed with coffee grounds and used Q-Tips and even some used condoms.　A DNA test might have been interesting, Jack thought, but he had neither the time nor the technology.　Among the docs were Empi's list of prospects.　Monstro had sorted all borrowers by the amount of equity left in their homes and their "remaining income."　Even under Janet's watch the lists were tossed unshredded each night.　"How stupid are these lazy fucks," Jack wondered out loud, waiting in the weeds for the office to close.　He was within five hundred feet of the bitch but so what.　He felt calm, he felt cool; he was chemically emboldened.　He'd gotten a prescription to calm his nerves.　Paxil, they called it, the made-up cure to the made-up affliction of Generalized Anxiety Disorder.　Ehrenreich chewed 'em like peanuts and now so did Jack.　They made him feel like a rapper, swaggering past the wild-haired teen on Olinville.　So too did the stun gun he'd bought used in Hunts Point.　The juice cracked blue between the pincers.　If you're gonna be a terrorist you've gotta have the props, Jack told himself.　The trial would be a slaughterhouse but he might fly the coop just before.　And Have-You-Been-Hurt Micah would defend him.　They needed to meet.

It was Micah who told him of the shoot-out in the Guzmans' basement.

"You think it's true?" Jack asked.

Micah shrugged.　"If it was, Kurt would have called the cops, I think.　Don't get me wrong -- I like the kid, the world needs more people like him.　But he's not stupid, from what I've seen.　Imaginative, maybe. He and Mrs. Guzman say they're going to call reporters.　We'll see."

Jack chewed on this like Paxil placebo.　Everyone was becoming a star but him.　*He* was the one holding the bag for a stupid fax, taking the risk of the dumpsters, making money for HomeQuik and probably for Micah one day -- he was like the village half-wit slut, giving it all up for free while his and Zalie's youths slipped away.　"You think *I* should call reporters?" he asked Micah.

This cracker and the press would not be pretty, Micah thought. The fax case was open and shut, yes or no: did Jack send it?　Micah thought yes.　The terrorism charge was a joke, could even be fodder for Sixty Minutes or in a pinch a cable legal show.　But he should be the one to talk, not Jack.　The poor fuck was only a cipher, the McGuffin caught in Ashcroft's police-state web. "I'd wait on that," Micah said. "It's better for you to lie low. Don't talk to anyone about the fax--"

"I din send it--"

"Just refer any questions to me. We'll go with the whistleblower defense. The more dirt you have on them, the better. Have you got any more?"

If the shyster only knew. "I'm workin' on it," Jack said. Three nights a week in the dumpsters and still the trial drew near. What would it take? Jack chewed a Paxil and considered his options. They were not pretty so he chewed another.

* * *

Amado said, "Fine, let's call that reporter. They come to my house, fire a gun at my wife--"

"I was in the doorway," Milly cut in.

"Fire a gun while my wife is here, who do they think they are, they're gonna scare *me*, buncha gangsters, *pistoleros*. Yeah call her and tell her."

"Milagros should be the one to complain," Kurt said without explaining. Candida might have deserved it but he still wasn't proud.

"*De acuerdo?*" Amado asked Milly. She nodded. Kurt dialed and handed the phone to her.

To Nicole it was fishy, that Empigroup would send a hit man to The Bronx. The downside for them was so big it was almost their defense.

"You're sure that's what he said? That he came from Empigroup?"

"Jes," Milagros said.

"And what did he want you to do?"

Milly looked at Kurt. They were using the speaker phone so Kurt and Amado were hearing everything.

Kurt wrote on his pad, "To lay off them," showed it to Milly.

"He say to lay off them."

"Like, not to file a lawsuit?"

"I guess," Milly said. "That must be it."

"But why did he shoot the gun?"

Milly looked at Kurt again. Their story was breaking down; there'd be no story in the Journal. Just a dead web site, Kurt thought. He cleared his throat.

"Uh, Nicole? It's me Kurt Wheelock. I'm here with Milagros. I was here when the Empi guy came too."

This doesn't add up, Nicole thought. Kurt was like the Guzmans' agent, their handler, telling them what to say. Maybe he'd told them to say there were shot at. She wanted Page One but this could be a set-up. "Why do you think they came?" Nicole asked flatly. "Did he mention a lawsuit or didn't he?"

"No," Kurt said. Half of the truth wouldn't hurt. "The guy told me to stop the web site. He was talking about trademarks while he kicked me in the ribs."

Martyr complex, Nicole thought. "Why didn't you call the police?"

It was a good questions to which there was no answer. Kurt bobbed and wove. "Even if the cops got him, Empigroup would denied he works for them. We thought that you could nail it down. I mean, just call Empigroup and ask."

"I need more than this," Nicole said. "I never call them until I have all my facts straight. What'd the guy look this?"

Kurt closed his eyes, tried to think of a better description than "black." "He was around fifty years old, his hair half-gray. African-American guy. Friendly-looking until he took his gun out. We still have the bullet. Maybe that'll help you."

Nicole'd been on the crime beat one summer, using a police scanner and using the words "accused" and "alleged" more than she'd liked. "It's better than nothing," she said. "Can you bring it down to me?"

"Yeah," Kurt said. When he'd fled Manhattan on the Two after slapping Candida, he'd thought he'd never go back. But now she'd come to The Bronx, with her EmpiGroup thug. "I'll bring it down now. You should call them though and ask."

Thanks for telling me how to do my job, Nicole thought. She hung up.

* * *

Chuck was fucked. He should have done the bed bitch first; that might have been enough for Rudehart. He shouldn't have brought his piece to The Bronx, or should have unloaded it. The Internet yuppie was a punk. He wouldn't have fought anyway. Now there was the chance they'd complain. He'd been using legit bullets, bought for him by Empigroup. The gun was registered in his name. He shoulda gone indirect and paid someone else to do it. And the picture came out too dark: you could barely make out a shiner 'round the girl's left eye. The delay for the flashbulb was bullshit.

To tell Rudehart or not: there still wasn't any easy answer. It would just give them time to scapegoat him -- they'd never told him, they'd never implied, blah, blah, blah -- anyway the web site fuck might not complain. Chuck could take sick time but that wouldn't look right either. They'd wanted some background on a guy they'd fired. He could pursue that and lie low. He'd like to go back and get the bullet but that'd just be another chance to get fucked. Skip-trace on Bender should be just the ticket.

* * *

Nicole was surprised at the slug. If this was a set-up Kurt had pulled out the stops. "I'll take it to a guy I know," she said.

"Have you called Empi yet?"

"No. But I guess I will."

Lena Jones had just finished blowing a BusinessWeek reporter about Sandy's most recent purchase of a hospital's research wing to conquer Death™ (his own). The questions were easy, the story would be positive, "Wall Street's New Social Conscience," hence it was a blowjob -- when Nicole Nour called. "I was just about to leave," Lena said. "Unless it's for tomorrow's paper."

It was an anachronism, this view of deadlines. What with Web exclusives, and the Journal's Asian and European editions, there was no single deadline anymore. Nicole wanted an answer so she pushed forward.

"I got a weird call today--"

"You're not the only one--"

"--and I just wanted to give you a chance to respond. The borrowers I wrote about, the Guzmans, they say a guy went to their house saying he was from Empi."

Lena sat back down in their hydraulic chair. Could those idiots have gone out again pitching a new loan, pointing out the need for aluminum siding -- was it a door-to-door insurance sale, offering a Financial Check-Up™ then some moldy mutual funds with high fees? "It's a big company," Lena said. "If anyone went it was totally unrelated--"

"They say the guy had a gun."

Lena make a coughing sound -- neither a laugh or a scoff, a loff perhaps. "That's preposterous," she said. "You're joking, right?"

"No. I was skeptical at first -- " she still was, but the point here was to scare Lena into actually asking around about this --"but they've shown me the bullet. I'm going to check it with a ballistics guy a know. I just wanted to give you a chance to look into it, a straight 'no comment' would give the story legs, as I'm sure you know."

How the hell was she supposed to look into *this*, Lena wondered -- send an e-mail to Empi's Department of Defense? She'd have to call Rudehart, she knew. She'd play it off that she was just covering all her bases. "Your sources are lying," Lena said. "I'm surprised you're even looking into this."

"I'm the one holding a bullet," Nicole said. "Call me with a comment as soon as you can."

"You're *writing* this story?" Lena demanded.

"We might." The plural tense was always better. Let them know that the combined weight of all of Dow Jones' units, its media reach in every time zone in the world and on hand-held devices from BlackBerry to Palm might soon be coursing with accusations. "Do you have my cell number?" She gave it, as well as a second-hand version of Kurt's description of the shooter.

Fuck, Lena thought. As if accounting scandals weren't enough.

* * *

Rudehart was re-reading a speech he gave at a World Bank meeting when Lena Jones' call came through. "I'm sorry Bob," she began. "I got crazy call from that Nour chick but I have to check it." Did he remember the Guzmans -- of course he did; had anyone been sent to shoot at them with a gun -- what the fuck?

"They live in a war zone," Rudehart said. "Why they'd think it was us--"

"They say that's how the guy identified himself. They say it was a fifty-something black man and that's what he said."

Rudehart scoffed, nothing funny about it -- he thought of Chuck. But Chuck'd been sent, if anywhere, to Riverside Drive and to Bertha Watkins' in The Bronx. "You're sure it's the Guzmans?"

"Yeah," Lena said, thinking what a weird question that was, as if sure Empi was shooting up the Bronx, everywhere except in the Guzmans' 'hood.

"Tell her she's crazy," Rudehart said. "And give me the number of her editor again. I'm going to keep them from making fools of themselves."

Lena opened her Dow Jones file, work home and cell of each reporter and editor.

Rudehart wondered who to call first: Chuck or the Journal? He didn't need facts to throw his weight around. And if Chuck had actually done it -- nothing was impossible, he'd learned that in the peso bail-out and the Asian meltdown -- he didn't want to know, at least not before he called the Journal. Maybe Sandy had a side deal with Chuck. They'd never done this at Treasury. But he hadn't been paid so well, either.

* * *

It was past ten o'clock when Nicole got the word: no more work on this story until she heard from her editor. He was out in the Hamptons and shouldn't be called. She still had the slug, and the tape she'd made of Kurt's account. She listened again, then idly surfed to WatchCorp dot org. They'd stopped updating the thing. If they wouldn't report it why should she? She called for a livery car and left the slug in the mug full of pens on her desk. As she walked through the canyon of cubicles for a moment she was scared. Then it passed.

30. Shyster in a Tight Blue Suit / Hampton Daze

Duwon was skipping another day of summer school -- the air conditioned was broken, he said, the only kids who went in where those too poor to eat at home, they went for the free breakfast and lunch, jamming packets of ketchup in their pockets like losers. Bertha refused to keep her kids cooped up this fine June day. "We'll go to the pool," she announced, turning off the TV and Duwon's wrestling video game with it. "We'll stop at Micah's office first, though. I need to ask him something."

"Like when he gonna take us to a Yankee game," Duwon said.

"You're too greedy," said Bertha. She wanted to ask whatever happened with that big shot downtown. She was paying the insurance but soon she'd have to buy new clothes: the girls were growing, their capris were tight and flip-flops were okay for June but not for school.

Micah saw the four of them out his window, carrying a bag from the Dunkin Donuts down the street. He wanted to have an answer for Bertha, especially if he'd have to perform in front of her kids. "Tell 'em I'll just be a minute," he said into his intercom. Then he dialed Swanker's office. "It's important," he said.

Swanker came on but his tone was weird. "You gotta go it alone this time," Swanker said.

"You're getting soft."

"Other fish to fry. There's a lender up in Rochester we've been getting a lot of complaints about. We're going to close them down, lock stock and barrel." Swanker paused. "Maybe you want a piece of that action?"

I might, Micah thought. But what about the great white whale? "Why go after pip-squeaks?" he asked. "You make a name taking down lions, not rats."

"I'm a *statewide* official," Swanker said pompously.

"Emi's statewide. Hell, it's worldwide."

"It's on hold for now, what can I tell you. Look, I gotta go." Swanker hung up.

Pompous fuck, Micah thought. Swanker had the cracker's tape if he wanted it; he had whatever he'd gotten with his subpoena. Some fleabag in Rochester? Swanker was shooting too low. And Bertha and her kids were waiting. Micah smoothed down his hair, shot some aerosol CleanBreath into the back of his throat. "Send them in," he told his secretary.

"Staying cool, I see," Micah said. The girls were in bathing suits; Bertha probably had one on, under that loose-fitting African print dress. Maybe it was time to play hooky. He punched Duwon softly on the shoulder and the kid pulled back.

"We're goin' to Crotona pool," Duwon said. "If you wanna come. The Yanks are in town this week too."

"Yeah I've been meaning--"

"Du-*won!*" Bertha said. Then to Micah: "I don't wanna keep you, I just thought I'd come and ask about that guy we met downtown--

"Swanker. I just called him. It's going slower than I'd thought it would. Actually, we might just do it the way I'd planned, just sue them ourselves. I'd meant to call--"

"Don't worry," Bertha said. Micah would complain about clients, how some of them couldn't wipe their asses without calling their lawyer, and she wondered if he meant her too. "I need the insurance knocked off by July, August at latest. School supplies and whatnot."

"We'll get more than the insurance knocked off," Micah said. "We'll sue for damages, we'll use that tape--"

"If you're gonna sue, maybe I'll stop payin' right now," Bertha cut in.

Micah shrugged. That could bring things to a head: *maybe* they'd file a case to repossess the bed, or collect on the debt; he'd bring up the defense of fraud and turn it into a class action that way. If they didn't repo it would just prove his point that the insurance was useless, of no benefit to the borrower. "Sure," he said. "Just be sure to put some of the money into escrow."

"Like put it to the side?"

"Yeah."

"Du-*won!*" Bertha shouted it again, because Duwon was looking through the framed photographs on Micah's bookshelf, had picked one of them up, Micah with the Yankees' owner, she recognized him from TV, dumpy looking white man with a whole buncha money.

"It's okay," Micah said.

"You know any a the players?" Duwon asked.

Micah nodded, lying. If he'd been smart enough to take Sports and Entertainment Law he'd be raking it in now. The money they paid for a mop-up reliever, for a backup catcher, was more than he'd won for a client, ever. "Why don't I drive you to the pool?" he said. "So you don't have to take the bus."

"We're fine," Bertha said. But she liked the offer, Micah's smooth ride. "Do you have a bathing suit here?"

"No," Micah said. To be the only white man in the Crotona Park pool, he didn't relish the thought anyway. He'd drop them at the gate, set a dinner date with Bertha alone. At some point he'd have to tell her he was taking the cracker's case, at least part of it. The terrorism part. He wondered if she got CourtTV. She should know what a big man he was, at least in that way.

* * *

Chuck drove the Bronx River Parkway with a bag full of dirt. This Bender was no big shot but like a slug he'd left a trail of slime behind him. The prostitution rap they already had, and the fax trial upcoming. But Chuck dug some trash up from Charlotte, had the number of the ex-wife, feelers out to previous colleagues all the way back to college. The poor fuck wouldn't know what hit him. Chuck would pass the shit on to Rudehart and hope for the best.

"In person," Rudehart'd said, when he tried to speak by phone. Normally he'd be the one driving Rudehart up here. But not today. It was a bad sign, like he was gonna get fired, demoted, scapegoated. He shoulda taped the bastards when they told him to go to Riverside Drive. Maybe they'd get him a lawyer. If that was needed.

Rudehart in Armonk was all business -- no whirlpool baths, no Sandy in sight. "It was you, I take it," he began.

Chuck didn't want to lie -- "insult my intelligence," as Rudehart often put it -- so he just stayed quiet.

"The bullets in the Bronx that was you, right?"

"Bul*let*," Chuck corrects. "The guy lunged at me and the thing went off."

"Real smooth," Rudehart said. He still hadn't told Sandy. And now he wouldn't have to. "You almost got us fucked," he told Chuck. "They called the Wall Street Journal, they gave them the bullet." Chuck shook his head. "But I called their editor, it's not gonna run. Close call. Why'd you go to that house in The Bronx, anyway?"

Chuck explained how one thing led to another, the dirt on Kurt, the brown Latin hottie with black and blue eye. This, Rudehart liked. "You took a picture?" he asked.

Chuck handed the copy he'd made to Rudehart. He'd paid for a color photocopy but it still looked dark. "It's a little blurry--"

"A little? What happened -- you didn't have a flashbulb?"

"It didn't go off." Photography wasn't Chuck's specialty.

"Well go take a better one," Rudehart said. "And be sure to use a flash, maybe some klieg lights."

"It might have gone down by now."

"Just get it."

Chuck thought. "The lady with the bed, you still want me--"

"Are you fucking kidding? We don't need anymore Keystone Kops routines. If they sue us on the bed we'll just fight it."

Chuck didn't like getting dressed down. Scraping and bending for this waif-like Massa. "I got some more on that Bender guy," he said.

Rudehart took the sack of documents. "We need to speed his trial up," he said. "Sandy doesn't like stuff like this hanging around."

"We can tell the D.A.--"

"Don't worry, *I'*ll handle it."

Chuck didn't like the tone. He winced and asked, "You need a ride back to the city?"

"I've got my own car," Rudehart said. With another driver, the subtext was. "Just get the photograph and don't fuck up again."

* * *

It was nice that the rich spent whole weeks of the summer in the Hamptons. Nicole'd spent the last 4th of July out there, sleeping on the couch of a house rented by a girlfriend from the American University in Cairo. The driveway was full of a six pack of leased luxury cars; yuppies fueled by hormones and passion fruit martinis trysted in the rooms upstairs. Strange that there was no luxury brands of condoms, no way to maintain class differences even in latex. "Ribbed for your pleasure" -- that's what a drunk day trader had whispered to her, sitting across from her couch on a bamboo beach chair while she tried to sleep. In the workplace you could file a complaint. But not in a summer-share. She told him she was a lesbian, to drive him away. But he said he didn't mind that, that he kinda liked it, actually. So she told him she had AIDS. He expressed concern then trod up the rugged stairs to continue his hunt up there. In the morning she took the air-conditioned jitney back to Grand Central, thinking on the LIE that her parents had perhaps not been wrong to be so protective. She hadn't called that girlfriend since. They were moving in different directions. One day that wench's lips would be covered with herpes sores, and Nicole would be a managing editor. That day was not yet.

Since her Hamptonite editor wouldn't be calling, not today not this week and probably never, with any green light for the Empi goon story, Nicole used the day to look into another angle. Bain's shorting Empi's stock just before she'd run her update on Swanker had grabbed her attention. People did it all the time, surfing the spread on inside information. But the topic was hot, Page One material if you could get the right bad guy. Bain was a nobody, a Section C cipher if that. But he must have passed the recommendation on, no? If the pressure rose on him he'd flip. There was a way to massage the story, to manufacture one simply by calling for quotes. First she'd call Swanker, then the SEC to ask -- just ask -- if they were looking into abnormal shorting activity at Bain's firm. They'd say no comment but they'd get right on it. Then she'd offer Bain a way out, an opportunity to explain why he'd done what he did. Bain bore some resemblance to the ribbed-for-your-pleasure guy from the Hamptons last summer. She could use that saved emotion to set the ball in motion.

* * *

It should have been easy for Swanker to back down -- he'd done it before -- but this time it wasn't. Maybe it was that the threat this time was delivered by a man he wanted to be. Respect wasn't the right word for what he felt for Rudehart. Envy, perhaps. A desire to go further. At least to equal. The smile on Rudehart's face when he said, *call and let us know you've decided to do the right thing* still haunted him. Carolyn didn't care; there was no way to talk to her. There was only his father, slumlord-*cum*-Machiavelli. What father would sell his own son out? And so Swanker dialed, his father's real estate LLP in Great Neck, where the phone lines were scrambled and the ends justified any means. The rumors of arson were a thing of the past. Now Swanker *père* financed other slumlords, all guaranteed by Freddie Mac and eligible for write-off under the Internal Revenue Code. Ernie Senior would understand. He always did.

"Take the House seat," the old man said. "There's nothing to be gained from fighting these people. You got some leverage now, take it. He who's not moving is dead."

Swanker *fils* vaguely remembered a song -- "if you're not busy being born" -- was that his father's reference? "It's the Senate I want."

"The time will come. For now you go to Washington, do a press conference every Sunday when there's nothing else going on. Carolyn and the kids will like it. I still don't understand why you put them in school in The Bronx."

"It's a *private* school, Dad. Rich kids from Manhattan take a bus up everyday." His father didn't understand that Horace Mann School was in The Bronx but not of it. Neither did Carolyn. But a populist like him needed to be able to say, when the topic was education reform, that his kids went to school in The Bronx. The reporters ate it up too.

"You'll make more connection in DC anyway," his father continued. "Have you thought about committees?"

Financial Services and Appropriations. "No," Swanker said. It was good to have a father even more vicious than you. He felt clean in comparison. No gasoline, just a silent back-down that no one would know about. "Thanks Dad," he said. He felt better already.

31. To the Red Room / Organized Crime

Gina contemplated her Franklin Cubby Planner just like they'd taught in the SoulTime™ class. A list of tasks -- not to be mistaken for her mission -- each ranked by delayability and relation to her ValuesStatement.™ She'd paid four hundred bucks of her own money; she felt better already. Who knew that Mister Nine Effective Habits had dictated a whole System for Life from his mountain in Provo? Orin Cubby was a new Messiah, unlocking the LifeTactics™ in each world religion. Her trainer had boiled it down to a PowerPoint slide, a single injunction: "To get where you want to go, recognize the power you have to make it so." Gina closed her eyes and felt her power. There were things she couldn't change but there were some that she could.

"I think we're out of coffee," Vinny called from the bedroom. Now *there* was an anchor, a weight that weighed her down. Cubby's third book, all in the package for four hundred dollars, applied the Nine

Habits to the realm of family life. She and Vinny weren't a family --
thank God -- but even for couples Cubby suggested a joint mission
statement. It was a test of the relationship, Cubby wrote -- you wouldn't
merge with a company without checking the books, would you? She'd
asked Vinny and he'd laughed. "You're gettin' too corporate," he said.
"Leave that shit in the mall."

But the shit she was preparing to leave was Vinny -- the mall as
well, perhaps. Habits, Cubby wrote, were all made in three weeks. On
day fifteen she'd seen the light: she could take the Series Seven herself,
not wait for Empi's empty promises, for Janet to give her back what was
hers, for a lateral transfer to Empi's Primusica unit, which pitched mutual
funds door-to-door to sleep-deprived suburbanites. She could study for
the Seven and take it herself. She'd surfed the NASD, there was only one
problem. You could only even *take* the test if sponsored by a registered
broker-dealer. Cubby said be proactive but this was a wall. It was a test,
like Jesus in the desert or that last night with the cup. Gina clung to her
power and ignored Vinny's suggestion that she walk out to C-Town for
another can of coffee. Let him get it, the lazy bastard. She was Quadrant
IV, a Cubby realm to which only the few were called and even fewer
arrived.

"You're still with that bullshit?" Vinny asked, walking into the
kitchen naked again, some disco boy-toy two decades too late, a man
without a mission, a man without values -- a man without a plan or a
Planner. "You're like a junkie to that book." He picked it up.

The Planner was covered in burgundy vinyl; its seven-ring
binder held Lessons for Life™ on cross-referenced pages of pastel green.
Cubby's partner said it'd all been based on that Father of Our Country
Ben Franklin, who carried a book of virtues with him along with a kite.
Frugality, Moderation and Temperance -- the last of these was hardest,
but Gina's been thirteen days without cocaine and saw the three-week
threshold in sight. Twenty one days and the habit would be gone,
replaced by ambition sharpened like tempered steel, even Clinton has
pitched it, flashing his Planner just like this one in the Rose Garden.
Now that Gina'd been initiated she saw her colleagues everywhere, using
their Planners like purses, like Bible briefcases, jotting their dreams and
their hopes and their tasks.

"Give it *back*!" she demanded. Vinny held it behind his back.

"We need coffee," he said.

"Why didn't you buy it yesterday?"

"I din know we was out."

Gina glared at him. He felt her Power and put the Planner back on the chair. "I'm just sayin'," he said. But when the soul is in darkness the mouth is full of trash.

"I'm leaving," Gina said.

"We got any tea bags?"

The man was blind.

* * *

Bain was playing DeathMarch™ when the equities chief came in. "There's some shit," the guy announced. "I can't talk to you but you're gonna get a memo."

"What shit?" Bain asked, pushing pause, scanning his Bloomberg for news of an attack, an Osama Bin Loathing sighting, anything that'd move the markets. The guy couldn't talk to him? After he'd given him the heads-up on the Swanker news, and profits to make up for the losses of the three weeks before?

"SEC letter," the guy said. "About the trades."

Oh fuck, Bain thought. Now he was glad that he'd spread the information. If he went down, they went down. Anyway the Bush II SEC wouldn't do shit.

"Thanks for the heads up," Bain said. "One hand washes the other." But the guy was gone. Tom Bain was washing his hands all alone, it appeared.

* * *

The swelling was down and the floozy hard to get. Chuck was in the hallway, speaking through a crack in the door, a chain between them. He had a fold-up lighting system in his bag.

"If he did it once he'll do it again," Chuck said. "I know the type."

Candida doubted it. But forgiveness wasn't her thing. But she hadn't asked the guy to fire a gun. He'd kicked Kurt in the stomach and that was fine and good. Her father deserved it too, maybe more so. But now they wanted to use her -- asking for a photo of her face when it looked almost normal again.

"What about the picture you took?" Candida asked. Chuck didn't answer. He'd made more copies but the flaws of the original could not be cured.

"I thought you were going to sue him," Candida said.

Fat chance, Chuck thought. Trademark law wasn't his thing but that hadn't been the point. He wanted a better photo not only for Empi, but to cover his own ass as well. This Candida Rivera could corroborate the gunshot. "I did what you told me," Chuck said.

"Not the gun part," Candida said.

"What gun part?" said Chuck. The neighbors might hear. It was time to go. He wouldn't fuck up on this Bender campaign. You want something done right get someone else to do it.

* * *

Nicole was waiting for Bain's call back, or the long-shot green-light from the Hamptons, when the call came through. It was the martyr with the dormant web site, asking about the gunshot story.

"They deny it," Nicole said.

"But you have the bullet."

"I have a bullet. That could be from anywhere."

"Did you have the ballistics run?"

She hadn't. She'd gotten the stop order and obeyed. "Look, I'm working on something else right now," she said. "If I need any more from you I'll call."

Kurt felt the blow-off. He was a batterer, okay. He'd done it once. But now he felt wronged. "There's a lot more to this story--"

"What happened to your web site, anyway? I mean, you haven't reported this. So I ask myself, why should I?"

"Uh, my computer is broken."

Typical. "Cheers," Nicole said before she hung up.

Kurt should apologize to Candida, or try to. So she'd spied for Empigroup -- she was a wacko Latino in the sway of corporations. No way he'd get back together with her. But it'd be better to set things right, plead for forgiveness and get it rather than have that loose cannon out there with a shiner and a heat-packing muscleman from Empi. He'd do it in person, without notice. Before the cops could come he'd have said his piece and slipped into Riverside Park. If she'd loved him once there must be something left. He could use it for closure or at least to make sure that he wouldn't be charged. He bought flowers on Tremont and jumped on the D.

Yuppies pranced on unconcerned down Broadway, buying fish on ice and leather luggage, preparing for vacations North or far South, Kurt imagined: Nova Scotia, Cape Town or Buenos Aires. Was it Candida he'd hit or a whole way of life? That was a cheesy way to think, he knew -- at a minimum he'd better not say it out loud to Candida. He needed a theory, some mitigating factor. Was he beaten as a child? Not really. Had he watched his mother smacked black and blue in front of his green eyes? Only once, and a closet door took most of the damage. Could he say he was drunk, or high, that he'd eaten too many Twinkies or had an adverse reaction to some anti-depressant he'd found in Candida's closet? That would be blaming the victim -- it might work; Kurt would play it by ear.

The doorman was distracted -- hauling a shipping trunk rolling on wheels for a GQ family decked out in Ralph Lauren -- so Kurt slipped through, up the stairs to Candida's floor, knocking lightly on her door.

"I told you -- no!"

Had she told him? She'd told him he was a racist Jesus. Lord take this cup away from me. "It's me," he said, standing in front of the peephole as pacifistic as he could. "I've been feeling so sorry, I just needed to talk to you." He sounded contrite, even to himself. The pause made him think she was calling the cops. Then the door opened, a fourth of the way, still held by the chain.

"You're a bastard," she said. "You think you're different but you're the lowest kind of man, a coward."

"Look, I never did it before, I don't know what got into me" -- your drugs, Kurt thought, wondering if he'd play that card -- "just let me in, I won't come near you, I just want to talk, I'm sorry, I'm so sorry." He held the bouquet of flowers up, felt the cliché, that he'd hit her again -- but he wouldn't. This was the exit interview; if it wouldn't be so crass he might even ask for a letter of reference. "He gave good sex or at least I pretended," she'd write. "You'd be lucky to have him."

"They should have buzzed me," Candida said. "I told the doorman not to let you upstairs."

"He was busy. Some yuppies paying him a buck to carry this huge trunk--"

"There you go again. Why is it that you think that everyone who lives here is corrupt?" She paused. "When *you*'re the one who beats women."

Keep your voice down, Kurt thought. That is not my self-image. "Just let me in for a second. Or we could go out to Broadway, get a coffee or something. Whatever. I just want to talk."

"Yeah, I don't want you in here," Candida said. Whew, Kurt thought. This might be for the best, unless she screamed in a restaurant that he was a punk. Maybe the park. She left the door open on its chain while she went in the bedroom. There was a phone in there and so maybe-- Kurt looked back down the hall. They had better things to do, the cops did. He wouldn't get trapped here for more than ten minutes. In the apartment he could get arrested. This was definitely better, hitting the streets to talk about why he hit her. He didn't have an answer but one might come to him.

Candida came out with absurd black sunglasses, a new set of sneakers and a pink velvet running suit. Like a tropical drink Kurt thought then scolded himself. He felt guilt but not really toward her. Generalized guilt, the kind you'd confess in a church if you were the kind who went there. Kurt wasn't, but he had a personal relationship with undirected guilt. "Put these in water," he said before Candida closed the door. She smiled -- almost smiled -- and went in the kitchen. The chain was off now but Kurt stayed in the hall. It could all be a set-up, he remembered. Sweet-talking with a deadly weapon.

Candida came toward the door with a clear glass vase, the flowers bunching up, the finest fruit of East Tremont vendors' shopping carts. The flower wholesalers made a good living on guilt. Mother's Day too, perhaps, but how was that different? Candida locked the door behind her and pushed the elevator button.

"Where do you want to go?" Kurt asked, his park-plan ready.

"No place they know me," Candida said. "I don't want them to see me like this."

Yeah those sunglasses make you look like an idiot, Kurt thought. His thoughts were cruel but it was just a sublimation. Guilt into put-down: this was the fuel that kept some marriages going for half a century. "We can walk in the park," he said. "It's nice out."

They crossed the speedway that is Riverside Drive, then turned the path lined with benches toward the south, the Hudson steaming down a cliff, the whiz of the cars on the West Side Drive, joggers and dog-walkers and a hundred contemptible people.

"Don't even *try* to justify this," Candida said on 88th.

"I can't," Kurt said. Disarming like. "I've been sick with myself since it happened." That was almost true. That garlic bread, the coffees too creamy, the kick in the ribs from the EmpiBank goon. Which reminded him. "Did you know the guy had a gun?" Turn the tables, baby: I slapped with an open hand, and you brought a gunman.

Candida didn't answer right away. Let him think what he wanted. Why was she even walking here? To hear what he had to say. To tell him something, maybe. But why?

"Look, I'm sorry," Kurt said. "I've always hated men who did that, I watched my father do it and I told myself, never, not me -- but something snapped, when I saw my laptop on the ground, the next thing I knew--"

"You're a fucking materialist," Candida said. Kurt let it go.

"It's a bad dynamic we got into, I should have noticed something, tried to make things different."

"You don't pay attention. I kept telling you that you were getting too wrapped up in that Jackal, in those stupid documents, that guy in The Bronx..." Candida's voice trailed off. She could see him, that Amado-like-her-father, in the basement she returned to with a gun, the wrong basement -- maybe it was time. "Let's go down here," she said, pointing to a path leading to the docks where people moored their houseboats. It was a quiet place, Rudy Giuliani had cleaned the homeless out and Bloomberg kept them swept; it was a place to confess, to say this thing and make Kurt see, for no reason anymore, no reason but truth, no reason but guilt, no reason but the upper hand.

They stood on the dock. The river smelled of PCBs and turds. Two men were fishing and Kurt wondered if they ate it. There were disclaimers everywhere; caveat emptor.

"We can never get back together," Candida said. Kurt nodded -- oh yes he nodded -- he put his arm around her. "I can never accept that," she said. "It'd be like suicide for me, or I'd end up killing you." Kurt lessened his pressure -- he'd like to take his arm away in fact. He could see her doing it, too. Riled up on a cocktail of conscience-suppressors from Metropolitan, sputtering purple-lipped with the sharp serrated knife she used for bagels. "There's a lot I haven't told you," she said. Kurt lit a smoke, gestured that they thought sit on the edge of the dock, the Dock of the Bay, that great song he'd rather be listening to than be here. There was a lifetime for music but only now to atone.

"When I lived with my father, in the basement in Queens -- remember?"

Kurt nodded. He thought they might be going there. The way she screamed *papi*, it curdled his blood and made his scrotum clench. It couldn't be by accident. There was something there.

"He used to drink, with these guys on the block -- they'd play dominoes, fight about women, wear those big white hats--" Kurt could almost see them, sitting on milk crates, their tall cans of Bud and sleeveless t-shirts, could see where this was going, nights maddened by the heat and boiler -- "he used to come in drunk. I'd be awake but keep my eyes closed. He'd stand over me."

Kurt was getting the willies. "How old were you?" he asked.

"It started when I was twelve," she said.

To Kurt that was too much. His anger now was genuine. "I'm so sorry," he said. But Candida was just getting going.

"He'd try to kiss me but I'd turn away. He'd say he missed my mother, he was alone in this country, that daughters sometimes took the mother's place." Candida's eyes were wet and far away; Kurt hugged her again, the stench of the river forgotten, the relation to his guilt less so. Had he played into this? Had he kicked her when she'd already been down, then worried only about himself? He had.

"I'm so sorry," he said again, again misplaced but less free-floating now. His debt was to her, and he'd miscalculated how much he owed. Was this why she lived so numb on Riverside Drive? Why she married a blatant fruit and still kept his clothes in her closet, played Channel 13 to erase the memory?

"It was never in the bed," Candida said. "He take me to the boiler, said he had to fix it and I had to come, said he'd show me about pressure, that I had to keep the door open because the fire bar was on the wrong way." Kurt tried to picture it, couldn't. For a moment it struck him like a Penthouse letter, some panting tale of "you'll never guess what happened." But this was incest, this was rape; this was pedophilia, the real deal that could fuck you up for life, *had* fucked up Candida - and he'd hit her.

"He'd block the door with a bucket of sand. The walls were painted red, I'll never forget them. The pipes on the ceiling were leaking. It smelled like oil. He'd take me behind the boiler, pretend to show me the valves and how they worked."

Stop, Kurt wanted to say. Stop I can picture it now.

"He'd lean me over, he'd raise up my dress. The first time I swear to God I screamed and I shouted, I don't know how the other tenants didn't hear. After that he put his hand over my mouth, even greased it up sometimes... He'd move slow, whispering about my mother, calling me *mami*, his little *mamita*, saying I couldn't tell anyone, it was a secret just of him and me--"

"He still lives there?" Kurt had never asked.

Candida nodded. "As if nothing ever happened. He even wanted to come to Stewart's and my wedding. That fucking bastard. I should have called the cops on him."

Why didn't you, Kurt thought. It wasn't a question to ask. His slap was now both less important and worse. His thoughts about ass fucking now made him feel sick. Which hole, he wondered. As if one would be better than the other. But still: which one?

"Tell me where he lives," Kurt said full of disgust. He wasn't a vigilante; he was, as Candida said, essentially a coward. But he wanted to see for whatever reason. If the room was still red, this fire door business. The valves, the whole nightmare. If it all came together perhaps he'd lash out to atone for hitting her. He was dog, he thought, but not yet old. He could learn new tricks.

"I don't know why I'm telling you this," Candida said. And she didn't.

"Just tell me." She did.

Kurt took the F to Jackson Heights, the streets all numbered by Junction Boulevard. It was a five-story building like any other, better than the buildings in The Bronx. The front door was locked but the intercoms worked. Kurt pushed buttons until the buzzer buzzed and the door opened.

He went down the stairs, no plan in his mind, drawn to this red hot room -- impossible that it would be the same but here it was, waist-high a fire bar, inside a bucket of sand and an ancient boiler with gauges like insects' eyes. He almost forgot and let the door close behind him -- he caught it before the thing clicked shut. Now he saw what Candida meant: from inside the room there was no way out. The fire door was required by law, but the handle, the bar you pushed to open it, was supposed to be inside. It swung the wrong way, the hinges reversed, slipshod basement construction of Jackson Heights. Probably the inspectors were paid off. Kurt blocked the door with the bucket of sand, went around to check the gauges. He knew something of boilers, having maintained FOCO's rotting heating plant in Flatbush. He'd gotten the license, a free class at Brooklyn Tech where they taught which kind of pollution was legal. No more than two blasts of black smoke a day. These gauges were old -- Kurt held on to them leaning forward, atoning in imagination, surprised and embarrassed by his own posture, sick with the smell of oil and sick with himself. Each day, he'd been told, provided a chance to begin anew. You could cleanse your past with an act and move on. When he went back upstairs he bought a roll of antacids and chewed them compulsively to a sweet white paste.

32. Orzata / The Haitian Campers

Micah got the note of issue -- Jack's trial date had been set and the district attorney wanted the whole thing sealed, no press or speaking out of court, citing the request to the PATRIOT Act. Micah looked it up and there it was: any indictment including allegations of terror triggered a closed proceeding. To keep Al Qaeda in the dark, Senator Chuckles from New York had said. As if this cracker were part of some multinational conspiracy. A one-man sleeper cell going by the name Tariq Noor, whatever that meant. That was the name at the bottom of the fax, and the pre-trial discover material the D.A. had sent, right at the deadline, claimed this was the name of a long-ago Muslim fighter, an invader of Spain whose name had become a code word for assassin. That word itself came from hashish. Micah remembered that from college, the sweet smell in his dorm room as his GPA hung in the balance. Tariq Noor's hashish made him go to Brooklyn Law School, where some long-haired classmate had dubbed him The Snake until the name stuck. Well fuck them he would make his own name now.

Lorraine Thompson said she had no interest. She was up to her *ass*, she said, in drug charges. "It's all yours Levine," she said. "Don't let the poor fuck down."

Micah called Bertha before he called his new client. "It's time to go to a game," he said. If he didn't do it now when would he? Five seats behind the Yankees' dugout cost him two hundred clams. So be it, he thought: this terror case would bring him more; the bed case was lucrative and he'd signed up two more paint-chewers just this week.

They turned his briefcase inside out at the gate. When he complained they said they could confiscate the whole thing, or make him check it with the bowling alley across River Avenue. He shut up. The changes Al Qaeda had wrought were too many to count.

The girls for some reason wanted Yankees' autographs. They leaned over the dugout roof, cute in their memorial thingees, probably being filmed as Faces of the Game,™ as examples how the love of baseball and ability to sit in expensive seats was not confined to any race, color or creed. Only the backup left fielder would sign. He flipped a batting practice ball to them, his unknown name scrawled illegible along the seams.

"Who the fuck is he?" Duwon asked.

"Remember what I said," Bertha scolded, "I'll wash out that mouth with soap."

Micah bought hotdogs and even a pizza. When money was no object junk food had no end. During the seventh inning stretch, when God Bless America™ was played and no one sang along, he bought a box of Cracker Jack™ and thought of his client, the terror defendant, the cracker with the comb-over and the faxing fixation. He told Bertha about the case while the game got out of hand. Million-dollar pitcher and the lowly Orioles hit five home runs.

"Sometimes the underdog wins," Micah said, loose with five watered-down six-dollar beers.

"It's jes one game," said Duwon. "The Yanks'll win the Series."

Bad luck for Jack, Micah thought. He wanted to knock on wood but there wasn't any around. A jagged bat flew into the stands but ten rows up. The fan was carried out on a stretcher and Bertha said, "Let's go."

* * *

Bain still had the hots for Nicole but now half the heat was anger. It must have been her who clued the SEC in to his trades. She'd asked him over Chinese lunch; now she'd left a message, "re SEC," the Post-It note said. Yeah *fuck* the SEC, Bain thought. Their SEC letter asked for all his phone logs and e-mails five days before and after his massive short of Empi. The e-mails were fine, they might violate the firm's policy on sexual harassment but that wasn't a crime. The phone log had Gina's number and that bothered him. He'd blown off her last call and the cooze was a climber, he could just tell. She'd been shopping for a job, betraying her employer -- the concept made him laugh -- so maybe she wouldn't. It made sense to touch base, though. The firm was getting grilled. They'd made bigger trades than he had in his own account. They hadn't suspended him because by that logic they'd have to do the same with the whole Equities desk or at least the chief. It was time to stonewall and fight. And to track down that diner hottie, make her an offer while he still had the chance.

Gina was desultorily closing a loan secured by tents and fishing rods -- who knew that Haitians camped? -- when her cell phone rang. With her life Organized™ by the Franklin Cubby system, she'd put in a lot of calls, to Dearborn / Kaplan crash course for the Series Seven, to the LifeCoach hotline she could call until her twenty one days ran out, to the half dozen people she knew on the Street, everyone except that bastard Tom Bain, the one who'd ignored her calls and made her redouble her commitment to Cubby.

"Hello," Gina said effectively, opening her Planner.

"Its me Tom," he said. "Look I'm sorry I've been hard to reach. I had to go to an analysts' conference in Boca Raton."

Gina didn't quite believe it -- it sounded credible though, she'd heard of those. Habit Five said Listen To Be Listened To;™ she gave it a go. "I was starting to wonder," she said. She was way past starting: she'd almost *finished* wondering. Almost.

"We need to get together," Bain said. "There's a lot of work here right now --" yeah, answering SEC subpoenas, he thought -- "and I'm needing an assistant, an associate, whatever you want to call it. I thought we should talk."

Dress for Success, thought Gina. And older wisdom: play hard to get. "No more calamari," she said. "I'm busy these days. You'll have to come to The Bronx."

What the fuck, Bain thought. Wasn't that where she wanted to get out of? "Just name a place. Any time tonight."

Gina paused -- she'd read Zagat, the only restaurants it listed in The Bronx were on Arthur Avenue. Vinny knew some people there but she no longer cared. She named a spot she'd seen with three tables outside, umbrellas advertising Italian sodas not even sold here. What *was* chinotto? "Seven o'clock," she said. She had to do the paperwork for a car repossession -- it was Janet's office now so that wench could go along on the repo ride, she wouldn't. She could still call her LifeCoach and get herself focused. Good things happen to those who are prepared.

* * *

Jack left HomeQuik with a big commission check -- he was making fifteen hundred dollars on every mortgage he closed, if he could stay out of jail Zalie's and his future was set. He needed to cash it to pay the shyster, a little earnest money before the trial began. He'd double it, he'd kiss that fucker's skinny ass, if he got acquitted.

The check casher on Morris charged one point eight percent. Mother *fuck*, thought Jack. When you needed cash you had to pay. That's how he made his living but he still didn't like it. He asked for the cash in twenties, looked up and down the block before leaving the air conditioning for Micah's neon office. "Have You Been Hurt?" the sign asked. You better believe it, thought Jack. But I'm still standing.

Micah didn't mind cash. He had to report every settlement: the companies reported them and probably wrote them off so he had to pay. But on side cases like this, cash was king. He kept it in a safe behind his set of Kornright's Civil Practice. He gave it to the cracker straight: "If there's no press you're going to lose."

"What'm I payin' you for, then?" Jack asked. He was making it again but to see a stack of twenties disappearing into this guy's wall safe rubbed him wrong.

"I'm going to oppose their motion to seal it. Them accusing you of terrorism, I think we can get press on that, I really do. And the whistleblower charge, we need it to be public to make Empi squirm. The complaint, do you have anything more on her?"

Jack'd listened in on the bitch's conference calls, boring as all hell; he could prove that she under-reported delinquencies to make her ass look good to Home Office. But real leverage? He had none. He was gonna take a final shot with Ehrenreich, trail Janet for a day but what would that prove? "The Kinkos guy who i.d.-ed me, have you talked to him?"

"Not yet. I'll definitely go there before the trial. It'll start in ten days. If we get a preliminary hearing on their motion to seal, I want you to come. Let the judge see you're not --" Micah paused, searching for the politically-correct word though it made no difference -- "an obvious Muslim or something."

"A rag head?"

Micah rolled his eyes. The less the cracker said the better. But he had one more question. "This Tariq Noor business, do you have any idea--"

"No," Jack said. "No fucking idea at all." He smiled and held out his hands, palm up.

* * *

Bain used a livery cab -- he'd seen the word "Bronx" as the terminus of subway lines when he took them to 96th Street, didn't like the look of the crew who stayed on for the journey north. But the driver was asking him directions. Where *was* this Arthur Avenue, above or below the Cross Bronx Expressway? Bain had no idea. "I thought you guys got paid to know the city," he said.

"We work Manhattan," the turbaned driver said. If Bain thought about it he'd admit he'd thought of the Towers and Al Qaeda when he got in the cab. But he didn't think about it. He was smoothing his hair, trying to prepare to appear to have not a trouble in the world. Assistant wasn't the right word. Associate or something even more hopeful. He needed to know if the SEC had called her -- he doubted it -- and if she'd talk with them if they did. This he was less sure of. Maybe she'd think that talking would get her to the Street. He had to offer another route. He could put her on per diem to deal with the subpoena. He'd tell them he chose her because he could trust her. Wink, wink; shred, shred.

They were driving between two raw-sheered cliffs, stuck between 18-wheel rigs. Up above Bain caught glimpses of apartment buildings. Some of their windows were blank and black; through some he saw the sky. "Don't you have a radio?" he asked the driver.

Suddenly a speaker by Bain's right ear blared sing-song Araby music. "You like?" the driver asked. Smart ass.

"I meant a radio to your base," Bain said, wanting to add *asshole* or something more ethno-specific.   There was a crackling sound, directions exchanged.

"We look for Webster exit," the driver announced. The next one said Jerome and the ramp was grid-locked anyway. The traffic got lighter; glimpses of liquor stores and storefront churches, a sign for Clay Avenue and then the ramp.

The Sikh driver drove past Webster Avenue, to a bleak street that fronted some railroad tracks. The signs said Park Avenue. There was a police station; there were kids playing in open spurting hydrants, rows of attached houses that looked like prisons. Bain remembered Nicole Nour's article, the Mexicans who got fucked on -- where else? -- Park Avenue. Which house was it? He hadn't brought it with him. He needed to get better organized. The thought came and it went.

They hit 187th Street and the driver turned right. "You're sure?" Bain asked.

"This they tell me," the driver said. There was a tall building that looked like a housing project, then incongruously a garish Italian men's store with fake gas lights in front, a bakery with a sign for biscotti, a mural on a tenement saying "The Good Taste of Tradition." "It is here," the driver said. He stopped in front of what looked like a social club; Bain saw Gina sitting at a table outside staring down at a book.

"You pay cash?" the driver asked. "Or charge to company?"

"Charge." Bain signed the receipt, added a ten dollar tip, why not. The perks of Wall Street. Bain wished Gina'd seen this. You might work to midnight but you rode home for free.

"Sorry to keep you waiting," Bain began. "The driver got lost, I felt like I was in the Bonfire--" He stopped. It wasn't a book she was reading, it was one of those cult-like Planner things. The lower-downs in Bain's firm were required to take some Time Management™ course and write all their dreams in this little red books. It was pathetic Bain thought. "So you're a Planner," he said.

Gina nodded, noting that Bain's reaction was different than Vinny's. "It's an amazing system," she said. "It helps you put the Nine Habits into practice."

Bain remembered the book she was reading in the diner. He hadn't know that these Planner-heads were connected. Over orzata and chinotto -- it was a vile tasting soda made of citrus and herbs, Gina found, and they said it key-noto like keno -- she explained the FranklinCubby company, how two Mormons had merged in Provo and the rest was history. "They're publicly traded," she said. "They have contracts with school boards and some stores in China now."

"Stores?" Bain asked.

"They sell audio tapes and even the Planner in electronic form, for the PalmPilot or any hand-held device."

She sounded like a press release, Bain thought. It was time to ask. "Uh, remember when you told me that the A.G. was nosing around?"

She nodded. She sure did. That was supposed to have gotten her a job, then he blew off her calls.

"Well there's some stupid stuff --" he kept himself from saying shit, if she knew the effort she'd appreciate it -- "down at the firm about it. Some trading was done, typical every-day stuff. Now the SEC is asking for records. It's probably nothing. I just wondered if you'd heard anything else." There. He'd tipped his hand about leverage, or at least that these weird sour drinks were not just about an assistant position. But he'd asked without asking. He was proud of himself.

He's still digging, Gina thought. The SEC part caught her attention. Stupid stuff, he'd said -- it didn't sound right without "shit," but the guy looked wimpier than before, more scared, younger -- that must mean an investigation. Was this an Opportunity™ presenting itself to her? Cubby would say so. He said the rewards started showing up even before the twenty-one days. "What *kind* of stupid stuff?" she asked. This was delicious as the soda wasn't.

"Just a letter. They want our e-mails and phone records from the days around the trade. I thought about because... I realized we spoke around then, I just didn't want you caught up in this bullshit." There was no other word; stuff just didn't work.

"I didn't do anything wrong," Gina said, emphasizing the I, watching him sweat. She raised the heat: "I mean, I didn't do any trades in Empi's stock. Not then, not since."

The ball buster, Bain thought. If she hadn't know the leverage, now she did. But the tipster -- or was it tipper? Bain couldn't remember, from his NASD ethics class -- got in trouble just like the trader. Maybe she should know this. It wasn't time for the Godfather yet. "Let's eat," he said. "Do they serve food here or just these, uh, drinks?"

Gina'd committed Zagat's four squibs about The Bronx to her Planner. "There's a place around the corner that got reviewed in the Times," she said.

"That's my Bible," Bain said half-serious. He paid for the soda, if you could call them that, and they walked two blocks east on 186th. Here were tables outside too. The inside was packed. They sat on white plastic chairs; Bain was surprised when the menu showed the entrees were thirty bucks. He had his company Gold Card, what did he care. "Get whatever you want," he said. "The firm lets us charge it."

Gina chose swordfish just to run up the bill. Bain settled on venison to feel like a man, like the gators in the Bayou, the fantasy camp of masculinity he'd begun to miss.

"So they haven't called you, did they?" he asked after they were served.

He's got it bad, Gina thought. There was that song about "and that ain't good" but in this case it was. At least he had a plan. A task if not a mission. "I'm returning my calls in order now," she said, lying through her fish. Cubby said to prioritize everything, A1 to C10, focus on the big rocks. A call from the SEC would blow her Planner to smithereens. Let him sweat, the deer-eating frat boy.

Bain was getting annoyed. He looked out at the street, a mundane scene of two-family houses and a fenced parking lot. There was an apartment building with a crowd on the stoop, babies in pampers and women in bras or what looked like them. Bain had done Asian but nothing darker -- the thought made him laugh and he poured some more San Pellegrino.

"What's so funny?"

"Nothing," Bain said, "just something that happened at work."

"The SEC subpoena?"

So she knew the word. They must teach it in night school. It was time to make a deal. "So about the job: I really need someone right now, the firm's said it's okay. It's be per diem at first--"

"What's that?" Gina asked before thinking.

"By the day. It'd be more than your making in a week, if Empi's financial statement are true. It'd be a first step. People start that way then go full time."

Gina cut another piece of fish. Don't show your excitement, don't pant; play hard to get. He'd dangled this carrot before. This time she'd wait to have it in her hand. "It'd have to be in writing," she said. "I'm a branch manager at Empi. Once people leave they don't let them back." That much was true. It was like a cult in that way. Cubby was more forgiving, with the stores offering a second chance to anyone who fell off the Planning wagon.

He could doctor up a per diem contract, Bain thought. All employment was at will so what the fuck. "No problem," he said. No way she'd talk to the SEC when she'd just got her first foothold on The Street.

"And one more thing," she said. "I'm studying for the Seven--" she'd read that saying "Test" just exposed you as a newbie --"and I need a broker dealer to sponsor me. So they'd have to do that."

Brassy, Bain thought. He should have known from her diner reading. He remembered how pretty he'd thought she was, that day after waiting in Elizabeth's weeds. She was dressed more severe but the full package, it was all still there. Ambition turned him off -- or maybe it was competition. That vicious Nicole was nothing if not ambitious but she belly-danced in his dreams. He'd have to cut that out at the root: pathetic pining for two women at once would be too much. So why not this one? "No problem. We've already got a block of seats for the test ten days from now, but it's probably better you wait for the next round."

"No, I'll take it this time. I've been studying."

She could always take it again, Bain thought. "They used to get ringers do the Seven for us--"

"I don't need that--

"I'm not saying you do. Anyway, they take fingerprints now." He paused. "I could even help you study."

He wasn't bad, this bozo. He was like a different species than Vinny. "Like I said, I've been getting ready for this for a long time. I've already got the textbook," she said. But she smiled. A final round of studying would be okay. Bain was no stud but the man had a mission. What would their statement be? To run a hedge fund from a boat. And goodwill to men, why not.

"Hey." A guy in a muscle shirt had stopped by their table. "Hey ain't you Vinny's girl?"

Bain was hoping no violence was called for: it wasn't his thing. Gina seemed to know the guy. Jesus she was really coming up out of the swamp.

"We're *eating* here, Tony, can't you see that?"

The guy looked them both up and down. "Yo who's this?"

Gina paused for a moment, squeezed her Planner and rolled the dice. "He's my boyfriend, stupid. My new boyfriend. And you can tell Vinny that. I know you will."

"Skeezer," Bain heard. "Skank and skanky whore." This Tony needed a thesaurus. Bain wanted to pay and leave. He'd been daydreaming about this Series Seven-hungry climber but this was a little much. White trash street thugs he could do without.

"I hope you don't mind," Gina said regally. "I was just joking."

"I hope Vinny-whoever-he-is knows that. Unless you're trying to shake things up."

"He's my boyfriend, or was. And yes I'm trying to shake things up. Here's my fax number." She gave the West Farms office: let them see it, who cared, it was time for a Change.™ "Send me the contract, per dios or whatever you called it, and we'll take it from there. I want to take the Series Seven the next time they give it. It's in the Javits Center. I already have the application, just need the sponsor part filled out."

Bain paid -- a thirty dollar tip and the greaser didn't even look happy -- and they walked back to Arthur Avenue. Bain had the number to the livery cab place. "You're driving?" he asked Gina, more out of habit than as a come-on.

He'd tried it in Greenwich but this was different. "Yeah I'm driving," Gina said. "Where do you want to go?"

33. Mister Bliss / His Precious Cargo

The red room was calling Kurt's kaleidoscope mind but there was a play that he had to make first. Micah'd told him that Swanker was backing off. Kurt didn't tell Micah why -- he almost did, with his link to his web site crushed with his modem he had to tell someone -- but the time to play the nanny card had come. He went to 120 Broadway just like any citizen can. He was ready with that whole spiel, how he'd come to see his elected official. Swanker's secretary, not half bad, was nonplussed. "If you'll tell me what it's about, you could see an assistant. But you can't just--"

"Tell him two things. W-Two and nanny. Maybe mention Zoë Baird. I'll wait."

It was amazing how clear this code language was. The secretary came back shrugging. "He'll see you. But he only has ten minutes. He has a speech to make." She summoned him back past file cabinets to a door. Nice view of Ground Zero.

Swanker's mouth went dry when he heard the three phrases. W-Two could be anything, some bullshit complaint about off-the-books waiters in Chinatown, cement-mixing sandhogs on Tunnel Number Three. But nanny cut closer, and Zoë sealed the deal. She'd lost Ashcroft's job under Clinton for negligent child care. She was fifty but he would have like to see her in a negligee. He hoped Carolyn held up so well. But if this nanny crap knocked him out of the box he might not even have Carolyn. It might be better but it was unimaginable. She'd been the one who'd hired the Mexican. Fuck!

Swanker stayed silent, looking out the window, looking past Vesey Street and tragedy straight into Jersey. Kurt stood too, suddenly not so sure. Was this blackmail? But what of what Milly described? If Swanker was taping so what. He'd never use it.

"So you know Zoë Baird," Kurt began.

Swanker's hopes rose then fell. Who was this fucker with his shirt untucked? Some undercover bagman for Rudehart? "I know most of the higher echelons of the Bar--"

"And you know some lower echelons too," Kurt cut in. "Save a little money hiring undocumented--"

"What do you want?" When Kurt didn't answer, Swanker asked, "Are you from Empi? You can tell Rudehart to stop fucking with me." Swanker stopped, seeing no reaction on this ridiculously bearded face. "Who the hell are you?" he demanded.

"Here's the deal," Kurt said. "I'm somebody who knows the squeeze play Empi put on you, and that since then you've backed down. I also know that you haven't paid taxes or social security on your domestic help for years. You saw what happened to Zoë--"

"We can cure that," Swanker said. "If it's even true. There's more recognition now of how difficult it is to handle on the paperwork on household employees--"

"So you're a libertarian. A nice Democratic slave boss who's father was a slumlord--"

"This is extortion," Swanker said. He was the state Attorney General Goddamn it. Blackmail was a crime, the mirror image of bribery, no different.

"I haven't asked for anything," Kurt said. He was thinking of the red room, he was thinking of Gene Ramos for some reason, his shattered laptop, the whole disgusting fuck. "I just want you to know, Empigroup has one threat over you to back off, but there's some other reasons you should do the right thing. Indict the bastards and whip Basso's ass in the primary. In the long run it's the clearer route." That line, Kurt had prepared. He appealed to Swanker's conscience not just his fear. Either way it didn't matter.

"*I* know who you are," Swanker said. "You're the web site guy, Corporation Watch or whatever."

Why not. "WatchCorp," Kurt corrected him. "The nanny tale will go up by next week if there's no indictment." He paused. He didn't mind bluffing with the web site, even if he could reconnect, was too obscure. "We can get it in the Journal too," he said.

Swanker thought of the day's calls and remembered one from Nour that he hadn't returned. Did she already know?

"I don't like extortion," Swanker said slowly, as threatening as he could muster. "I've prosecuted it with a vengeance. But I've heard what you said. Give me two weeks -- I'm not acknowledging anything, I'm just saying, give me two weeks." He wondered if this creep was wired. It was too late for that.

"Ten days," Kurt said. He had to get FrontPage Express. His web site was dying but he wouldn't take it lying down. He heard the call of the red room as well, again. It was like an exorcism. You had to cause pain to the right people. When you slipped up you had to redouble your efforts. Double or nothing.

* * *

Ehrenreich was one of those mediocre fucks who didn't even wanna make money. Jack had his own reasons to want to trail Janet. But Ehrenreich should too. "Lemme show you how they do it," Jack'd said. "I may not be here much longer--" he didn't tell him why -- "but if you get the system down HomeQuik will be throwin' money at you to keep you on their team."

Ehrenreich waivered; Ehrenreich chewed Paxil. "Mister Bliss," Jack'd taken to calling him, along with "Mister Second Rate."

Finally Ehrenreich agreed, but only if Jack drove. "It just feels kinda sneaky," the Bliss-man said. "I'm not used to tailing anyone around."

That's why you're in the bottom rung of managers in a second-tier company, Jack thought. If he got demoted from The Bronx where would HomeQuik send Ehrenreich -- Rwanda? They set out at three p.m. with the sun still high. "It's almost quittin' time," Ehrenreich said. "They must be knockin' off for the day."

"You don't know these people," Jack said. "Their real day's just starting."

In the West Farms Mall parking lot Jack couldn't find Gina's car. Maybe they'd fired that bitch too, or she'd seen the light and gone to the dark side. She could take Ehrenreich's job in a minute, even with her coke habit and her days cut short by the dago's demands. But maybe she'd taken her high wire act somewhere else. Today she was not here. They parked and Jack slumped low in his seat, sent Ehrenreich out for two three-meat tacos. Before he got back Jack saw the posse start to form. Janet came out with two guys in blue overalls, the muscle they used, such as it was. They walked to the back where the guys had parked their car-hauling truck. It was a repo run. This Ehrenreich had to see. "Come on you stupid fuck," Jack said inside the car, watching the Bliss-man wander through the lot with his sack of Jack in the Box.™ Jackal in a hot box; Ehrenreich's air conditioner was almost a heater. Jack rolled the windows down, and started moving the car as Ehrenreich got in. "We're rolling," he said. Nothing but jungle music on the radio. They headed north on Boston Road.

The truck up in front managed to catch two yellow lights one after the other. Jack burned them on the red, Ehrenreich making scared blissed-out noises through his taco. "Take it easy," Jack told him. "I come from the heartland of NASCAR. These fuckers couldn't shake me if they had a rocket on that truck."

They turned west on East Tremont, the north again on Mapes. There were ticky-tacky brick houses, the band aids on the moonscape. The truck stopped by a hydrant and no one got out. Jack drove to the end of the block and double-parked. "They wait, we wait," Jack said. Ehrenreich was slurping his Doctor Pepper like it was his mother's tit. "This is how they do a repo," Jack added. "I think it's the SUV that those people are gettin' out of."

In the middle of the block a woman was unloaded plastic bags from Pathmark into an asphalt walkway. Only half of these houses had driveways. The rest of the homeowners parked on the street, which had once been lined with tenements but was now a low-rise Levittown. It was Anywhere U.S.A. and so was the scene. In the rear view Jack watch Janet, who in turn was watching the Spanish lady struggling with her grocery bags. The lady opened the door to her house -- there were pathetic steel lions on each side, Jack noticed, as if this was a library or something; the door closed behind the lady after she entered. The truck pulled out, backed in again in front of the SUV, raising the thing up onto the ramp, like picking an apple or popping a zit.

"They can do that?" Ehrenreich asked, down to the ice now, sucking like a kid.

"They're doing it," Jack said. He'd brought along a camera with a telephoto lens, cheap knock-off from Taiwan but through it he could see the cow-like look on Janet's face as the men in blue raised up the car. Janet got out and taped a notice to the mailbox in front of the house; Jack got her in slow motion, click and click and click. For what, he didn't know. The repo hall of fame.

They piled in the truck like gangsters and squealed off down the block with the SUV on the flatbed. Jack turned the key in the ignition to follow, but Ehrenreich grabbed his shoulder. "The lady," he said. "She's out on the sidewalk screaming."

Jack turned back around and took a few shots. The lady was shouting, "My baby! They took my baby with the car!"

Jack laughed. "What a cluster fuck," he said.

"Oh Christ," said Ehrenreich, as if that would do anything. Jack handed him the camera and jogged back to the frantic lady.

"They're from Empi," Jack told her, pointing to the notice taped on the mailbox. "You should call the police."

"My Luisita! My baby!"

"She was in a car seat?"

Yes, the lady wheezed. Then, "Who are you? How could you watch and do nothing?"

Jack thought for a moment of the photo-journalist's quandary, some gruesome shot from Vietnam: a gun to a man's head then the man's head gone. A skinny naked girl running down the road with her back on fire. It was pure Americana, all of it. "Let's go inside and call the cops," he said. He'd love to see that bitch Janet in cuffs.

* * *

Gina had missed this fiasco for the first day of the Series Seven crash course. It was Dearborn / Kaplan, the one she'd called -- but Bain's firm was paying. The offer had firmed up as had Bain's nether regions too. Gina noted his come-ons in her Franklin Planner but did not give in. She'd taken a room in the Comfort Inn by Co-op City, hiding out from Vinny, checking her voice mail at Empi without giving notice. She had sick-time built up; it ran through the day of the Series Seven test. Keep your options open Cubby'd said, or should have. Gina felt her power and remembered the phrase, "to get where you want to go, recognize the power you have to make it so." She was making it happen, and jotting down every step in her Planner, as her LifeCoach had said, cataloguing "elements that denote success" for her morning meditations.

The class was like SoulTime, in a way. Tomorrow would be Options Day; two days after that would be Market Structure. It was beautiful, Gina thought, the way these Systems meshed and were transparent, climbable like a web to those who opened their eyes. Let Bain pant and fear the secret she had, the Swanker tip-off, the SEC subpoena. Let Vinny comb The Bronx with his half-wit friend, trying to corral the horse when it had already gone. She'd been called a filly and this she didn't mind. The markets made her frisky. Her Plan and Planner were working, together, for the best of all possible worlds.

* * *

When the cops arrived on Mapes they laughed, then wiped the smiles from their face. This was a hot one, baby stolen, might even be federal. "It's a kidnapping," Jack kept saying. The woman muttered the name of a bank. Some storefront in the West Farms Mall. Let Ten-Ten WINS get ahold of this one and it'd be on the cover of the Post and News tomorrow. Jack wanted to call 'em but the cops said no. Ehrenreich waited in the car chewing Paxil.

It was Janet who first heard the baby's screams, as they lowered the car in their lot on Zerega. They stored repos here, on a landfill lined with razor wire, until the deadbeats paid or they auctioned on Webster. "What the--" Janet began, opening the driver's side door and seeing the car seat in the back.

"Waa!" the baby screamed.

"You fucking idiots!" Janet shouted. She hadn't checked the car while the blue men worked, had only taped the notice and borne witness to a clean repo. Now they were kidnappers, with the customer's baby on a lot in Zerega. Janet checked the docs on her clip board. There was the self-executing contract, non-judicial foreclosure with Empi's name on the title, it all checked out except the baby. On a bottom sheet was the customer's number. "This is the last time we'll use you," she told the men while dialing the cell.

"I am *so* sorry," she began. The lady was screaming, that was understandable. A man came on the line, said he was a cop and she better bring the baby back, right now, or there'd be an All Points Bulletin for Empi's repo truck. "Right away," Janet said. "It's a terrible screw up and I'll accept responsibility." She thought of Mudnick and Yonkers and the possible fall-out from the blue men's blindness. Then behind the cops she heard a voice she recognized: The Cracker. "Tell the bitch she's a kidnapper," he was saying. He was laughing like a nightmare and Janet clenched her eyes tight shut. "We're taking the car back too," she announced to the men. Make kissy-kissy with the customer and refi the loan. If the customer understood what could The Cracker do?

34. LazyBoy™ / The Ice Queen

With the cat still in the Hamptons the mouse Nicole was eager to play. She'd set the wheels in motion on Bain. Before writing the SEC story she wanted to give him a chance to sing, to implicate any Page Six client he'd tipped off about Swanker's interest which since had waned. Bain wouldn't return her calls but she knew where he worked. She was not a paparazza but stories were made, not given. Even dead stories could be used to dig around. So she called Lena Jones, to rattle her cage about the bullet and see what came out.

Lena'd been briefed by Rudehart: the story was dead, she knew, and she knew something else. She even had a photo to prove it. A dark photo but the ring around the eye showed through.

"I'm gonna fax you something," Lena said. "But first let me explain it. The incident at the Guzmans, you know what it was about?"

"That's what I've been asking."

"Nothing to do with us," Lena answered. The guy who runs WatchCorp--"

"Kurt Wheelock--"

"Yeah, him. He beat up his girlfriend. That's what's behind this. We have a photograph."

A dirty tricks campaign, thought Nicole. It was a mean city but for reporters it worked quite well. Let corporate targets dig up the dirt on their accusers. Report it as your own work; shake and *voilà*, a Pulitzer. Facts were facts. Their provenance was not the point. She got the name from Lena, checked the spelling of Azuela. "Fax away," Nicole said. The accounting scandal could wait for a while.

* * *

Bain worked past eight redacting his e-mails. The compliance officer said it was fine: anything not work-related could be blacked out. It was the *Securities*, not the Sex, Exchange Commission. The only real problem was the phone notes from Gina. But he'd bought her silence with per diem checks -- he was paying it himself for now, getting back whatever he could be using the company credit card. From the diner to the Street, she'd used him well. It was worthy of Steve the Sleaze, but the woman had style and that hungry look in her eyes. She was Babe Dickerson, not Emily Dickenson. Each and every use of the word dick he blacked out with a pen.

He was loosening his tie as he walked out onto Park Avenue. He hadn't called for a livery cab, would probably skip the subway. He could walk south on Broadway eating fruit from the ice of Korean bodegas. From behind came a voice. "Bain! Tom Bain!"

Tony and Vinny were still in his mind but the voice was a woman's. He recognized it, some previous fetish now dead in his heart. There she was, the turn-coat princess, the SEC's tipster, Nicole Ice Queen Nour.

"I have no comment," Bain said, pulling his tie through his still buttoned collar. "Call the press office if you got a question."

"The SEC monitors shorts," she said. "Options especially they watch. I just report -- I don't *make* the news."

Bain knew it was bullshit. Arbs shorted stocks every day of the week; people traded on the inside every minute and the feds didn't care until the press took an interest. Sure she was hot, this Nicole. But so were a thousand other girls in this town, including Gina.

"I got nothing to say. Can't you people take no for an answer?"

When Nicole heard "you people" she thought of Islam. Osama Bin Petulant, couldn't wait for the Saudis to screw up their American concubinage on their own so he blew up the towers. But it was the paparazzi angle Bain was playing.

"It's that I know it's not just you," she said. "You're just doing your job but you might take the fall."

"I'll take my chances."

"I want to tell your side," Nicole said.

"*My* side?" Bain asked. He was a goof-ball at heart. "This is my side." He raised his middle finger and even Nicole was surprised. Frat boy would be a step up for this doofus.

"Can I quote you?" she asked.

Bain might have mooned her. He could see it now: "Mister Bain, reached outside his office, flipped the bird declining comment." He could black out his finger. It was nobody's business.

* * *

The Mapes grateful mother declined to press charges. But Jack had the photos including three snapped by Ehrenreich of the baby's return. Janet told the cops of the order of protection, so he'd retreated to Prospect and let the Bliss-man play shutter-bug. He'd paid for three hour development and here they were: the baby with Janet, like Mary Magdalene. He could smell freedom now, remembered the smell of his own baby's diapers, his Zalie in Charlotte, the princess for whom he fought with these turds in the Bronx-land ballet. Where to go but the shyster? He'd know what to do.

"This has to be the most colossal collections screw up ever," Micah said. Jack knew of worse: Empi'd foreclosed on an iron lung in Charlotte that had still been in use; they'd auctioned off the wrong house once and had to buy it back. But kidnapping a baby wasn't bad.

"It gets me off, right?" Jack asked. Micah didn't see how. "I mean, we call them, saying we'll take the photos to the newspapers unless they drop the fax case and now."

"Did you get the officers' names?"

He hadn't. "But I'm sure you could get 'em. And the Mapes lady might be happy for now, gettin' her daughter back and all -- but if you tell her how much she could sue for I'm sure she'll jabber like Oprah to the press."

The cracker knew a bit, Micah thought, about the way the world worked. "Let's go up there."

"That's what I like about you," Jack said, "at least as my lawyer. You got the heart of an ambulance chaser."

For now, Micah thought. Like sowing wild oats, you couldn't chase ambulances forever. Eventually you wanted a Bertha, accepted her kids in the mix -- eventually you wanted to work on appeals and not have to look the braindead babies in their rolling eyes, smell the fruits of the sphincters without constraints. "Let's go." And so they drove.

Mrs. Peña, Micah thought, needed schooling in the American way. Here she was sitting on a million dollar claim, false imprisonment on behalf of her child and egregious infliction of emotional distress on herself -- to say nothing of the Fair Debt Collection Practices Act -- and she just shrugged and served coffee. "I so happy she is back," Mrs. Peña said, showing snapshots of Luisa, the real thing sleeping in a crib in a room upstairs.

"You can sue," Micah said. "Think of it this way -- if you don't, they'll do this again to another mother, another baby, and maybe not bring her back. They have to be held accountable."

"The lady she say they cancel my loan. Forgiven, all of it. This I like."

"Did you sign anything?"

Mrs. Peña smiled, still euphoric, and went into the kitchen. "Yes," she said, "I sign this paper here."

Micah read over it and groaned. A full release and even a gag order: if Mrs. Peña ever disparaged Empi or any of its affiliates the loan would be re-instated, with interest, and she could be sued for all damages occasioned by her breach of the contract.

"What this mean, dis-porridge?" Mrs. Peña asked.

Micah didn't answer. The cracker was still fucked, but he had a good photo album.

"We don't *need* the lady," Jack said as Micah drove him to Olinville. "We got the photos and I can explain what they mean."

Yeah the whore-monger of credibility, Micah thought. The death-threat faxer with this photos and his tales.

"Ehrenreich could do the talking," Jack continued. "He's a little blissed out but he's got no rap sheet that I know of."

"Yeah whatever," Micah said. "Just get ready for the trial. No monkeying around from now until then."

"When in Rome," Jack said. He'd heard that at SUNY and he'd always liked the phrase. It was racist without a single racist word. The shyster'd said monkey and he'd said Rome. The joke might flop in Charlotte but he was proud that he'd made it. And he felt like calling Zalie tonight. He had nothing firm but he had to tell this story to someone.

* * *

Micah called Bertha, since for once he had a joke to tell. He parked by the Zoo, by the Bronx River's ramp, and dialed on his cell. She was screaming at Duwon but that was par for the course. He didn't tell the story quite right and Bertha didn't laugh.

"Those bastards," she said. She was thinking of Penny Zade, that moment in the hospital knowing she was gone. Mrs. Peña was lucky but still. "You thought that was *funny?*" Bertha asked. Micah was almost like a cop, she thought, taking pleasure in other people's pain, numb to it since it was his business. This side of him she didn't like.

"Not funny, exactly. Just, you know--"

"I have to go," Bertha said.

"But I thought--"

"I have to go." She hung up and Micah felt empty. He wanted to whisper "you bitch" but the words wouldn't come. She was right. He'd lost his feeling -- his "caring," she called it. Maybe empathy was the word. But if you couldn't laugh, in the face of braindead babies, what could you do? He had a trial to prepare for and a life to sort out. He turned on Steely Dan but found it cynical and sick. Songs about pedophilia? What had he come to?

* * *

Gina was driving just then to Vinny's place. It was his softball night so the coast should be clear. It was her apartment, really. She'd found the place and signed the lease. But Vinny could keep it, install some hair-sprayed bimbo in her bed. The road for her was looking up: from the Comfort Inn she would move to Manhattan. She would never drive these streets again and she would not miss them.

The light was off, she could see from below. She bought a box of garbage bags at the all-night bodega and climbed the stairs. One for the bathroom; two or three for clothes. Then *arrividerci* Vinny. Tomorrow was Options Day.

She knocked on the door just to be sure, but only silence. She slipped in her key, turned but fuck: the door wasn't locked. She pushed it open, saw smoke in the darkness, the flickering of a candle from the bedroom. Was Vinny already boinking some bimbo? She wouldn't put it past him. And she wouldn't waste this night, either. This would put her on the moral high ground again, as if she needed it. Cubby said aspire and that meant bye-bye Vinny.

She walked toward the bedroom. No music she thought was weird, but Vinny'd always like to hear, to kid himself that sighs were real and all about him. She stood by the door frame and snuck a peak. Then she turned to leave but too late.

Vinny was slumped on the LazyBoy™ by the window, the ashtray smoldering, a dozen bottles on the floor. "You bitch!" he screamed after her. She heard his footsteps, turned to throw the box of garbage bags. He got to the door before her and pressed his back against it. "All I wanna know," he said, "is who this bastard is. 'Cause he's a dead man. You get me? He's a mother fucking dead man walking."

Gina thought of Bain and wondered how fast Vinny could take him. Vinny wouldn't go alone. Tony was a loser who liked to cause pain. They'd beaten a black kid for a television set and left him tied up in Arthur park -- Vinny never stopped telling that story, no matter how much the TV spoke of hate crimes, mandatory sentencing, aggravating factors and the rest. This was Vinny's main claim in life: other men were afraid of him and women, he thought, couldn't resist him.

"It's not *about* him," Gina said. "It's about *you*. Or us, really. We don't want the same things in life."

"Yeah some bastard whisperin' in your ear about Wall Street while you give him a hand job--"

"Stop!" Gina said. "Your mind's in the gutter and that's while you'll never get out--"

"Just tell me his name is all. Tony said the bastard don't even have a car."

"Oh so he spied on me."

"Yeah he watched your ass. What kinda friend would he be if he din?"

"A friend with a *life*," Gina said. Take control, Cubby said. So she tried. "I'm here to pack up my stuff. You can go back to drinking. Just don't burn the place down, at least 'til I leave."

"You're a *cunt*, you know that?"

She'd said never say that word and now he had. "You're a *loser*," she said, emphasizing it the same way. "You'll be just like your father, even worse."

"Leave the old man--"

"It's you I'm leaving." Gina turned to the bathroom, trying to project her power and feeling it, throwing her make up and tampons and Q-Tips and bath oils all into the bag, Vinny standing in the doorway, a zipping sound -- she turned around. He had it out, waving it like a mad man, pathetic and sad.

"You *know* you want me," Vinny said. "You know you wanna piece of this."

Gina thought of the lady who'd cut her man's dick. She'd gotten what, probation? But she'd said the guy had hit her, had affairs right in their bed. Vinny at least kept his chippies in his car. "Put it away," Gina said, feeling her power. "We're through." It was a Planner moment and she'd later write it up. It denoted success and good luck, this desperate flaccid penis.

Vinny was smart enough not to hit her or even try. He'd find this bastard himself, he said. Him and Tony would give the guy what-for. While he vented she wrote him a to-do list. Take her name off the lease, off the phone and Con Ed bill. It wasn't worth a Planner page so she wrote on a pad from the hotel. Gina handed it to Vinny, felt Power™ and left for the Comfort Inn.

35. Mister Rogers / Code Red™

Bain flipping the bird was the next-to-last straw for the SEC story. Nicole has the numbers on the trades, for Bain and his firm; she had a quote from an unnamed source in the SEC that the matter looked serious. All she needed now was to check in with Swanker, make sure his investigation of Empi was ongoing, maybe get a sound byte from him on his outrage of people inside-trading on his work. He hadn't returned her earlier call but these things happened. You had to let them know what was in it for them.

"I'm working on a profile of his office," Nicole told Swanker's secretary. "So I really need to run it by him."

"Just a moment."

This Nour had served his purpose before, but now silence was golden, silence until the Rochester press conference. A profile about his office? That was different. Spun right he could use it in mailers for the House race.

"You didn't return her call from before," his secretary said.

"What would I do without you," Swanker said. He waited until she closed the door behind her.

"I'm sorry," he began, making him self breathless and important, "we're working on an investigation and we're into the ninth inning." "The investigation of Empi, right?" This was all she needed. Her finger were poised on her keyboard, ready to type yes.

"No it's something different, something more pressing," Swanker said, back peddling fast, ready to spill the beans on Rochester, tell her she'd have an exclusive for the day the indictment was announced, as long as she'd wait.

"More pressing than Empi?" Nicole asked, disappointed but excited at the same time. "Tell me about it."

"It wouldn't be fair to the target for you to print anything yet," Swanker said.

Like that's ever stopped you, Nicole thought. "We can do it on background for now," she said. "But I need a quote on Empi. Just that the investigation is continuing. Something's come up."

Swanker had hoped it would just die out, her previous story about his subpoena, leave it hanging, blame it on his successor that it never came to fruition. As if he'd be leaving a single file for that puppet Basso. "What do you mean, something's come up?" Swanker asked. He was ready to say Rochester. Let's move on.

"The SEC has caught wind of insider trading, started just before I reported on your subpoena. It's for tomorrow's paper but I just need a quote from you. Two things: that the investigation is live, and your feelings on insider trading." This should be easy, Nicole thought: it's a scourge on America, as insidious in its way as terrorism. It had been said before but she always liked to report that ludicrous comparison. Go ahead, make the quote.

"You know my views on insider trading," Swanker said weakly.

"Freshen 'em up a bit."

"No better than terrorism," Swanker said by rote.

"This time with feeling," Nicole said. His silence on Empi was weird. It undermined her story. This new pressing matter was no compensation: a bird in the hand. She had Bain and his firm dead to rights, this bird-flipping had sealed the deal. "And yes or no on Empi."

"I don't accept the dichotomy," Swanker said, reeling. He should have blown off this call like the last one. He remembered. "We do not comment on ongoing investigations."

"*That's* pretty weak," Nicole said. "It's also not true. I've already quoted you about the subpoena. So that won't work."

"Read it however you want to," Swanker said. "I'm not a press whore," he added, more to himself than to her.

Bullshit Nicole thought -- you're a press *pimp*. Swanker's backdown might be a story in itself.

"Let me ask *you* something," Swanker said. "Your story about the couple in The Bronx--" he was thinking of Milagros, whose thigh he'd squeezed without W-2s -- "it had details in comment with a web site I've been monitoring--"

"WatchCorp," Nicole filled in. The world was getting smaller. She thought of the bullet and looked at the photograph again. Not a bad looking woman, this victim.

"Yes, that's it, WatchCorp." Swanker wanted the question to come off casual, so not knowing the name of the site was a start. "What's your experience with them? I have my reasons for asking," he added defensively.

"Funny you should ask," Nicole said. Maybe a trade of info would loosen Swanker's lips. "I've learned something about the founder -- I mean that web site is basically him, you know -- that maybe he'd find interesting, if only you'll give me a straight yes or no on Empi.."

"You first," Swanker said, thinking of forked tongues and crossed fingers and how phones could disconnect when you least expected.

The bullet story was effectively killed so why not. "The guy beat his girlfriend. Pretty bad, it looks like. I have a photograph." She looked at it.

"How long ago?" Swanker asked. He told himself to stay cool. He hated domestic violence almost as much as impotence.

"Recent. How I got the photo is a long story, one I'm not going to get into before your yes or no."

"Finish your part of the deal," Swanker said. "Either the story--
"No--"

"Or fax me the photo. I could send someone to pick it up."

"I'll fax it." Why not. "Then it's your turn, yes or no."

"Go ahead and dial." Swanker gave her the number of his personal machine, watched as a page with a black square in the middle came out. He could barely make it out: a surprised-looking woman with a black left eye. "Who is she?"

"Candida Azuela," Nicole said. "She's in the Manhattan book, there's only one." She paused. Enough was enough. "Okay, I'm all ears."

"I'm sorry," Swanker said and pushed on his telephone's black plastic tongue. Fucking Verizon. Swanker jogged to his door, ripped the Walkman headphones off his secretary's ears. "Tell her I've had to leave," he said. "Tell her it's Rochester." Somehow that made it right. "And get me the address and number of a Candida Azuela, in Manhattan."

His secretary was still rubbing her ears.

"Now," he said. He'd get new eye candy in the District.

* * *

The Paxil undermined one of Bender's main drives: the hunger for sex or at least to beat off. Nightly now he sat in the Olinville half-light, cruising the 'Net with a troubling calm. He'd bookmarked three dozen porno sites, downloaded ten second M-pegs to his hard drive but now the salt had lost his favor. He stared at the gyrating bodies as if they were Martians, or bugs or deep-sea fish like you'd see on PBS. He tried, Lord he tried, to rekindle his interest. He spent more time on the sites than before, because nothing was happening.

The penultimate of his bookmarks was a post Nine-Eleven site, "Bitches in Veils" it was called. Before the plane attacks there'd been Asian sites, interracial sites, Ebony sites, Latina sites -- even some sites that specialized in Eastern European refugee whores or at least capitalized on the rumor of white slavery. But now there was this Muslim site, sure to drive the rag-heads crazy. In slow-motion downloads a woman slowly removed each piece of her black garbage bag -- she was excellent-looking, vaguely off-white like you'd paint your apartment. The last to come off was the headdress, those black eyes fluttering behind.

This almost got Jack Bender up. Almost.

He wondered if the CIA or Homeland Defense was funding this, just to drive Al Qaeda crazy, to flaunt the First Amendment™ in their face, monitor the Internet traffic, especially the long visits, from the Middle East. Perhaps to show that within the Palestinian Authority or what remained of it there were slacker proto-suicide bombers slobbering over their culture's demise. The site has stories too, breathless accounts of hand jobs in the camel train, supposedly translated from the "Original Arabic," both words Capitalized. One tale that mixed sex and violence mentioned this guy called Tarik Noor. Jack wondered about Carnivore, he'd heard of it, some monster which monitored everyone's surfing. And didn't every keystroke leave a ghost on the hard drive, that couldn't be erased, no matter how you de-magnetized, no matter which landfill you dumped the shit into? If these rumors were true then the die was cast. Might as well re-read the story, feel the Paxil slip away.

It was a fantasy of warriors on horses with scabbards, riding through flamenco lands defiling any maiden in their way. It was pure revenge, something about the rip-off of the abacus, the looting of some library in Alexandria, conversions by the sword and now this. The meat-swords were described in some detail, their movements in and out -- Jack was drawn in, felt Arab, felt this listlessness morph hard as a rock. Maybe it was these pills that made Ehrenreich an idiot. Jack'd wean himself off. To lose the ability to pleasure yourself was the ultimate fuck. They won't take me alive: Jack blurred John Dillinger with this Tarik Noor, wondered about myrrh and frankincense, thought back to Star Wars, spilled his seed on the dull hardwood floor. Jihad, he thought, remembering that word from the rap music downstairs. Holy mother fucking war. The world revolved around a Hole and he wouldn't fall in, not him. He wiped the floor and himself with toilet paper, lit a smoke and dialed Charlotte. His next call'd be the New York Post.

* * *

George had left Kinkos and his last name was Wilson. Micah pled his case to Kinkos' H.R. -- he needed to depose Mr. Wilson for an upcoming trial, did they know his home address or at least his new employer. We protect our employees' privacy, was their rote response. Even our ex-employees. Micah spun some mumbo-jumbo about subpoenas and obstruction of justice and voilà: George now worked for Megalopolis Messenger Service in midtown. Micah hung up without saying thank you. Have a good old bureaucratic day.

The dispatcher at Mega -- that's what he called it -- asked what it was about, whether Mr. Wilson had some trouble with the law. No, no, Micah said quickly. Getting George to recant would be Jack's only way out. To get him in trouble before they even spoke wouldn't help.

"Tell you want," said Micah. "I have a pick-up, it's very important, I want George Wilson to come get it, I'll pay your company double and give him a tip."

"Sounds pretty fucking fishy to me," the dispatcher said. Maybe he thought drugs. Maybe he thought male prostitution.

"I'll pay double," Micah repeated, offering his credit card number. These sixteen digits spoke. Micah sat back to wait. He wondered idly if Empi or the D.A.'s office had gotten the George a new job, to lock his testimony in. But messenger was still the bottom rung of the ladder. For a lousy thirty bucks Mega was breaking its own rules. This wasn't a no-show job like Clinton gave his Little Rock pals. Warren Hubble, like the telescope. He thought about Bertha and his sick sense of humor.

George was on the crosstown bus when his Nextel went off. Some lawyer in The Bronx wanted a pick-up, forget the architect's drawings he was holding and head uptown. It was weird but what the fuck. They'd given him an unlimited MetroCard so the city was his. He took the Five train and walked toward Lincoln Hospital.

He looked like a kid, Micah thought -- maybe some lead in his childhood diet. But that wasn't the point. Micah shook his hand vigorously, had his secretary bring him any soda he wanted.

"Really?" George said. "Usually I just pick up--"

"Really," said Micah. "I'd offer you a beer but then I'd need to see I.D."

George smirked. He was old enough to drink, had been for two and a half years now. Maybe he should pump iron or get a tattoo. Wear a doo-rag and smoke Philly Blunts. He was an Afrikan prepster and he always faced this shit. "Code Red," he said. "It's a kind of soda."

"It's red Mountain Dew," his secretary added. "My son drinks that stuff like it was water."

"Sit down," Micah said. "I want to be up-front."

That'd be a first, thought George. When the customers offered you soda and beer they had shit on their minds. It was true for a messenger as it had been at Kinkos. Usually he entered faceless Manhattan office buildings through the service entrance, the separate windows for the youth of color with their wrist-thick bike chains and their carry-bags slung over their necks. Two bikers got hit by cars last week and the company fired them the same day. Worker's comp? Get the fuck out of here. George took the train and watched his back.

"I'm a lawyer--"

"I can tell--"

"And I represent a man named Jack Bender."

So that was it. George remembered the night, the white lady and the burping brother with his forms to sign. He'd gotten a summons, certified mail with the promise of a witness fee, especially if he'd meet with some Tsai guy next week.

"Do you remember--"

"Sure," George said. "It's like I told 'em -- it could be the guy, maybe not, probably is. They showed me a photo and I thought I recognized it."

Micah nodded, smiled, waited while his secretary came in and poured the bright red soda into a Brooklyn Law coffee mug. "Go ahead and drink," Micah said. "You must be thirsty."

George was thinking of truth serum as he kicked the Code Red back. He wasn't lying then and he wasn't lying now. How the fuck should he remember? The secretary left.

"We just want you to tell the truth," Micah said. "Has the District Attorney asked to see you before the trial?"

George put the mug down. "They sent me a letter, I had to go to the post office to sign for it."

"A summons."

"Yeah. That. They said they'll pay me witness fees. I'm supposed to go talk to 'em next week. I don't know what Mega will say about that."

If the kid didn't testify that'd be best, Micah thought. They'd call the affidavit the best evidence, but it was easier to try to shoot down a stationary target than a moving one. "Are you going to go?"

"I guess I got to."

"Okay then. If you weren't totally sure then, that's all you have to tell the court. Just the way you told me."

"The guy came in later."

Micah remembered. Loose cannon Jack. They had to get this straight. "Be sure to say that. Like, if you recognize him, it might be because he came in later."

"In the letter they sent me the photograph again. A better one this time."

Slick fucks, Micah thought. That was suggestive but probably not illegal. Maybe Jack should shave his head like Aryan Nations and screw the whole thing up. "Be sure to say that on the stand, too. What I want you to understand is that it's the District Attorney, not Jack, who's making you go to court. You understand that, right?"

George nodded. Sure the white man would rather he didn't go. Was there money being offered?

"So first the district attorney will question you. He'll ask you to point at Jack, he'll be in the courtroom, he'll try to make you sure you were totally sure. All I'm asking is that whatever doubts you had, whatever doubts you have now, you say them. Can you do that?"

It sounded like Mister Rogers' Neighborhood, like some kid's TV show, talking down to him like he thought he was dumb. "I think I can handle it," George said.

"Then they'll ask if I have questions. I might have some, depending on how the first part went. It might feel like I'm trying to trick you -- I want you to know now, it's just my job, I'm trying to help Jack, trying to make the truth come out. It's just--" Micah pauses to think -- "a game. Except for Jack it has high stakes."

"That it?" George asked. The soda was finished and he'd had his fill of condescension.

"You're busy, I'm sure."

"Yeah."

Micah handed him two twenty dollar bills. "Since I slowed you down."

George pocketed them. There were a couple CDs he'd been wanting to have. "I thought you had a package," George said.

"No, this is more important. After you speak with the district attorney, if you have any questions, any at all, you can call me. Will you do that?"

If you pay me forty bucks, George thought. "I might. Well I gotta go."

They were street-vending bootlegs by the train at Third Avenue. George burned a twenty on a video and three CDs. Maybe he would call this Mister Rogers again, ask for sixty this time. Kinkos withheld his last check but he'd make it back now.

36. Bea Pissed-Off

Zalie was really counting on him now -- he'd even said the word Mexico, talking about horses and waves you could body-surf, how it was better than Disney World but not to tell her momma nothing, it was just their secret, just between them. Diane wasn't as much of a bitch as usual; he'd paid her a child support in advance this time, for just this purpose. He needed to hear those words, not guilty. Or to hear no words at all.

Jack read the Post, on the can or on the train, even the sassy business section. They had a page called Bull's Eye™ that made fun of business. This was like the right "john-ruh," the word they used at SUNY. Last year they'd skewered a SUNY Oswego graduate, that's why he remembered it: the bookkeeper for WorldCom, hid four billion bucks and built a mansion in the Florida Keys before taking the Fifth. The Post had a column called Winners and Losers -- WorldCom moved from one to the other -- and there's where he wanted Janet's tale.

The bitch was called Beatrice Piskoff and she wasn't hard to reach. She was looking for losers and that's when Jack called. He told about the repo-ed SUV with the baby on board, the stupid yellow sign suction-cupped to the back window even said that but Janet'd paid no mind. "I got photos," Jack said. "Of when they brought the baby back."

Beatrice Piskoff -- "Bea" to her friends, who were few -- liked the sound of this fuck-up. It wouldn't fit in a sidebar, what with the photos. It might get her out of Business and onto Page Six. "Can you messenger them down?"

"I can do better," Jack said, happy to say this. "I got 'em developed like on a CD-Rom. I can e-mail them to ya." She gave her address -- losers@nypost.com and sat back to wait. This was like something from the Eighties,™ stealing a baby to collect on a debt. Some movie called "Tin Men," very Southern like the guy who'd called. It beeped with the mail arrived and there they were: shot after shot of a blonde lady holding a baby, a darker lady crying and grabbing it, two cops staring at their feet then an empty front yard. What it proved she wasn't sure. Nothing in the photos said Empi. And the Post *liked* Sandy Vyle, as a trash-talking New York success story. They liked to trash Ivy League MBAs from Houston. Still this story was too good. She blew up the pictures in her PhotoShop program, bigger and bigger until she could barely make out the names on the cops' shields. This was her back-up, the thin blue line like a vein on-- she dialed Lena Jones.

She should work in the White House, Lena thought -- if it wasn't cooked books it was stolen babies, it was gunshots in some loser's home, it was wife beating Internet crusaders brought low by Polaroids. This time the photos cut the other way. Piskoff said she had pictures, it was comic, really, they brought the baby back. But she wanted a quote.

"I really doubt this happened," Lena said. "But give me a day I'll find out."

"Bulls Eye moves faster," Piskoff said.

Loser, thought Lena. This Bronx office must really be a piece of crap. First the bed loan, then Nicole Nour's exposé of the Guzmans' rip-off. Now this. They'd fired that jackass from Charlotte but things just kept getting worse. She'd call Baltimore first to try to find a *homo sapiens* to speak with.

* * *

Mudnick had to laugh. West Farms was in his region; it was giving him jokes that made him the toast of the Club Chuck, almost got him laid last week and maybe this one would.

"Protocol is to check the interior of the vehicle before towing it," Mudnick told Lena. "But I'll check with those bozos and get back to you. You think they're really gonna run this story?"

"Wouldn't you?"

He had to admit he would. Even the forex yuppies in the Club Chuck read the Post, delivered like junk food to every train station between New York and DC. They loved a scandal, whether the Saudis paying death benefits to the families of suicide bombers or some shit about a baby stolen by the biggest bank on earth. "I'll call West Farms," Mudnick said. Emerging Markets was looking better all the time. They probably didn't even *return* the babies there. And any journalist who reported on it would be shot. Nice work if you can get it. And Mudnick would.

Janet'd been sitting on her humiliation like hemorrhoids. Grin and bear it, it'll pass. The Cracker snapped photos, then some washed-out guy who coulda been his dad. WatchCorp was dead -- she checked it daily -- and how else would that loser get the news out? Anyway Jack'd signed a contract not to disparage Empi. So Janet told no one. Her work load had doubled since Gina'd disappeared. Sure she had sick days but she was like a deserter. She'd called Gina's home but heard only curse words from the drunken dago. These were personal days, then. Maybe Gina's had an affair, or caught that gigolo who eyed even her up and down.

The e-mail from Mudnick put Janet on edge. It was short and on Monstro but it didn't bode well. "Need to talk about a repo. Call me asap." This would remain in Monstro. There was no turning back.

"I think I know what this is about," Janet began. Always better to disarm them, start with admission, blame it on the hired help. "I want you to know that we're changing car-tow contractors."

"The baby -- that's true?"

Janet sighed. "It happened. They didn't check the car and as soon as we saw--"

"Didn't *you* check it?"

"I was taping the notice. The way we do it here, it's the towers who do the check."

The captain goes down with her ship, Mudnick thought. "The press office says they have photos."

That Cracker bastard. "It's the same guy, Bender. He's been following me around. He got lucky that day."

"Don't you have an order of protection?"

"Yeah. When I told the cops they made him leave. But he got this other guy to continue. He stood across the street and the cops said so what. He signed a non-disparagement--"

This Bender was recruiting an army, Mudnick thought. "You got the cops' names?"

She had. She might screw up once but generally she was organized. The cops about the fax had been assholes. But to have their names was better than not. She told Mudnick, asked if she should call.

"Executive office is handling everything." He paused. "They're not going to like this, Janet."

"You think I do?" This bland prick -- she'd driven him to Penn Station, he probably didn't even tell them how good she did in Yonkers.

"Let's hope it blows over," Mudnick said and hung up.

* * *

Rudehart wasn't going to like this. Lena'd gotten him on the cover of Newsweek when he first joined Empi's army, something about the three white men who saved the world. Alan Greenspan looking like a cartoon; Larry Summers -- they called him Springtime there -- fat like a walrus, and Robert Rudehart, thin, trim and making fifty times more than either of them. How soon they forget. Now Lena was the messenger of bad news and she knew it.

"We got another P.O.S.," she said, standing in front of his desk, he didn't bother to ask her to sit. It was short for Piece of Shit, it was their juvenile shorthand but Rudehart didn't smile. She explained the photos and Baltimore's confirmation.

"Those fucking zeroes," Rudehart said. "Can't they go a week without making us look bad?"

"Baltimore says that Jack Bender was involved, remember him?"

Rudehart did. Of course he did -- Chuck was supposed to be handling this. This one dumpy good ole boy was kicking them drunkenly in the balls every day. It had to stop. "The Post loves us. It's Bea Pissed-Off, right?"

Lena nodded. Even Rudehart read the Post, to see his name in the Sightings™ squibs on Page Six, dining at the Four Seasons, signing a book contract, traveling on the U.S. Air shuttle without even bodyguards (they hadn't noticed Chuck).

"That Bulls Eye page is independent, more than the Journal," Rudehart said. "Bunch of gossip columnists who don't understand business. But I'll try." He paused. "Sometimes I think we're not playing the press right over here." He let his words sink in. Token flacks were a dime a dozen. They could bring Howard Rubenstein in-house and read nothing but Carnegie Hall all summer. "For now, give her the dirt on Bender. Tell her we'll give her the scoop on something else. Sandy's daughter's wedding, Jaime Dimwit's peccadilloes, whatever it takes. Fuck!"

* * *

So her source was a loser -- so what? It took one to know one. Piskoff fought with her editors, ending up winning by showing the photos. They could play this as a whole page spread on pages 4 and 5, even get the cover on a slow news day, if no bombs went off in Tel Aviv, no quote from Bloomberg about smoking pot. "Baby Snatchers!" wouldn't be a bad headline, though it lacked the Post's trademark poetics. "Empi Cradle" was closer, but still no headless body in topless bar. That was the grail to which they aspired. It had been decades and it had still not been topped.

Piskoff didn't speak of the cops' pervasive silence. Even with the badge numbers, even with the names, even with all that the Post had done for New York's Finest™ since they lost 23 in the Towers' fall, the baby was a dead-end. "No charges were filed," was all they would say. She e-mailed back to this shutter-bug Jackal and let him think it wouldn't run -- always the best way to get more info from a source, she'd found -- and asked for the name of the babyless lady.

Jack had seen Micah fail with Mrs. Peña; now his leverage would be lost when she blew off the Post. "That's not important, is it?" Jack asked desperately, rhetorically they called it in his English class at Oswego. "I mean you got the photos."

"It's got to be confirmed. And we need the wah-wah quote to close it."

Jack told her of Mrs. Peña, and that Empi'd cancelled her loan. "They bought her fucking silence," Jack said, wishing they'd do the same with him. What could it take? How many times did he have to tag these mother fuckers before they just dropped the charges and paid him some walking around money? He thought about the skinny guy who'd walked across the country for cancer. There was wackos in this world but he wasn't one. He just did what he had to do. He thought of Zalie. "I could take it to the News," Jack finally said. You had to talk these people's language.

Drawling schemer, Piskoff thought. "I'll call the lady and see what she says. It's been a pleasure." She hung up.

* * *

Rochester was a ruse, Nicole had been thinking. Swanker's hang-up had been transparent like the markets were supposed to be. He'd let Empi go and she didn't know why. But she had Bain dead to rights and a nice SEC story. No censor in the Hamptons would stop her on this one. The batterer? They could shoot him for all she cared. Only in America.

There was one final piece that she'd like to nail down: where did Bain get the tip from? If from Swanker there'd be no way to prove it. But he clearly had a source in Empi's Executive Office. He'd known about her call to Lena. Well let him know this one.

"Will you leave us *alone*?" Lena began. Did the Journal have the baby-grab fuck-up too? It wasn't their style. Just nothing more she'd have to take to Rudehart, that's what Lena was hoping.

"This story's not mostly about Empi, necessarily," Nicole said. "The SEC is looking into a firm that shorted your stock around my Swanker update. The trader's name is Tom Bain--"

"He *covers* our stock, doesn't he?" She saw the guy at every briefing on the quarterly earnings, vaguely remembered some stupid question he'd asked at SIA.

"Yeah he always says buy, but then he sold you short. The SEC's all over it. I have two questions. One, I'm trying to nail down who tipped him--"

Fat chance, Lena thought. I'm not touching that one with a ten foot mole.

"And two, I need a quote about Swanker's investigation."

Dead in the water, Lena knew. She could spin some horseshit about Empi's respect for the honorable Attorney General of the State of New York, and his heroic campaign to keep the markets clean for everyone. She did.

"Is it live or not?" Nicole demanded.

"I think you'll find we've been exonerated, that everything checked out. Mistakes occur, like that Guzman thing --" she was thinking of the baby stories which she hoped Rudehart could get the Post to bury -- "but on balance we are a leader in the consumer finance industry, the lodestar of compliance to which all our competitors aspires." Damn I still have it, Lena thought.

Get a job at Hallmark, thought Nicole. "Heard anything about Swanker and Rochester?" There was no reason not to fish. A reporter's main asset was her source, and working at the Journal they always took your call.

Lena thought of Basso, the squeeze play Rudehart proudly told. Was that what Nicole meant? "Nothing comes to mind," Lena said. "But he'll attack market fixing wherever he finds it."

Definitely Swanker's investigation of Empi was dead, Nicole realized. This praise was as thick as the honey on the baklava in the AUC snack bar.

"It's been most illuminating," Nicole good-byed.

Fuck you too, Lena thought. The life of a flack was mostly shit.

37. The Inverse Floater

The Five train from Co-op City to Manhattan was laughably slow. Gina got a seat thank God and she studied the textbook on her knees, Solomon's and Meyer's NASD Exam Book. Options still befuddled her, no matter how much she prayed in her Planner, made this the Big Rock™ task on which she would focus. Bonds, commodities, the double-talk ethics on churning and money laundering, all this she got. Options were a bitch: equity open interest, today's topic, was like Chinese or Arabic, some language she didn't understand. But she would.

The train was elevated. She looked up at Tremont, thrown left by the curve in the tracks into the sleeveless Jamaican next to her. He had on a WalkMan. She heard dirty lyrics, toasting they called it, "Murderah" was all she knew. The guy smiled at her and she looked back at the book. Vinnies came in many hues. She would not be sidetracked. She'd left her car in the Comfort Inn lot since the parking by Ground Zero was ridiculous. Train full of Vinnies but she would prevail.

They passed 174th Street and the West Farms Mall. Gina stared down at it, Janet's car in the lot and the gate already up though it was still before eight. They must be freaking out about something. Gina no longer cared. If she passed the Series Seven she'd make it her business to find Tom Bain's boss, make a pitch to stay at the firm whatever happened to him. Self-reliance was one of Cubby's touchstones, unless you had a partner you could trust which she didn't. They passed Freeman Street, the cinder block row houses extending to Intervale; they took the hairpin turn at Simpson, judo and check cashers. No more low-ball finance, Gina vowed. Options and stocks; pork bellies and inverse floaters. She loved these terms like an incantation. The train went underground and her eyes glazed over.

The crash course was in a faded and now fated hotel in West Street, three blocks from Ground Zero and three-fifths vacant. In the conference room were rows of long narrow tables, her classmates already here, sucking cheap mints and doodling on the table cloths with the water pitchers' sweat. She'd meant to buy the papers but'd had to run from Bowling Green. The instructor was tuning his PowerPoint up. It began as fate would have it with just the information that she'd sought.

"Equity open interest is the total number of options contracts not yet exercised or allowed to expire." She was writing that down, repeating the duality to herself, the double E mnemonic -- "exercised or expired" -- when the next slide came: "It is seen as an indicator of longer-term interest in these instruments." She loved this mumbo-jumbo, felt like a doctor getting to know her instruments, scalpels and saxophones, cymbals and symbols and ticker-tape hypnosis. Was credit insurance on a bed an *instrument*? If so it was like a hacksaw, a pair of brass knuckles, a contra-bass kazoo. Bertha Watkins was a commodity -- she snickered at that -- bouncing on the bed that first day in Sicilian Furniture. Only that crap had now brought her here, prepping for Series Seven on Bain's firm's dime. She said grace, unwrapped a mint and glanced at the cover of the Post on the seat next to her.

"Empi Cradle!" the headline screamed. The page was cut in half, a plane crash in the Philippines getting its due as well. But she recognized the blonde wench -- Janet, on the cover of the Post! "Do you mind?" she asked the nerd larvae two seats down, not waiting for an answer.

The spread on 4 and 5 was more pictures than words. But it nailed Janet Peel by name -- just like the Journal'd done to her, Gina thought -- and quoted Empi's flack to the effect that mistakes will happen. The PowerPoint slides were a blur, equity options volumes for the last five years flashing by as in a dream. Let 'em find a new branch manager, Gina thought. She wanted to serve youth -- at least the kids of those with disposable income -- not steal them in their SUVs. She wondered if the Journal had this story as well. They had no photos so maybe not. She picked up the nerd's three-part copy -- the guy was a walking newsstand, probably had Barrons in his briefcase along with his cheat sheet -- and flipped to the Index of Companies. Empigroup -- B4, it said. She opened the section, found an article by Nour that confirmed what Tom said and said more.

"The trader, Thomas B. Bain, responded with an obscenity. SEC sources last night indicated that the timing of his trades are strongly indicative of his use of non-public information for profit. 'It's classic insider trading,' said John F. Latte of Columbia University's business school, who has written two textbooks on the topic."

She had Bain by the balls, Gina saw. The timing of trades made for probable cause -- this was right in her study aid -- but they'd need to show the insider scoop he'd traded on, and how he got it. I'm right here, Gina felt, feeling her Power. She glanced at the drones and the slides and stood up. Nobody cared. The classes were paid in advance. She went out into the empty red-rugged lobby and dialed Bain's number. Per diem no more, she thought. And about that ringer...

Bain had gotten reamed, in a call to his house before the sun was even up. The contents of Nour's story were no surprise. "But what did we tell you -- all inquiries are referred to the press office!" That the bird was his quote was Nicole's little trick. Bain felt sick in the shower, and sicker still here by the ticker, reading Bloomberg News' recap, grafs filled in with further quotes, "another black eye for Wall Street," that stupid Latte spewed. His fate would be decided today. If he went down he'd burn the whole Equities desk. He wondered if Elizabeth had read this, some e-mail forwarded by a Greenwich day-trader, her old boyfriend become symbol for a day. She's always said that he lacked for ethics. Now he'd proved it, or had it proved.

He took Gina's call while he thought of all this. "We need to talk," she said.

"Aren't you in class?"

"This is more important. You saw the Journal--"

No I'm fucking illiterate, Bain thought. At the first sniff of blood all the vultures swooped in. He thought of those hunting birds, falcons, that the Arabs jammed hoods on and trained for the kill. They tried to cut your arm but wearing pads made it okay. "I could use a drink," Bain said. "You want me to meet you downtown?"

"I'll come there," Gina said. It'd be more convenient to talk to Bain's boss or threaten to. This was the day for the options contracts to be exercised. Use it or lose it: it was true of all instruments. She'd take a taxi. She could afford it; this profit was as good as booked. She'd write in her Planner in the cab ride uptown.

* * *

Parked on the shoulder of West Street was an El Camino, the miniature pick-up truck that all the test fuel junkies loved to collect. In the driver's seat was Vinny. Tony rode shotgun. Tony'd trailed Gina from the Comfort Inn to here the day before. Stupid cunt wrote her stupid instructions on the cheap stationary of the cheap hotel. The Post lay unread on the backseat's floor. On Broadway Nigerians from Fort Lee sold thesaurus and Black Power books from the back of a windowless van.

"There she is!" Tony yelled. But Vinny'd already seen. He followed the yellow cab past the Chelsea Piers, east past the Javits, the hookers sick in late-morning light, on the ramps through Grand Central and up Park Avenue. He double parked by a Con Ed truck and watched. His delicious filly dialed her phone, appeared to argue. He'd like to get closer but she knew the car. It stood out like the Beverly Hillbillies in this get-over canyon. She stood by a white marble waterless fountain.

"That's the guy," Tony said.

Bain had talked her out of coming upstairs -- "I need a drink, remember?" he'd said, then simply ordered her to wait, saying the walls had ears -- and on the way down in the elevator he'd considered his options. Everyone knew now. Even from the building's other floors, people got on and smirked at him. At least I had the balls to flip her the bird, Bain thought. He stepped onto Park Avenue with a sense of foreboding. That Arab bitch had fucked him and now the Habits girl from Greenwich would do the same. Which way did her ambition cut? Silence or squeal?

Vinny powered the El Camino forward, burning some rubber like a Mob hit or something. He left the car running, charged around the wide sidewalk toward Gina and her fruit. Tony stayed in the car with the back-up. Thirty eight caliber with the serial number filed off.

Bain saw the workman approach -- it was beyond on-the-clock, he thought, some ceiling tiles must have cut a T-1 line or something. But the guy was looking at him. Gina saw his look of concern grow and turned back. "Vinny!" she yelled. "Vinny get the fuck out of here!"

Vinny ignored her. His beef was not with her -- it had been *inside* her, Goddamn it, and still would be except for this Brooks Brothers Svengali. Vinny had rolled a pipe up in the New York Post and now he swung it at the yuppie's face, the crowd pulling back and no cops in sight. Tony'd changed seats -- that was the plan and even he could unnerstand it: they could be on the FDR Drive in three minutes, take the 59th to Queens on continue uptown depending.

Bain ducked and felt his shoulder break. It was like a baseball bat; his hand went numb. "Vinny you stupid fuck," Gina yelled. Bain fell to the sidewalk -- safer this way he thought through the pain, as if it were a choice -- and Vinny stood over him. "You leave my girl alone," Vinny said, spacing the words nice and slow, sensing the crowd drawing back in, knowing it was time to go. Shatter a knee cap? He'd wanted the face but the way the guy was holding his shoulder he wouldn't be strumming nookie for a good long time. Not Gina's anyway.

"C'mon," Vinny said to Gina. "This pussy don't deserve you." He grabbed her arm but she pulled away.

"You're pathetic," she said. This was Options Day and this deadweight lug was screwing it all up. She looked at Bain on the ground, crying he was, she felt contempt and empathy, all mixed -- Vinny could kill him, Tony probably had a gun and could be coming.

"We'll turn you in," Gina said. This would be the second of Vinny's three strikes and it focused his mind. Hers, he figured, would realize through time that two pussies together are less than zero.

"C'mon!" Tony yelled from the car. "I ain't gettin' arrested for this shit!"

Vinny jogged to the car, looking at the fruity glass towers that blocked out the sun, happy to hear no sirens coming, just the suit-and-tie crowd shocked like a mother fucker. "Let that be a lesson to you" was a line he'd heard but that wasn't his style. "I'll do you again, pussy," he shouted at the supine Bain. The same applied to Gina. Vinny wouldn't wear the horns for no one. Tony pulled away from the curb with Vinny's door still open.

"Fuck yeah!" Vinny screamed as they burned the light on Lexington. Ahead was the FDR, the open road to the big bad Bronx. He dropped the pipe on the floor, let the pages of the Post flap crazily out the window.

"You broke that fucker's arm," Tony said flatly.

"I shoulda stomped his balls."

They crossed on the Willis and headed to Gino's in Allerton. Fuckers made a mean pork chop. They could stash the El Camino for a few days and then lie low. The bitch would come back, Vinny was sure. They always did.

38. The Poster Child

The rent-a-cops were strutting and clucking like chickens. Their radios squawked too. By the time the real McCoys showed up, Gina'd told Bain she'd explain it all later. No names for now. The press always screwed things up.

There were two dozen witnesses but no one saw the plate. "I think it's called El Camino," Gina offered cagily. "But I didn't catch the color. Something dark."

Bain's arm was throbbing. Through the haze he'd seen the guy in the car, with his "c'mon the cops are coming." It was the guy from the sidewalk café in the Bronx, the double-skank Tony. The animal who'd hit him was Vinny, then. He had no last name and that wasn't the point anyway. He could amend his complaint when the pain killers took hold. Gina rode with him in the ambulance, clutching her Franklin Planner like a pipe, he thought. These gutter whores were plain bad news. They could take the Series Seven but still their pimps would hold them back.

"It's separated," the Pakistani doctor told him. Maybe Indian, Sing with an h. "Get ready." The sawbones pushed up and Bain's mind caught fire, like an electric fuse box that sparked and clicked and smoldered all at once. Bain felt a pop, bones grating on nerves like a shredder gone wild, pain like lightening right down to his middle finger. I'll never flip the bird again, he thought, insane jokes through the agony, begging for morphine, settling for Celebrex.™

"Do I stay overnight?" he asked.

"No reason. You still gotta fill out the insurance forms."

Bain's firm had MetLife, let 'em pay. Gina did the paperwork, grateful somehow that Bain hadn't fingered Vinny.

"Where do you wanna go?" she asked as they stood in the Discharge line. "We still need to talk."

Park Avenue was out. "Do you think they're still following us?" Bain asked. If he saw that white trash pickup truck outside he'd call the cops, whatever she said. She'd led them to him. But she hadn't fled. This Gina knew her Options, better perhaps than he did.

"They're long gone," Gina said. She could imagine them now, chowing down at Gino's, laughing at the powder puff they thought she fucked. What they didn't know was that Vulnerability™ was okay. A sucker-punch with a pipe in a paper didn't make you a man. She had Bain by the balls and it was kind of cute, the way his eye balls rolled on Celebrex. "I'll take you home," she said. "I'll tuck you in and we'll figure it out."

But didn't she live with that Vinny, Bain thought through the haze. Maybe he should call the cop over, blow the whistle on this gutter rat trio. "I don't wanna go to The Bronx," he mumbled. "*Your* home, silly," Gina said. She'd never called Vinny that, but on Bain it fit. "I'll call us a cab and we'll go."

Maybe they were going to rob him. Maybe they'd switched cars and would use the service elevator of his condo and rip off his Blaupunkt speakers, steal his computer password and make a day of it. Still he needed this Gina, he needed her silence. The rent-a-cops must have told his bosses he'd been waylaid on the sidewalk in front. It was still afternoon and he wanted to hide. "Fine," he told her.

The cab stop-and-started down Broadway, the streets more demonic now, the city not his. He felt her hand on his thigh, not sleaze but chaste, precise like a poem by Emily Dickinson. He closed his eyes.

* * *

Swanker surfed to the now-dead WatchCorp, found the founder's telephone number: it was 718 like his home in Riverdale but probably not like it at all. The nanny extorter was a lowly practitioner of domestic violence. Why call this Candida Azuela since he could hit the guy direct with his knowledge, describing the photo and the things that might happen? If the guy had any pride, Swanker was free. He could normalize the paperwork for Milly or could just cut her loose. She'd rebuffed him in the car so it'd serve her right. Like his father had said -- he remembered one time when a grand jury had voted not to indict on an arson charge -- you just have to start over. Leave a scorched earth behind. In this case not some run-down buildings with half-assed tenants who wouldn't pay rent, but Basso in Rochester, Milly the turn-coat maid, and most of all this WatchCorp moralizer, this batterer with a web site, this private attorney general who thought he had Swanker's balls in his hands. He was wrong. These gonads were already spoken for.

* * *

Kurt in the basement was groping, not flesh but his soul, not Milly but her mind, not yet the future but the past. "Forget the coffee," he said. "I need to ask you something."

Milly'd come down to deliver some news but it could wait. "What about?"

How to put it? He wanted her story not his. "Uh, don't take this wrong, but I wonder if you think that a woman if she's hit should call the cops, if she should ever..." Kurt's voice trailed off and Milly thought she understood. The day of the gun, that Latina girl -- she looked South

American, that much Milly had made out through the half-light -- probably Kurt had hit her.

"I don't make rules," Milly said. "Every couple is different, that's what my mother always says."

"But Amado, has he ever--"

This bothered Milly but given the news, why not. "Yes he hit me. Only once -- after that I told him I would leave him if again it happened. He's thrown plates, one time he broke the barbecue in the back yard with a baseball bat. But never has he hit me again. Like I said, every couple is different."

Kurt considered this, tried to picture Amado smashing the Mexican crock pots upstairs, his chance of losing Milly -- Kurt remembered his sick idyll dream with this woman, considered making a play even, saw he had no chance. He needed to talk to someone and no one else had come to mind. It felt like a confessional, this basement with a phone line and a broken computer, the fold-up cot in the back. His life had come to this for now.

"If a woman's abused, I mean really abused, how far do you think she could go to get revenge?"

The kid was scared, Milly thought. The South *Americana* had brought a gunman but perhaps it wasn't over. He'd brought trouble to their house, more than EmpiBank perhaps. But soon it would be over. She'd answer the question then give him the news.

"The abuse, it depends how serious it was."

"Very serious," Kurt said.

Had he raped her, Milly wondered. He'd always acted sweet but with men you never knew. When the phone rang she took the chance to go upstairs, on the pretext of coffee.

"Yeah, WatchCorp--"

"Look you little bastard, I *know* what you did to Candida Azuela, I got the pictures right here in front of me."

Kurt's mind reeled -- at first he thought Empi then the voice's rhythms made it clear: Swanker. Milly should have been down here, so she could use the leverage of the nanny threat, not him.

"That's none of your business," Kurt said, hearing the pathetic defensiveness before the phrase was done.

"Yeah just like my contract with Milagros Guzman. Just like my conversations on the terrace of my home -- they're all confidential and I'll have you know, I could make you the poster boy of domestic violence, string you up by your balls and your own cowardice."

To note a mixed metaphor was worth precisely nothing. Kurt wondered if he cared, about being exposed -- it wasn't that, but jail he couldn't stomach. Had Candida gone to Swanker, even after she sent him to Queens? The more obvious link was Empi. They'd killed the Journal's story and now they were closing the loop. "So Empi handles all your problems," Kurt said, trying to regain control, wondering what options he had, seeing: none.

"A photo is a photo," Swanker said. "And you should be aware that they can bring D.V. prosecutions without the victim's cooperation. I don't even have to talk to Candida Azuela unless I want to. It's a crime against society, a crime against a whole gender."

Kurt's mind went back to a euphemism Milly'd used: Swanker'd driven her to Broadway and he'd tried... to drive her home. "*You're* the lecherous fuck," Kurt said. "You rip off Milagros Guzman and try to feel her up on the side." Kurt wondered if he'd gotten any. No. It couldn't be.

Swanker thought of the pols who'd gone down on this rap. Senile Bob Packwood, pressing himself on his secretaries and keeping a *diary*, the stupid fuck. But Clinton'd survived the blow job and Teddy Kennedy was a florid face of nature. No reason to let on. "You can stew in your own sleaze all you want," Swanker said. "If I so much as catch wind of you taking any of this to the press, or even your bullshit web site, I'll have you indicted as a batterer. You got me?" He'd seen his father do it, seen one crusader after another give up and fold. Reporters from the Village Voice, the head of the state's housing department, even the Bronx D.A.. This Kurt was a nobody and he had the photo.

"I'm taking that as a yes," Swanker said and hung up.

"Milly!" It was the kid calling her from the stairway. She'd put the water on to boil but wasn't going down again.

"*Estoy haciendo café*," she called down. "*Subete si quires hablar.*"

Kurt came into the kitchen, lighting a smoke like she'd asked that he not. He was no one to be afraid of. But to bring bullets to this house, that could not continue.

"The thing I asked about revenge, I was serious. If the woman struck back, or someone did it for her, do you think that'd be wrong?"

"Are you afraid?" Milly asked.

"Yes," Kurt said. He was sick and he was angry but he was also afraid.

It was time. "Look, I needed to tell you -- Marcos is coming home from the Army, they give him time off. We thought he would go to see my mother, his *abuelita*, in Tijuana. But he come in to east coast, he will come here. He will need the basement to live in, like we said before...".

Kurt nodded, numb. "When does he arrive?"

"Tomorrow," Milly said, trying to dress this lack of notice up. "We thought *Los An-hell-es*, Tijuana, west coast. But he will be here. We will move a second cot down, but...".

"I understand," Kurt said, more afraid now than before, seeing his actions before he would do them, seeing the future but only short term.

* * *

Jack bought ten copies of the Post at the newsstand on Fordham, gave them out to his boys at HomeQuik. "This," he announced, "is how you fuck yourself royally." He slapped Ehrenreich on his lizard-like back, pointed out the photo credit, which the Post had magnanimously given him. "They should pay you for that shit," Jack said. "You're a fucking photojournalist."

Ehrenreich felt calm, chemically calm, but nonetheless was nervous. "Empi is bigger than us," he stated the obvious. "If they dig into our loans they could find problems too."

"But the Post doesn't give a *shit* about HomeQuik, don't you get it?" The hook here was Sandy Vyle, the chance to put him in the Loser of the Week sidebar, if only this week, if soon to return to winner when he bought a new bank.

"Be sure to check the cars before you tow," Ehrenreich instructed Jack's Boys, fumbling in his desk for the antidote to this Generalized Anxiety.™

Down North, Jack thought. Bubba-land in The Bronx. He had to call Micah and see how this could help.

Micah read the Post, of course he did -- his clients from Lincoln Hospital brought it or the Daily News in with them, unread and rolled up and sweaty, the waiting room prop. Usually only the back sports page was visible but Empi Cradle, even his secretary had seen that this was relevant, left scroll unrolled on his desk when he arrived. So even without Mrs. Peña's consent they'd run it. He wondered if she could sue for invasion of privacy -- but no. The photos were taken in the public street, the Athenian agora of that false Levittown. There must be a police report; it was fair game. It could be an exhibit to a debt collections lawsuit. But how it helped the Cracker, if at all, was unclear. It didn't even mention him by name. Just "a source who calls himself The Jackal." The Post loved this cloak and dagger shit, even when it made no sense. Jack could have gone on the record. What did he have to lose now?

The Cracker, the Jackal, whatever one called him he showed up at Micah's at noon with a stack of the Post. "They're fucking going *down*," he said too loud. Micah closed the door once he came in.

"Nice move," Micah said -- he couldn't quite peg this Cracker who wheedled a story when WatchCorp Kurt couldn't, even with a bullet. "But don't get overconfident. And when you're in the court at trial don't gloat." Micah wanted Jack to come off as a slow Southern fuck who got caught up in the terrorism hype like a turtle in a tuna net. One of those endangered species. The problem was there'd be no jury: the terrorism charge assured that. He was lucky the venue wasn't changed to a Navy destroyer offshore, or to the remains of the camp on Guantanamo Bay.

"Gimme some good news for once," Jack said. "I'm out there bustin' my hump, screwin' Janet from five hundred feet without grease and you're all doom and gloom. I don't see why they don't just drop the charges now before they look too stupid."

Because you shot your little leverage like a sailor with a Filipina whore, Micah thought. But that didn't matter now. "I talked to the Kinkos kid," he said. He explained the back and forth, the kid's new job at Mega but not the forty bucks. "He might help us," Micah said.

"Might's a little shaky."

"I gave him my card." Micah paused. "I don't want you talking to him, in case you had that in mind."

It's *my* life, Jack thought. My freedom. "Do you have a suit?" Micah asked. Jack did but hardly ever used it. The non-conforming customer didn't expect -- didn't trust -- a man in a suit. Especially a white man. A black pastor could get away with it. Jack nodded.

"I'd like to see it, before the first day of trial. You may need to get another one."

If the trial would come down to suits then his goose was cooked. The Kinkos kid was their weakest link. Jack'd go to Manhattan, first time in a *while*, and track him down.

39. The Full Head

Gina'd gotten all the accoutrements of a yuppie convalescence for Bain: the Haagen Dazs ice cream, the microwavable tortellini from the Food Emporium, the full prescription of Celebrex and even a Cuban cigar. This frat boy made money, she thought, looking out through the curtainless floor-to-ceiling windows at the Statue of Liberty™ and the oil refineries of the Arthur Kill smoldering behind. It was time to put on the squeeze.

"So the SEC wants to interview me," she announced.

Bain groaned. His boxer shorts hadn't been clean that day and she'd seen them. He'd given her his keys to go out and do the shopping -- she could have made a copy; Vinny and Tony could be on their way to strip his condo clean. "They can't make you," he mumbled.

"That's no way to start a career," Gina said. "Taking the Fifth or whatever."

The word career brought Bain back to himself: his was probably over. The firm would keep him around for a bit, to make sure he wouldn't flip on the Equities desk. If he kept his mouth shut they'd give him severance and then sayonara. No one on the Street would hire him. Maybe he could hook up a job with some second tier brokerage in the Midwest, help them start a private banking unit for the grain silo heirs of Des Moines and Kansas City. It made him sick. He hated the fast lane but what else was there?

He watched the toy-like silhouettes of planes complete their descent into Newark, New Jersey. Slowly a plan took shape. "I have an idea," he said, noticing for the first time a half erection in his day-old boxer shorts. Double or nothing was the way of the Street. He hadn't slashed his way through all those Jap video games for nothing.

She liked Plan with a capital P better than idea but what the hell. Would he split his annual bonus with her? Guarantee her a transfer to the derivatives and synthetics desk as soon as she was ready? "Run it by me," she said. She knew Options now and was burning to churn.

"I'm thinking of starting my own firm," Bain said. "Going indy like they call it."

This Gina liked, down to the last entrepreneurial strand of her American DNA. "That costs money," she said.

"They'll pay me when I go, if I keep quiet. If *we* keep quiet," he added, since that was the plan.

"Yeah and once you go they'll fire me," she said.

Per diem, Bain thought. They wouldn't even have to fire her. To date per diem out of *his* pocket. "I thought you'd come with me. You pass the Series Seven, I can teach you more as things go along."

"I'd be like what, your assistant?"

You should be creaming in your jeans, Bain thought, looking at her skirt. She was glaring and the sky was orange. All good things, however they turned out, began with risk. "No," he said. "You'd be my partner."

Gina longed for her Planner, wanting to jot this element that denoted and promised success down on a brand new page. "Sunday and Bain," she said.

"Bain Sunday," he replied. "It has a better ring. And I'm the one with the Series Twenty Four."

She'd studied all these NASD numbers -- but which the fuck was this? Four was Options, Registered Options Principal, she'd learned that today. Eight was branch manager, and Sixty Three was blue sky laws. "Supervisory," Bain clarified. "General Securities Principal."

"I knew that," Gina said with peeve. "I was thinking about the money, the back office, how it all would work."

"It's not overnight," he said. "There are places that sell franchises, or do the back office on an á la carte basis. Wallstreet Exotonica has the lower ticket charges." He remembered that Elizabeth's father had a near-dormant Broker Dealer license. With that the net profits would all be his. His and this Gina's, this right-place right-time diner girl. "We'd have to hang in 'til you pass the Series Seven," he said. "And we'd have to sign some gag agreements--" this was the part he liked best -- "to get my severance, the funds to start up."

Gina knew the statistics on restaurants. "These things fail most of the time, don't they?"

Bain sat up in bed. "Hey, I'm good," he said without an ounce of conscious doubt. "I'm the fucking wild man of the Street. At least half my book would come with me in the first week."

Gina liked this in Bain: it was the thing she liked best, perhaps the only thing. "If I do it we'll flip for the name," she said. "But I still have to think about it."

Bain wanted to laugh but he didn't. Coming in as his partner straight out of that gutter in The Bronx? The one thing she wasn't was stupid. This he'd learned without pleasure but now he was ready. "You do that," he said. "Now what about those tortellini?"

* * *

The baby-napping fuck-up was the last straw: Sandy'd had enough. He made his views known to Rudehart, replete with profanity and reminders of how much the prick was getting paid. "If Lena's gotta go so fucking be it," Sandy said, stringing a tux tie around his reptilian neck. "And make sure this Bender shithead gets thrown in the clink 'til Dow Jones fifty thousand. I'd like to sue his ass for disparagement but Blowman says it wouldn't work."

The fuck-up wasn't Chuck's so Rudehart let him drive, circling their island on the FDR and West Side Highway. "What do we have on Birnbaum?" Rudehart asked.

"Don't need much," Chuck said. "He sucked up to Giuliani to get appointed, his term is almost up. If the Bronx Dems don't nominate him he's fucked and he knows it."

"They know our views?"

"They will." Chuck was glad to be back in the fold. His strike force pension was okay, but to move down south he'd need a second one from Empi. They'd work the judge first then fuck this Bender directly if the need arose. Green Onions played in his mind, Booker T. and the M.G.s, they used it in ads now but what did they know. "You wanna see where Bender lives?" Chuck asked. He'd already cased the block, a dozen likely suspects just the way he liked it. He'd snapped photos of Bender and sent them to the Bronx D.A..

"Spare me," Rudehart said. "Drop me at the club then check it out yourself. That is your bailiwick."

Baily my ass, Chuck thought. Or Bali or whatever the fruit was talking about.

* * *

But Olinville was empty -- Jack was in midtown, not far from Rudehart's club, standing across the street from Mega's faceless entrance. He'd remember the kid, he felt sure. He had a way with faces.

George was working late, hauling camera-ready advertising copy for some Japanese soda that was sure to tank. By opening the sacks he carried he got a preview of next year's failures. He had on his Walkman, the bootleg CD he'd bought in The Bronx. White rapper rhyming of raping his momma. Fucker lived in a mansion in Dearborn while in the projects kids made do with cheap Korean keyboards. Another Elvis Presley rippin' off the black man but George Wilson liked the bass.

"Hey yo!" It was the white man, no rapper, crossing the street in George's direction. The second photo they'd sent looked more like him. It was in color so it captures the boozehound redness of his face.

"My name's not yo," George said, taking off his headphones.

"Yo I'm sorry." Jack watched too much TV. It was better than boy but a similar sickness. "You know who--"

"Yeah, I know. Your lawyer, Levine or what's his name, he already talked to me. Unless you got more--"

"I just wanted to make sure. These fuckers are tryin' to string me up."

The reference to lynching left George Wilson cold. "What'da *you* know about stringing?"

"They set me up. The way they showed you that picture--"

"Whoa," George said. "The district attorney said I'm not supposed to talk about the case." With the double C-note wink they'd asked him to report any contact.

"It's my life on the line," Jack said. "I mean, I got a daughter, she lives down in Charlotte, I need--"

"Hold the sob story, chief. I'll call it like I seen it." George put his headphones back on. Now the white rapper's mother was being drowned, his favorite part. "I got another delivery to make," George said loudly and entered Megalopolis Messengers Center, slamming the steel door behind him.

Four hundred years and I'm the one who'll pay, Jack thought. Wasn't that the shit.

* * *

As Swanker prepared for his Rochester play he noticed again his receding hairline. It made him look smart, Carolyn said. Kind or maternalistic, either way it wasn't true in DC. In the House, hair was power. Bush II was dyeing his all the time; Clinton had that Arkansas mop and Reagan wore shoe polish and gel in his Alzheimer's years. Only Bush I's hair was thin and Swanker saw where that got him. This Doctor Boneley could transplant from the Donor Zone,™ put three-hair strands as far down as your eyebrows if you wanted. A one-day operation, nobody had to know. He'd do it before the campaign poster; he wouldn't tell his dad although the problem came from him. The sins of the father were visited on Swanker's pate. Before the Fall he'd fix this shit.

Artful Homes was a bucket shop in Monroe County. They ran ads during the black TV shows on the WB, saying "Praise Jesus, I finally own my own home -- and you can too!" The ads showed Artful's founder, a white man like Swanker in the latter stages of pattern baldness, embracing SEIU matrons and giving them keys. Aspiring homeowners had to plunk down five hundred dollars to attend Artful's Pathways to Freedom™ seminar. They gave their social security numbers and then nothing. The applications were never ruled on. Artful would move on to Syracuse when it had finished draining the Monroe pool of dupes. They could use the same ads with no further filming expenses.

This shit was beneath Swanker: an ordinary con the cessation of which led nowhere. But the point here was to prance on Basso's stage, imply he slept in bed with Artful. Swanker might decamp, but he should choose who would succeed him. Him, not Empi. He wasn't for sale, not Ernie Swanker nor anything he controlled.

The town was cold as hell in winter; hot and drab in summer's sweat. When he ran statewide, Swanker had read up on Rochester to drop historic fiddle-faddle into his speeches, pronounce right the all-purpose brand name Genesee. The beer, the river; the useless port. The word to avoid as taboo was Xerox: they'd ditched Rochester like a first wife for Hartford. Kodak was doing the same; the future with Bausch & Lomb was murky. East Avenue was lined with mansions, including a few by Frank Lloyd Wright. There were more people in Mount Hope Cemetery than anywhere else in town. A real Rust Belt shit hole, Swanker thought. His last dance in the boondocks, his final flex with upstate politics until a Senate race. Some fleabag airline flew prop planes up there. Land in the morning and pull out by dusk, with Basso sucking in his dust, the D&C asking why why why. Why had Basso let Artful slurp the dough from the nineteenth ward and the entire zip code of One Four Six Two One? (Swanker had a map.) Why was crack sold openly on Conkey Avenue on Basso's watch; how could he hope to police the state when even the Chesters Plaza strip mall seemed beyond him? Swanker'd leave questions in his prop plane wake, show Empi who the fuck was who. Then he'd schedule the hair transplant. WatchCorp was dead. Of this he made sure.

* * *

Kurt needed the green light to see in the red: he outright asked Milagros about her father, wondering racist if this was a Spanish thing.

"He died when I was young," Milly said. "My mother raised us, working three jobs to do it. Now it's her we must raise up." When Marcos got married the basement might house her *mama*.

"If a father did something to his daughter, do you think--"

"That is evil," Milly said and meant it. "Nothing would be too much for such a man."

Kurt needed a laptop. But there was something in Queens that he needed even more.

40. Doo-Wop

The sun was barely aloft, a weird weak-looking ball in a hazy humid sky, when Marcos' bus pulled in to Port Authority. He was wearing camouflage fatigues with his name, Guzman, stitched in black on the left side, over his heart. The assortment of bleary-eyed nightriders and homeless and hustlers in the bus station's bowel eyed him with what seemed respect.

"Atta boy," an old man waking up on a bench by an all-night hot dog stand said to him in the second sub-basement.

Marcos nodded, noticed for a moment that the compliment included the surname of one of the plane-jackers who'd started the madness which had dictated the itinerary of his tour of duty. He'd eaten baked beans and dust at the Bagram air base, looking for Taliban in every muffled rifle shot. Sometimes it was a wedding -- it was these people's custom to fire in the air like in the Old West. Sometimes it resulted in weddings and whole extended families cancelled due to Smart Bombs,™ denials from Rumsfeld at the Pentagon, promises to investigate, and then nothing.

Marcos was as patriotic as anyone. He'd enlisted at the recruitment center on Fordham Road, cut his hair, made his forearms big with pushups and steroids from the health food store. At Bagram the idle talk about kicking ass and revenge for the Towers didn't bother him. But the wizened dirt farmers he'd seen blown up, the remaining descendants bombarded with fliers of Osama Bin Laden airbrushed in a business suit -- Marcos wasn't so sure any more. The choice was still his about a second tour. He'd stay at his parents' house in The Bronx for a while, maybe travel south and west to his *abuelita*'s shanty in Maclovia Rojas and consider his options. At Bagram and here they told him that he was a hero. He wanted to believe but wasn't quite sure.

The morning scene on 42nd Street was surreal. The porno theaters and smoke shops had been replaced by closed-shut palaces to Disney and, in Times Square itself, Reuters and Morgan Stanley. "We Will Never Forget," a billboard screamed, next to a forty foot tall white rapper in his underwear. Marcos walked to Bryant Park to catch the D Train. When it came it was air-conditioned and clean, the advertising space all seized by a single company: skeleton-skin white models playing hide and seek on a beach selling a lifestyle. Whatever it was it wasn't his. He got off at Tremont, smelled the piss on the stairs up to the Concourse. Already the old men out selling *malanga* and *yautija* from their metal shopping carts; a guy selling drugs to the cars that passed on Carter Avenue, a residue of shattered bottles on the sidewalk in front of the welfare hotel. He'd like to move his parents out of this neighborhood but they said they liked it here, they were proud of their house, their little yard that his father's sweat had bought. What good was a yard if the junkies clamored at the gate?

He turned north on Park Avenue. The first thing he noticed was a weird yellow sign in the window of the basement, WatchCorp it said. His mother had told him they rented the basement to a white kid, something about the loan they'd taken out then cancelled -- some loan shark screwing them while the signs screamed "We Will Not Forget." Marcos stood at the fence and rang the bell. His mother must have been waiting, because she came right down the stoop throwing open the gate and her arms, reaching up on tip-toe to kiss his cheek.

"*Ay, mi hijo*," she whispered.

"*Mama,*" he answered back. Inside Amado hugged him too, more masculine with a slap on the back. Milly'd made hot tortillas, the strong coffee he'd missed during boot camp and in Afghanistan and what seemed like a half dozen other 'Stans. He told them war stories, mostly second-hand, but not of the erroneously-killed villagers, not yet. The boarder came up, *un blanco* with sandy blond hippie hair, trim but not in fighting shape.

"I'm Kurt," the kid said, and got himself a cup of coffee. He was more than a boarder it seemed. He listened to Marcos' stories, nodding but not joining in. "I moved all my stuff to the back," Kurt said after breakfast. "I'll be moving out soon. I don't want to--"

"Don't worry about it," Marcos said. "I'm used to sleeping in barracks with thirty, forty other guys, stinking and sweating and farting all night. Even with you in it, this shit feels private, like--" he tried to remember then did -- "a sensory deprivation tank."

While Milly grated yucca for *pasteles* upstairs, Marcos unpacked. Kurt told him about the Empi loan, the story in the Wall Street Journal. He told him about the bullet, because of course his mother would.

"Those fucks," said Marcos. He'd been out defending the country while sleazeballs were shooting off guns at his mother. He demanded the whole story, whether Kurt knew the name of the guy who had shot. "He was from Empi," Kurt said, sensing that the story's twists might come back to squeeze him. Marcos was clean-cut but Marcos was a killer: he had 'roid rage written all over him. Kurt didn't want to question the mission for reasons both large and small. He'd go up to the Fordham library and try to download the free come-on version of FrontPage Express. He'd look in the Daily News for ads for rooms for rent; he'd study the map of Queens. Let the homecoming son have quality time with his parents so proud.

* * *

Bertha took the kids to hear doo-wop in Crotona Park. To edutain youth on a limited budget was not easy. The Parks Department paid faded stars to croon in the back of an eighteen wheel truck, one side open like a bandstand, the barbecues smoking and old folks dancing on the grass. They were playing a cover tune, Why Do Fools Fall in Love -- it was a good question, Bertha thought, often sung but never answered to her satisfaction. With Arthur, she'd known: he'd croon *Save the Last Dance for Me* in her ear, gyrating past midnight by the baby's cradle in Concourse Village. But Pall Malls and heroin and the general crap of life had taken that from her. *Why Do Fools Fall in Love With Micah* was the better question, or the question before: Do they?

Micah was supposed to be here. He'd said he'd take the day off work, buy some burgers and briquettes at the Pathmark and let it all hang out. Then he called and cancelled, the case of his terrorist cracker client: he was meeting with the ACLU, he was lining up witnesses. Now Micah wanted Bertha to testify at the trial, background about Empi's practices he said, if the judge would let it in, whatever that meant. The better question was whether she would or should let Micah's it in. Micah would never understand, not Arthur nor Duwon as the boy got older. Micah could buy him for now, with a WalkMan or a Yankees' game. But Duwon's Afro-centric days were coming. Last week he'd asked, as if hit for the first time, "Micah *white*, ain't he?" She'd scolded him on diction but the answer was right: Micah he white; Micah from the tribe that Professor Griff and Farrakhan denounced. When his BMW was parked on St. Ann's she felt from time to time like a whore. He wasn't paying but that's what people thought. Mrs. Morales cross the hall thought it a good match. But she didn't like the jokes she got, at the Burger King across the street, at the discount stores on 149. If they were gonna get together for real they'd have to move, to an integrated neighborhood if one could be found. Crotona wasn't it: other than in storefronts like

Empi's in West Farms there wasn't a white face in miles of here. Still they sung Dion and the Belmonts from the stage and most people stopped dancing. Next was Under the Boardwalk and it started again. Bertha closed her eyes and sang along, "down by the see-ea-ee-ea-ee." Maybe she'd testify or maybe she wouldn't. The question of letting it in had yet to be resolved.

* * *

In the West Farms branch the beat went on. Janet'd been placed on the Critical Watch list, like some rookie loan officer who'd unluckily been caught forging docs. She called Mudnick to complain. He didn't care about the non-disparagement clause Jack had signed. Photos weren't disparagements they were facts, he said. "The Critical Watch is just for now," he told her. "The Empi Cradle business has to die down first."

Mudnick was idly surprised that Janet was still around, that she hadn't been ordered to fall on her figurative Freudian sword. He'd seen Branch and even Regional Managers fired for less. That hard-ass in Austin, caught by the cops while beating a customer up to get paid. The branch in Syracuse where the loans had all been fake, no money actually owed to Empi, just a branch manager high on RocoPoly masturbating in the ruins. Mudnick did the cleanup: a Styrofoam coffee cup had been left on top of the guy's computer so long it rotted and left its contents sticky on the screen.

Some bozo in Spartanburg last year got the boot for selling counterfeit watches in his branch, making all employees buy them. When Home Office looked into it they found deeper problems: the guy was holding interviews with new female hires on his motor boat, telling them to wear bikinis if they wanted into Empi on the ground floor. He got 'em on the floor alright, sloshing around with gas and chum for deep-sea fishing. Finally a lady complained, made a threat about calling the E.E.O.C.. The guy got severance, set sail and had not been seen again. Not like this landlubber Bender who hid in the weeds for revenge.

That's why they kept Janet on -- to nail Bender at the death threat trial. If they fired her now she might not testify. Or Bender's lawyer might dig around into her firing, drive her mad on the stand or even flip her to his side. Mudnick got e-mails about the coming trial: there was a chance, their outside law firm said, that Empi's practices might become an issue. They were getting the judge to make the case closed-door only, no TV or even press. But things had a way of getting out, like the babynap fuck-up or that Guzman loan.

"Anything about loans, you don't answer," Mudnick said. "The reason you fired him, you say it's private. Proprietary, that's the word."

Janet wondered: I'm watching their back but who's watching mine?

* * *

Behind the windowless wall of the storefront Bender crept. As the trial got closer the Jackal got crazier. There must be a doc, he thought, that would solve all this shit and get him out of this hellhole, down to his Zalie and then maybe further south. He had to look through last night's garbage. Dumb fucks still weren't shredding, just put clear plastic bags in the dumpster and closed the metal top.

Jack reached in and grabbed the two top bags, dragged them back into the weeds. Without a car he had to read them here -- so it had to be daylight. He dug through the first bag: some "All Staff" directives that he'd take to WatchCorp Kurt; a bunch of pay-off docs; some originals which meant that the forms had been forged. Mister Light, they'd called him, holding the last round of docs up to the window to trace the signature. If you looked close enough the differences could always be seen. They'd get rah-rah memos from Empi's Home Office repeating Sandy's supposed motto, "Always Do the Right Thing." Jack'd used to laugh down in Charlotte, how they talked high and mighty but made you rip the customers, jack them right at the closing table to get your Roco-bonus. Now they wanted to fucking crucify him, to get him cornholed in some jail -- well not him. The Jackal was hungry.

There was a breeze, which made the humid slop of the day better but blew the docs around, further down the weedy hill. End over end the loan papers rolled, across a service road and onto the Cross Bronx Expressway. There were social security numbers, copies of driver's licenses and answers to questions about pre-existing medical conditions including AIDS and venereal disease. It was a crime, Jack thought, that they threw this shit right out in a dumpster. It was him digging through but it coulda been anyone. Just like the so-called death threat fax.

41. Tex-Mex / Sunny Delight™

Kurt headed to the Guzmans' at dusk and he was not alone. After downloading the web publishing software and doing a WatchCorp update as a test -- it worked -- he'd stopped at HomeQuik to check on Jackal's trial.

"Jes *about* to begin," the Jackal howled, handing him crumbled-up pages covered with coffee grounds. "You back in the publishin' business or what?"

Kurt nodded. It would be slower without his laptop but it still could be done. The Jackal seemed restless, speaking strangely nostalgic about Charlotte and especially his daughter. It made Kurt think: let Marcos hear of Empi's dirt from Jack, so the blame in Rambo's 'roid-filled head would fall on them and not Kurt's d.v.. Jack shrugged but came along, muttering something about idle hands and the Devil's work, thinking of that Arab porno.

They walked along the Metro North tracks: a canyon of ominous tenements, the sheet metal fences of junkyards and janitorial supply houses. "I wantcha to testify," Jack said.

"What about?"

"Me n' Micah, we're tryin' a turn the case around on 'em, make it about Empi and the way they fuck their customers, like the Guzmans."

"What's that prove about the fax?"

"That they got a *motive* to accuse me, to set me up. I'm a whistle-blower, that's what Micah says." Jack paused. "It's better'n a lotta other kind a blowers."

A train roared by. "Hey, if Micah wants me to testify, I'm there," Kurt said. With his web publishing access restored, if only from the library, he could report on the trial. WatchCorp would rise from the dead, like a Dominick Dunne for the Rent-a-Center set.

They passed a storefront church with its door open: older Puerto Ricans shaking tambourines with their eyes closed. "You believe in God?" Jack asked out of nowhere.

Kurt didn't answer right away. In his backpack he carried a crumpled copy of the Tao Te Ching. How the man with power didn't show it; how being content with the bare minimum was heaven. Candida had hated the Tao. "I believe in something," Kurt finally muttered. If he was going to talk theology it wouldn't be with Jack.

"I had this teacher," Jack said, "down in Charlotte. I'd always gone along, at least going to church with my momma. Then he read me some German shit from like 1905, how God was dead but we bubbas was the last to know. I'm gonna find me that book and read it again someday." Kurt doubted it.

Jack stared at a vacant lot with a weeping willow in the middle. "He was a strange fucking dude, Mister Cromartie. I think he was gay."

They arrived at the Guzmans' without another word. Marcos had the basement door open; he'd brought down the TV set from his parents'

bedroom and watched a Venezuelan comedy show while he unpacked his
duffel bag into a chest of drawers that Milly brought down.
"*Que tal*," Kurt said.
"You speak Spanish?" Marcos asked.
"Yeah."
"Well there's no need with me. I'm just watching this station
'cause my favorite band is supposed to be interviewed on the next show."
Marcos looked past Kurt at Jack.
"This is the guy who helped your parents," Kurt said. "He used
to work at Empi but after he left, he got 'em a better loan."

"My mother told me about you," Marcos said slowly, shaking the
Jackal's hand. What she'd told him was that she didn't trust this hot and
cold loan shark, nodding while she got had that first day in West Farm,
then coming door-to-door with his song and dance.
"Is she around?" Jack asked. "I need to talk to her."
"Yeah," Marcos said coldly. "I'll go up and get her."
"I'll go up," Jack said, starting for the stairs.
"No," Marcos said in a voice that made Jack stop. "I'll tell her
you're here."

While Marcos was upstairs, Jack looked around the room. "So
you're gonna have to move, right?" he asked Kurt.
"They said I could stay, but, yeah."
Milagros came downstairs with Marcos behind her.

"Mrs. Guzman, hi, it's been too long," Jack said. His accent was
lighter, forcedly Northern. Six words without a single swear: the Jackal
was smooth when it counted, Kurt thought.
Milagros smiled thinly. "How have you been," she asked
without a question mark. Jack half-explained the coming trial, asked if
she'd testify about the loan that Gina made.
Milly didn't answer but Marcos did. "I'll testify, *mama*," he said.
"If they came to the house and fired a gun, we need to say that."
"Uh, that's not what the trial's about," Jack said.
"I will testify," Marcos said. Milagros took the chance to say
goodnight.

On TV a band was playing, accordions and congas and a
keyboards that played Germanic techno sounds. "That's my boys,"
Marcos said, bringing his half-cocked bulging arms up and down in a

dance that neither Kurt nor Jack had seen. "They're from Monterrey," Marcos drew out the r as long as it would stretch. "It's some Tex-Mex acid rock. The shit is dope."

Kurt said he liked it; Jack didn't. "I'm gonna split," Jack said. "This guy called Micah will wanna talk to you about the trial."

"Any time," Marcos said, not taking his eyes from the screen. Kurt was watching too. The lyrics were Spanglish, new school to the max.

When it was over Marcos switched to CBS, a War on Terror™ report by a used-up anchorman posing rhetorical questions in a flak jacket. "They don't know shit," Marcos said. "The people we killed when I was over there had nothing to *do* with Al Qaeda."

Kurt's ears perked up. He wouldn't be the first one to broach politics but he wanted to hear. A quick vision of an as-told-to-memoir did a Tex-Mex two-step in his head. "Who were they?"

"They were like farmers and shit. They don't even have cars over there, most of 'em. They use horses. They're like Mexicans, like the *indios* in the south except they drop down on the ground five times a day to pray."

"I hear you," Kurt said, waiting for more. WatchCorp was silent about the war. If you fought corporations you didn't need another battle. But Marcos had the right to speak: he'd given two years, had the crew cut to prove it. It was like the Vietnam vets who turned against the war, or the ones from the Nineties who got sick after Desert Storm and sued. "Are you like on leave?" Kurt asked.

"I'm between tours." Marcos paused. "I might not go back in. I haven't told my moms."

Kurt nodded. "Do you drink beer?"

"Are you *kidding*? Beer, rum, vodka -- whatever it is, bring it on."

"I'll go to the liquor store."

"I'll come."

In the dark Park Avenue was quiet; Tremont had some people, clustered in front of the Korean Liquors in the storefront of a two-story house. Kurt ordered through plexiglass, a two-liter bottle of Russian-named vodka from Georgia. "Bullet'd crack that shit easy," Marcos said, pointing at the inch-thick plastic. The Korean owner smirked, took a half-step back as if unconscious. Marcos watched and said to Kurt, "I want my parents to move. They like the house but this shit's probably more dangerous than Kabul."

"It's not that bad," Kurt said.

"What would you know."

They got a half-gallon Sunny Delight™ at the bodega; Kurt mixed the drinks back in the basement. On TV were reruns of a Boston bar, the theme music about everybody knowing your name. It was interspersed with public service announcements by the Ad Council,™ different takes on the theme of freedom. Marcos watched them closely. The camera panned down a supermarket aisle, showing the two dozen brands of fruit juice then toothpaste. "America's freedom," a voice-over said. "Don't let them take it away."

"What *shit!*" Marcos said, slamming down his plastic cup. "That's what we're bombing for? Crest and AquaFresh and Colgate? I always thought that shit was a waste, twenty different tubes of paste to clean your fucking teeth."

On the sitcom they joked about refills; in the basement Kurt poured them, mixing each drink with his pen. The next Ad Council spot showed a kid in a library, asking for a book. "That's no longer available," an ominous voice said off-camera. "I'll need to see your I.D.."

"That's more like it," Marcos said.

"They already do that," said Kurt. "Ashcroft and the FBI can already search library records, and the librarians can't even say when it happened."

Marcos swallowed the rest of his drink and grimaced. "You smoke?" he asked Kurt. The answer was yes.

* * *

"I might need to fuck somebody up."

It was hours later; the vodka was gone. TV was all paid advertisement for flat bellies and hair transplants. You could become a computer technician in three easy weeks, six easy payments.

"I'm yo man," Marcos slurred. "Thas what they trained me to do."

Kurt outlined the basics. He had a girlfriend, an ex-girlfriend now, who told him last week that her father had raped her. Repeatedly. In a boiler room in Queens.

"Let's get the fuck," Marcos said. "I can't stand a short eyes."

Kurt had read the play, by the now-dead Nuyorican. "You wanna go to Jackson Heights?"

"Let's go, bro," Marcos said. They walked to the D, getting two more half-pints on the way.

* * *

The train cars were empty except for the homeless, a few yuppie club-hoppers and night-shift zombies. They changed to the F Train under Rockefeller Center, Kurt riffing drunkenly on the irony, the monopolist memorialized in drab stone slabs, too short to be targets for Al Qaeda, a blessing but a loss of face. The F became an El, the sun rising far out over Queens and Long Island, Daily News and Post trucks burning the red lights and throwing their bundles on the grocery stores' sidewalks. "Next stop," Kurt told Marcos, who had finished his half-pint and was doing pull-ups on the strap-hangers' bars.

"You're sure about this, right?" Marcos asked in the faceless streets. "That he raped her and all."

"You could hear it from her herself," Kurt said.

"I might need to."

They got to the building, waited until a sleepy eyed Latin guy came out through the door. They went in. "Her father's the super," Kurt said. "He did it in the boiler room and that's where he's got to go every morning."

"In this heat?"

"Gotta turn it on for the hot water."

Marcos nodded. "In Bagram the shit was cold. How those fuckers live there I don't know."

"They get used to it."

They hid in the basement, behind a bedroom set and a stack of green bathroom sheetrock. Marcos finished the dregs of Kurt's half-pint. The exits of residents upstairs were becoming more frequent. The moment was being lost.

"Yo, it's him," Kurt said. There were footsteps, the rattling of keys on a key chain. Kurt peeked out around the bed's headboard. Candida's father -- it must be him -- was shorter than he'd imagined, like a flyweight boxer in his white sleeveless T. Whistling, the motherfucker was, on his way to the boiler room and all its memories. He pushed the door open; before it snapped back on the hinges' spring he blocked it with the red sand bucket. There was some clattering, then hissing, then the banging in the pipes above their heads.

"My idea--" Kurt began but it all became moot. Candida's father came whistling out of the boiler room, kicking the sand bucket back in to shut the door. After his footsteps faded away, Marcos lit a smoke.

"I wanna hear the story," Marcos said. "In Afghanistan they just said 'bomb here' and that was that. This has gotta be different, if I'm gonna do it."

That wasn't Kurt's plan. But the sky was now light, and the fun of the drunk had begun to fade. "I'll set it up," Kurt said. "But it might not be necessary."

42. The Sand Bag

D Day had arrived and it was just as Micah'd hoped. Sunny but not humid, good suit-weather he called it, leaving his car windows down as he sped down the Concourse, left on One Six One, right into the Concourse Village Mall parking lot. They charged by the hour but this wouldn't take all day. Judge Birnbaum had begrudgingly agreed to hear arguments on why his decision to close the trail to the press should be reversed. What Birnbaum didn't know was that there was a plan afoot to blow him out of the water, courtesy of the wily Lorraine Thompson.

Jack was smoking his third cigarette of the morning and reading the Post by the cop saw horses on the corner of Sherman. "You better get in line," Micah said. The criminal courthouse had only two metal detectors: one for the lawyers, the other for the great unwashed. There the guards wore rubber gloves as they patted down women with electronic wands, lingering too long by the crotch, by the breasts, sexually harassing from a distance and all authorized by the need for security.

"I'll meet you in the basement," Micah said. "Lorraine Thompson is already down there."

Jack stamped out his smoke and loosened his polka dot tie. "Don't start without me," he said.

"I don't think we're starting at all today," Micah said. He walked past the line of unwashed, wives and girlfriends come to watch their men arraigned.

"Hey hey, Mister Levine," the lawyers' line guard greeted him. "What's the good word?"

"Removal," Micah said smiling. "Or maybe recusal."

"You shysters never stop, do you."

There was no pat-down; the buzzer went off but the guard didn't care. What lawyer is going to bring a gun into the courthouse? The women, sure: they might try to sneak in a Tech 9, have a final shoot-'em-up and spring their man free. But the lawyers made money no matter who won or lost. No reason to shoot; no reason to pat-down.

Lorraine was waiting by the OCA office, counting the pages of her motion. Micah'd called her last week and made an offer she couldn't refuse. She'd play bad cop, the peremptory strike; in exchange, Micah would refer her some slam-dunk lead-eating cases, to diversify her practice beyond crack-slingers and whore-mongers like Jack. The collegiality of the Bar, Micah called it. For a Jew he wasn't bad, she thought.

"How many'd you find?" Micah asked.

"Almost two dozen," Lorraine said. "Birnbaum just sits on cases, figures the skels won't complain, can't afford to appeal. I got four of 'em signed up."

"Should be enough," Micah said. "After you." He held open the door to the Office of Court Administration sub-station. They were supposed to monitor judges' productivity and basically did so only when complaints were filed. Today twenty-two complaints would flood in about a single judge. Birnbaum was asleep at the switch, Lorraine's motion argued. Justice delayed is justice denied and all that crap. He should be removed for any active trials until he ruled on the prisoners' *habeus corpus* pleas that had languished in his in-box since the last decade -- the last millennium, in fact.

Micah sat in the rickety chair, its plastic upholstery ripped and graffitied. Lorraine wasn't bad herself: she talked her way back the clerk, to the second-tier bureaucrat who was shocked at the bomb she'd assembled. "We had no idea," he said. "I'll have to call downtown."

"My clients are rotting upstate," Lorraine said. "Losing faith day by day in our system of justice." You go, girl, Micah thought. Birnbaum wouldn't know what hit him.

"Come in as soon as you hear," Micah told Lorraine. "I'm already picking out the cases I think would be good for you."

"Good luck with the cracker," Lorraine said, adding, "that's what they call him."

"I know," Micah said. Bertha heard it and the name was right on.

They'd made Jack take off his shoes -- black sneakers with their heels worn down so he walked like a penguin -- as if this were an airplane. "Wanna smell my ass?" Jack asked. The guard glared at him. A white boy skel was the lowest of the low in his view. A four hundred year head start and you're in Bronx Criminal Court? Please.

Jack took the escalator down, met up with Micah in front of Birnbaum's. "Nice tie," Micah said dryly. Jack shrugged. They went in.

Birnbaum was getting dressed in his chambers, no bigger than a toilet stall, really, but this was a big day for him. Until this, he'd been just another Giuliani appointee, a judge whom demographics would condemn to the scrap heap. An operative -- bag man was the word but why go there -- for the Bronx Democratic Committee had called him up, saying it was important to the Committee that this Bender case go smoothly. No circus, no press; no grounds for appeal. If all went well they'd give him the ballot-line; he'd win fourteen years of judicial independence. There was law to support it, they'd reminded him: the terror charge should not be aired, to school those who'd take all our freedoms away. Bring it on, Birnbaum thought. He tossed his gavel from hand to hand.

Wing Tsai was prepared but this wouldn't be his day. His ultimate boss the Honorable District Attorney of Bronx County Robert Jackson would argue the motion, would make the opening statement and take credit for the terror case. Tsai would manage the trial's middle: direct examinations of the Empi target and the Kinkos kid. It was open and shut, really, except for Levine's witness list. Birnbaum would strike most of the names, limit the case to the fax, just the fax ma'am, one terroristic cracker upstate moaning.

"All rise!"
Birnbaum sauntered in, squeezing the gavel's handle in his sweaty pink palm like a gun. He sat; they sat. Two court officers locked the door. This was like military justice, just the way Birnbaum liked it.
" Mister Levine, I've read your brief," Birnbaum began, pronouncing it Lah-Vine like wine just to rattle the guy. "I'm not inclined to grant your motion -- the law is clear with regard to the terrorism charge. But you've asked for oral argument and I'll grant it. You may begin." Birnbaum sat back and smiled. All the trappings of justice with none of the headaches.
"Thank you, your Honor," Micah said, also smiling. Let this hack have his last smug moment. Micah could wax poetic and buy time until OCA dropped the bomb. "The courts, despite rumors and recent developments to the contrary, belong to the people. When a man -- or woman -- is charged with a crime, he is faced with the extensive machinery of the state, which ironically he or she, him- or herself, has

paid for." This awkward gender-correctness made Birnbaum sick. Micah continued, "There are only two protections. The first is a jury, which my client is being denied in this case, given the state's cynical invocation of the anti-terrorism statute. The second and last protection is the press -- that the trial, even if only before a judge, be open to the public, be reported to the public--"

"Hold on there, Mister Levine," Birnbaum said. "Have there even *been* any requests from the press to cover this trial?"

Micah was ready. "Yes as a matter of fact there have. There's a reporter at the Wall Street Journal who has closely followed the lead-up to the trial. There's another reporter at the New York Post who would like to attend." Micah did not mention WatchCorp; that flimsy web site was their last defense, their deuce in the hole.

"Your Honor, that's just not true," Wing Tsai spoke up. Robert Jackson was watching him without a smile. Don't fuck up, his blood-shot eyes were saying. Tsai continued: "The articles to which Mister Levine is referring have *nothing* to do with this case. The Journal article was about a loan -- nothing about the faxed death threat at issue here. The Post article was even more remote, about an occurrence at EmpiFinancial long after the defendant left their employ, long after the death threat--"

"It's *all* related," Micah said. "As we will show."

"Mister Levine, I'm not inclined--"

"Let me finish." Micah needed to draw this out, get his lifeline from Lorraine and the OCA before this hack judge could issue a ruling. "The brief we've submitted cites cases that stretch back through the decades, on the fundamental right of the defendant to be tried in open court--"

"Those are almost entirely *Federal* cases that you cite," Birnbaum pointed out. "I am bound to follow the New York Court of Appeals. Federal decisions may be persuasive, but in this case--"

"They've included a Federal charge," Micah cut in. "By tacking on the anti-terrorism count they've opened the door."

"*As* I was saying," Birnbaum prissily proceeded, "that statute explicitly allows for trial in the state courts, where state law applies. I've given you your chance but I'm not moved."

Oh but you're gonna be, Micah thought. You're gonna move or be moved. Your lazy negligence is about to explode if all goes right.

"So I'm denying the motion," Birnbaum ruled. "The case will proceed with a sealed courtroom, in the interest of national security. If there are no more motions, let's discuss your witness list." Birnbaum sneaked a glance at Robert Jackson, like, how'm I doing, how do ya like me now. "Frankly, I'm not convinced that the majority of these witnesses will provide testimony even remotely related to the facts at issue here. Marcos Guzman, for example. Or Kurt Wheelock. Explain to me the relevance."

My shyster sucks, Jack thought. He talks a good game but he's losing every point. Jack thought of Zalie, felt his future slipping away. "This isn't fair," he said out loud, standing up, pointing at Birnbaum. A court officer came his way, an enormous Hispanic with tape over the name on his shield like some torturer.

"Be quiet, Mister Bender," Birnbaum commanded. "Or I'll have you locked up right this minute for contempt."

Jack'd heard the word and it felt like it fit. "I'm being railroaded," Jack said as the guard grabbed his arm. Just then the courtroom door shook in its frame. Birnbaum stared over.

"Tell them to go away," Birnbaum told the guard. "The sign outside says it clearly, Do Not Disturb."

"I believe--" Micah started, thinking of motel rooms, but already Lorraine was shouting through the door.

"There's an order," Lorraine said. "It has to be served on Judge Birnbaum right now."

Birnbaum squeezed his gavel. This was not the day for some vulture to take advantage of his peccadilloes, like the way they sued Dick Cheney just as Bush was giving his post-Enron pabulum speech. "It'll have to wait," he told the guard.

A white piece of paper came under the door like a tongue from a mouth. "Bring that here," Birnbaum directed. Whoever this process server was, he was going to see that their license was stripped, reduce them to handing out handbills for strip clubs. The guard brought it over. Jack and Micah watched as Birnbaum's face went flat, cold hatred and fear like a burned-out sun. A white dwarf, Micah thought, remembering astronomy. A big bang on a mean little man.

"There must be some mistake," Birnbaum said. "We'll take a short recess and I'll call OCA."

Micah held his tongue and thought of the braindead babies he'd bequeath on Lorraine Thompson. For an 18-B she sure got things done.

"What's the play?" Jack asked Micah in the hall. Lorraine had slipped away, to the soul food on Gerard Avenue where the beef patties burned your mouth.

"Judge Birnbaum, unfortunately, has other matters to attend to," Micah said fake-pompous, looking around for a better audience for his jokes. Jackson had followed Birnbaum out, thinking their combined micro-might could flip OCA one-two-three. But the rule was the rule, in this case at least. When the volume of cases unruled on got too great, the remedy was to make the judge sit in the corner, make him write on the blackboard one hundred times, "I will be productive. I will be productive." It was like market discipline in the gulag.

"How'd you--"

Micah brought his finger to his lips. "The next judge could be worse, you never know."

"I doubt it," Jack said. The shyster was alright. He could see Zalie again, in his mind; he could hear her little girl's whine for toys and glee at fries. I'm coming, baby, Jack thought or even whispered. This sleazy snake will set me free.

43. Bitter Melon / The Rocket Docket

"Scumbag's luck," Rudehart said, to himself more than Chuck who was waiting for orders. Rudehart had Ivy up to his eye balls: law degree and MBA, even a Ph.D. in economics from the time he'd wanted to replace that Greenspan scrooge. Now some Brooklyn Law School shitbag was playing his tricks.

"At least he ruled," Chuck said. "About the press and all."

"Who do we know at OCA?" Rudehart asked. His contacts were in the Federal courts, and they went high. But he'd never even heard of this bullshit rule, that pending motions could take a judge off a case.

"Too late," Chuck said. "They already assigned to another judge."

"A player?"

"Usually. It's Burton Wolfson. He did the Eleanor Bumpers case." Chuck thought back on that: a three hundred pound African grandmother shot to hell by Emergency Services Unit cops. Wolfson had cleared them. Good for Empi, probably, but bad for The Race.

Rudehart had been too busy making money during the Bumpers case to remember what it was about. Some deadbeat with the I.Q. of a mushroom charged the cops with a knife and some roach-killing spray.

"Gimme something more recent," Rudehart said. "I've got to tell Sandy and I want to sweeten the news."

"Well he's white," Chuck said, not without irony.

"Enough of your mau-mau shit," Rudehart said. His Ivy was but a veneer. If the game was in the gutter he was there, as long as he had muscle, preferably black, to watch his back. "What's his link to the Democratic mafia?"

"They got him elected. But now he's like a free agent. He's got twelve more years on a term of fourteen. He'll retire or die before it runs out, so he can pretty much do whatever he wants."

"Get me Martindale-Hubbell," Rudehart said. "He'll know someone who knows someone, it always works that way. If push comes to shove, it's Bender time on Olinville, right?"

"Yaz, boss," Chuck said. He'd like to have Wolfson's insulation. But to take orders from this pampered fruit, without even a come-back, would be too much. Chuck would do the dirty work, sure -- he already had a plan. But Rudehart should have to smell the shit too, at least some of it. Let the fruit earn his money, the old fashioned way, as Vyle's middle-man.

* * *

Gina'd moved back to the Comfort Inn for her last round of study. Bain was mad with desire but this he relieved with his good arm. Their first time should be memorable, he'd decided. He'd need full mobility and none of the slacquor that came from Celebrex. Viagra, perhaps, to over-determine the outcome. In the interim it was time to hit up Dickinson Liz for her Daddy's dormant Form B/D. He'd won the coin toss: Bain Sunday, he liked the sound of it. The last remaining step was to exorcise this otherworldly cunt. He took Metro North to Greenwich, strode confident down the road in his Armani Exchange Casuals.™

She'd agreed to meet him; the time and place had been nailed down in terse e-mails with neither showing what they felt. Be brash, Bain told himself. Be cocky like she said, cocky like she misses, the cock she coulda had but had fumbled now to a younger and hungrier version. Gina's poetry was pure numbers and ambition. It had rubbed off on him. No peeping Tom this time: straight to the door, straight to the jugular.

Liz had bought lunch, French melons and prosciutto ham. The dining room table was dark-stained wood. Outside the sprinklers squeaked and sprayed.

"You look well," Bain said, puffing out his chest. "How's the real estate game? How's the ex?"

If Bain had known what Liz was thinking, his cockiness would have gone flaccid. Liz was lonely, sure -- but not for him. She went now to weekly meetings of Sapphists on Spring Street. She had miles to go to free herself but the journey'd begun.

"I spoke to Papa," Liz said, as if she were English, as if this were Masterpiece Theater and not the pulpy last time they'd see each other. "His license is still valid -- you're lucky you called, because the two years had almost run and it would have expired."

Her father had always liked Bain, at least it had seemed during the summer Bain had interned at his wood-paneled boiler-room brokerage operation. He'd expected Liz and Tom to be married, even referred some accounts to Bain before they broke up.

"He said you'll have to pay."

Tom put down his melon, running his tongue on the glossy near-porno flesh of the prosciutto. "Right now I can't do it. There's start-up expenses,   there'll   be   rent--"

"He figured as much. Don't worry, *he* still likes you." Liz emphasized the word, staring at this mousse-haired idiot and wondering why? how? as if it had been another life. "Pay him through time. He'll want a monthly cash flow statement, that's what he said. And that you'll have to file your reports under his name until the whole thing's paid off. The license is like -- there's a word he used -- his collateral."

Cheap old bastard. Maybe he'd die before Bain Sunday broke into the black.

"He'll fax you the paper work, but he needs to know where. To your work, I figured."

Bain shook his head. "I've got a home office now," he said. "Like you, I guess." He looked to the left, toward the computer room den he'd stared into, tip-toe in the flower beds, pathetic. It seemed a long time ago.

"I doubt it," Liz said. "Go ahead, eat up." She wanted him gone; she wanted her peace and not these warlike random looks.

Bain chewed the greasy meat feeling as insufficient as ever, maybe more so. He reminded himself that he'd gotten what he came for: the NASD Form B/D, license to broke and deal, Bain Sunday's license to hunt and steal. They'd be different somehow: no bogus advice to halfwit Internet investors from the Midwest, no fake research reports full of puffery. They'd screw by night and trade by day, making their money the new fashioned way. The thought cheered him up and the melon was crisp. When he finished he left with a ham-handed volley of false bravado. Elizabeth took a long shower, luxuriating in the beta-versions of the New Technology.

* * *

They called Burton Wolfson's the "Rocket Docket," like the federal court in Virginia where they tried-and-fried terrorists without the presence of the press or even defense attorneys. Wolfson was old now. He'd had enough of lawyers' tricks. He didn't need press coverage: his career had ended here, the crotchety sage of the Bronx Supreme Court. He'd dreamed of the Court of Appeals, or of a federal judgeship, when Clinton was in. None of it had come through. His rulings were too quirky. Sure he'd let off the cops who'd blown away Eleanor Bumpers. He'd put himself in their shoes, busting down a door and finding roaches everywhere, bug spray in their eyes, the glint of a knife. Some rookie pulled the shotgun's trigger. He would have convicted the police commissioner, or the head of social services. But neither was on trial that day. Only the rookie and a mob of off-duty cops drinking beer and chanting down on the Concourse below.

They called him a racist when he ruled the rook not guilty. The next year they called him anti-cop because he excluded evidence -- the fruit of the poisoned tree, he'd always loved that botanic phrase -- when a Street Crime Unit chased a Dominican teen for no reason and found fifty pounds of smack in his trunk of his Acura. It was the logic of his decision that ended his career: it was reasonable, he wrote, for a Dominican teen to flee a gang of white men with guns in the South Bronx streets at midnight. Perhaps he could have been more judicious. But fuck them, Burton Wolfson thought. You held a mirror to society and they blamed you for it. He'd ruled against a provision of Welfare Reform,™ got reversed on appeal. It was bullshit, the scapegoating of the least of these. Who *liked* being on welfare? If the schools were better, if the jobs were better, the problems would disappear. But without fixing those things, to make a single mother of three go pick up leaves in a park with a nail on a stick was a joke. The voters lived in la-la land, whipped up to resent some fantasy of people getting over, screwing on food stamps and lifting weights. Clinton gave free reign to this *ressentiment*, rebranded small-heartedness as tough love. Like the judges who preened for Crime & Punishment™ Court TV, outdoing themselves in trash-talk at sentencing. Vanity, all of it. The brutish war of all against all. Wolfson liked to read.

Wolfson knew Birnbaum, the sweaty climber always shaking hands at the Democratic Committee's annual dinners at Marina Del Rey in Throgs Neck. Birnbaum was pathetic: rather than a mirror what he held up was an air-brushed postcard of a world in which hardworking New Yorkers, all or most of them white, struggled to heroically put food on their family's table against the jungle-like backdrop of deadbeats and thieves. Birnbaum's politics were correct for advancement but he lacked a certain charm. He tried too hard and no one liked that, least of all Wolfson. Wolfson had become a geriatric James Dean in a black judge's robe, a rebel with an order to show cause. He'd always liked the Trickster character in African myths, or Loki in the Norse: make 'em laugh while exposing their small-minded greed. And now this.

He read through the papers they'd brought on a hand truck from Birnbaum's. What struck him first was the terror charge -- typical Bob Jackson, grandstanding opportunistic prostitution of the law. Any pol with ambition tied his cart to the Nine Eleven horse. An angle could be found in any case: this is not food stamp fraud, it's money laundering for Al Qaeda. This South Indian businessman must be a front for Saddam Hussein. Wolfson wasn't afraid to read -- he wasn't afraid of much anymore, in his ramshackle twilight, his high-ceilinged courtroom with its leaking ceiling and broken chairs penned-in with police tape. That the press was excluded by Birnbaum's last order might be for the best. Wolfson was as decrepit as his courtroom. Closed-door or open, it didn't matter any more. Wolfson was playing for a different audience now: a jury in a heaven he didn't believe in.

Wing Tsai the ADA he didn't know. But Bob Jackson was a cokehead. "The Snowman," they called him in the courthouse bathroom stalls. A man who'd had all the advantages and snorted them all straight up his vein-lined nose. The DAs in The Bronx had always been Italian, Merola then Foglia. Jackson rode the wave of demographic change, which was fine with Wolfson except that Jackson misrepresented his race, showing up high from last night's coke and flubbing his arguments. Well this time he'd work, Wolfson decided. Let Jackson *try* to link this Bender to Osama Bin Laden, with a straight face and a runny nose. It couldn't be the first issue in the case but he'd let it loom and see what happened.

The incongruous factoid in the case was the name on the fax: Tariq Noor. An Arab name for sure. But what did it mean? Wolfson knew Google; Wolfson knew Ask Jeeves.™ Half of the hits said you needed a program for Arabic script to view them. While he waited Wolfson wondered, idle and dry: if convicts from the Bronx took on

Muslim names in jail, what did Muslims do? Say you should henceforth call me Billy Joe Smith? This was Wolfson's kind of humor, deadpan for no one. If there was a comedy club in heaven - if there *was* a heaven -- Wolfson would give it a go. In his head he practiced endlessly.

* * *

"Do - *not* - fuck - this - up."

Jackson thought it funny that the world's largest bank sent a flunky black middle-man to give him this pep talk. He knew which side his white bread was buttered on, how outside forces gave the bulk of the money for election campaigns in The Bronx. But show him some respect -- give him his props like his ghetto slang consultant would put it.

"I'll do my best," Jackson snorted, "with the proof that there is. It's all gonna ride on the Kinkos guy's I.D.." He paused. "He's black, right?"

Fuck, Chuck thought, this brother ain't done his homework. "Didn't cha interview him?"

"My ADA did it."

The Chink. "And he gave him our offer?"

Jackson thought about it. It wasn't just plausible deniability: he didn't know. "Not in so many words. But he wrote me a note" -- where was it, Jackson hated cases with thick files -- "about this cracker's lawyer offerin' him a bribe. So that's even better."

"He'll say that at trial?"

"That's where you all's deal comes in."

"I'm not dealin' with the kid directly," Chuck said. The fuck-up in the Guzmans' basement was more than enough. He hoped the end-game on Olinville would not be required.

"We got it under control," Jackson said. Chuck doubted it.

44. The Gravy Tie

Kurt ran up the hill of East Tremont, sweating in his long-sleeved shirt. The tie, he would put at the courthouse. It was too hot to wear one outside, and it made you a mark for muggings too. The subway station smelled like piss. Kurt sipped the milky coffee he'd poured into a glass Snapple bottle, pick-me-up on the run, first day of trial.

Kurt had gotten himself on Micah's witness list so he'd have an excuse to be just outside the courtroom or better, inside. They could close it to the press, and had. But as a witness he could attend, then run at the end of the day to the Fordham library and upload an update to

WatchCorp. It'd be an exclusive, if anyone cared. He'd left three voice mail messages for Nicole Nour but she hadn't returned any of them.

The drunken dawn with Marcos in Queens had been weird. So too was Candida's reaction when he called: she didn't hang up, she apparently didn't find it strange that he asked her to speak to the Guzmans' son. He felt like a pimp for a moment, or like this was murder-for-hire. Marcos wanted to hear it from the horse's mouth -- and Candida hadn't said no. Marcos was on the witness list too but he wouldn't be needed today. The government had to present their case first. Marcos was already up and out when Kurt awoke. "Army clock," Marcos said the night before. Drink til dawn then grab your M-16 and PalmPilot.

The Yankee Stadium D Train station was under repair: two by fours with nails sticking out, light bulbs on pigtails on coiled white wires, a slew of signs saying "Pardon Our Appearance While We Renovate." It had gone on for years and was still a rats' maze. Kurt came up on the corner of 161st and River Avenue, under the El tracks of the 4, across the street from Yankee Stadium's faceless blue wall. The House That Ruth Built and that ruthless people wanted to remove from The Bronx. Well let' em. The trickle-down benefits to Bronxites were negligible. A few sports bars and jersey shops owned by Irish from Jersey.

Despite the foot traffic that the courthouses drew, there were still few restaurants around here. A Mickey D's with a prison-like fence; a delicatessen in an old vaudeville theater. Kurt got an iced coffee, still waking up, and jogged up the steps of the Art Deco courthouse. Carved on the frieze there were quotes about justice; there were figures from myth carved on each side of the door. The line at the metal detector was long. Kurt read through the court file that Micah had given: the badly-copied death threat fax; Micah's motions for press coverage and explaining each witness. For Kurt it said, "Expert in EmpiFinancial's lending practices." It did not say "reporter;" that was Micah's trick. There was Marcos Guzman and even Bertha Watkins.

"Yo, it's your turn."

Kurt looked up. A pudgy guard with rubber gloves beckoned. Kurt submitted to the scanning wand and took the elevator up.

Another guard stopped him at the door to Wolfson's courtroom. "Are you parta the case?" the guard asked. Kurt nodded, ready to point to his name on the defendant's witness list. "I'm an expert," Kurt thought to say but didn't. The guard stepped aside and Kurt went in. The room was paneled wood, with twenty-foot windows that faced the Grand Concourse. There was a carved wood desk where the judge would sit;

two rows of seats for a jury that were empty. Micah and Jack were at a table up in front.   At the other table was a flashily-dressed man Kurt recognized: the Honorable Robert Jackson, a hack in Kurt's view, and a younger Asian man whispering in Jackson's ear. There were a few other people in the front row of seats. The courtroom was like a Greenwich Village theater, with seating for a hundred or so. But three blocks of seats had yellow tape around them. As Kurt approach he saw why: the upholstery was torn off them, with screws sticking out. On the ceiling someone has drawn circles in white spray paint. The grandeur of justice, Kurt thought, committing it all to memory.

Jack came to the railing, pointing at a woman in the front row, whispering too loud to Kurt. "That's that bitch Janet Peel," Jack said. "The one who's trying to break my balls." Micah said "shh," but Jack didn't. "Micah made an action, a motion, whatever, to kick the terror charge but it ain't happening. What happened with the Guzman kid?"

Kurt didn't answer. How to explain: he'd hooked the returning hero up with his used-up ex-girlfriend, to get him motivated to commit a crime more serious than Jack's. "He'll be here tomorrow," Kurt said. "Micah said today he'd just waste his time."

"All rise!"

Wolfson pranced in from a door by the empty jury box. He gestured that they all could sit down. "I'm not a king," he used to say. "I'm just the schmuck who has to deal with children's squabbles." Today he didn't say that. He'd been surfing the 'Net for this Tariq Noor, took a detour crash-course on predatory lending including the articles from the Journal and Post. He felt ready. As ready as he ever felt, since his wife's death.

"Good morning," he said, looking at Jackson, trying to conduct a urine sample with his eyes. The pompous shvartzer was dressed to the nines, and ready to play the dozens.

"Good morning, Your Honor," Jackson said. "There are some preliminary matters that we'd like to address."

"We'll get to that -- let me say my hellos, okay?" Wolfson turned to Micah, a well-known snake of the slip-n-fall set. "Mister Levine, I didn't know you did criminal law as well."

"I see this as a civil liberties case, Judge Wolfson," Micah said. They couldn't have gotten a better spin of the wheel than this, when Birnbaum got bounced. Wolfson didn't punk out from Constitutional issues -- he'd been a member of the National Lawyers Guild at one point, if Micah'd heard right.

Wolfson looked at Micah's client. He sure wasn't an Arab. He had on an off-the-rack suit, from a thrift store it looked like. His face has red splotches; he had on polka dot tie with some kind of gravy stain near the tip. A man of international terrorist intrigue, it was clear. "Mister--" Wolfson looked down at his papers to be sure -- "Mister Bender, I'll try to treat you fair, especially since there's no jury here. If you have any questions about the procedure as we go forward, just ask Mister Levine and we'll take a break. Okay?"

Jack stood up. "It's not right that they're closin' the courtroom to the press," he said.

Wolfson, barely peeved, raised his hand. "We'll be getting to that. But try to remember -- it's your lawyer who speaks for you. If you have a question, ask him. That's what he's paid for." And very richly, Wolfson thought. The gravy-splattered loan shark was a real catch.

Jackson tried to speak again but Wolfson shook his head. "With a jury here I'd do this different," Wolfson said. "But since the statute you've sued under precludes a jury, we'll do it my way. The defendant has a question about the press, so I wanna take that first. Let's go on the record."

The court reporter was a mousy woman from the North Bronx, a failed cellist who used her finger skills to tap away on the stenography machine. They should have used a tape recorder but it was a union job and so it stayed. She flexed her fingers like a concert pianist, gave the sign and they were off.

"This is the matter of State versus Jack Bender," Wolfson began. "The case has come to me on referral from Justice Birnbaum of the Criminal Court. Present here today are the defendant and his counsel, and the Bronx District Attorney himself, along with his assistant Mister--" Wolfson consulted his papers again -- "Tee-sigh. Is that how it's pronounced? I want to get this right."

"It's t'sigh, almost sigh, Your Honor," Wing said. "But thanks."

"Butcher a man's name and you've made an enemy for life," Wolfson quipped. "Especially given the *international* flavor of this case, I think it's important to pronounce things right." The joke was lost on Jackson, but Micah got and liked it. He'd play the anti-xenophobe card whenever the chance arose.

"Before he was so suddenly called away"-- Wolfson smirked -- "Justice Birnbaum ruled that the proceedings should be closed to the press, in light of the sensitive matters of national security allegedly at issue here. I don't know what these might be, but I'm as patriotic as the next man. If Congress and the New York legislature tell us that even *invoking* a terrorism charge must lead to this result, who am I to disagree?"

Wise-cracking Jew, Jackson thought, a Catskills geezer. Fourteen year terms were too long. Micah was hoping Wolfson's set-up would lead to a punch line: Birnbaum reversed.

"So I'm letting that stand at this time," Wolfson ruled. "To put you on notice, Mister Jackson, I might change my mind later. But I always presume, at least in the first instance, that my colleagues' judgments are sound and have their reasons."

"Thank you, Your Honor," Jackson said. "But there's another issue."

"Oh, I'm sure there is."

"Given the nature of the charges, we think it's important that no one be in the courtroom other than the lawyers. And the defendant, of course." Jackson would try to exclude Bender too, but the Constitution got in the way: the right to confront your accusers, even if shackled with your mouth bound with tape. Jackson had requested and gotten that a few time, but never with Wolfson.

"You have witnesses, I assume," Wolfson said. "I mean it's not just you and Mister T'Sigh, *mano a mano* against Messrs. Bender and Levine."

Jackson smiled thinly. "We're concerned that with all the people on Mister Levine's witness list, some may be here just to listen. That's what the statute's intended to stop."

"The walls have ears," Wolfson said, stroking his now-gray beard. He looked out into his ruined theater: a perky yet somehow dumpy blonde in the front row, a black young man in his high school graduation suit, and a hippie-looking white guy, knotting his tie while this all went on. Comedy club dregs, Wolfson thought -- who are these people? He asked.

"*They*," Jackson said, pointing at Janet and George, "are the People's witnesses." He turned to Kurt. This was the one he wanted out -- Chuck Stewart from Empi said this was important so it must be.

"He's one of our witnesses," Micah cut in. No reason to say more unless Wolfson pushed it.

"I think it's fine," Wolfson said. There might only be three in the audience but it kept him on his toes, raised the quality of his quips. "Any more procedural matters, Mister Jackson?"

"Your   Honor,   we   think   it's   important--"

"I have *ruled*, if you didn't notice. Let's get the show on the road. Bada-bing. Opening statement, Mister Jackson. Or will it be Mister T'Sigh?"

Jackson wanted a recess, to regroup with Empi upstairs and explain for the record that this loss right out of the box wasn't his fault, that Empi had to give him a reason, some support for making these requests. He could also perk up at a recess, with the stash in his office and the dual-purpose mirror. Snorting then staring. He cut a sharp figure and he knew it.

"We may want to appeal your ruling, before we begin," Jackson said. "With all due respect, Your Honor," he added.

The Snowman wanted hardball, as if he'd change his mind at the mere mention of an appeal. "You're free to do so, Mister Jackson," Wolfson smiled. "But you better hurry and try. Because this trial's going forward at ten thirty, with or without you. See you then." Wolfson stood, noting their reflex to follow suit. Before they'd stood all the up way Wolfson said, "Cut the formalities. We have *much* more important things to deal with in this case." He went into his chambers and opened his browser.

* * *

Kurt called Marcos on the break, on the cell phone Marcos got in a store in Jackson Heights. "Uh, so did you talk to Candida?" he asked.

"Yeah man I did. She's an excellent girl -- older than us but I think you fucked up, dumping her and all."

Kurt wondered what she'd said. "She told you about her father?"

"Yeah," Marcos said, his voice becoming hard. "You're at the court?"

"There's a break," Kurt said. "They might not even get to your tomorrow. It looks like the DA is going to appeal every fucking ruling."

"Lemme know. I gotta run." Marcos hung up, and Kurt wondered for a moment if he was right, about the waste of cutting Candida loose. It was only a moment, because Jackson came out from the elevators, with three white guys that Kurt had not seen before. He followed them in to the courtroom.

45. The Flowing Juice

"Ahhh," Wolfson said when he came out at 10:29. "The more the merrier. Did you get me reversed?"

"We've decided not to appeal at this time," Jackson said. Wolfson stared at the three new faces in the front row. Two wore lawyer suits, Brooks Brothers or better; the third wore the drab uniform of corporate middle-management. "Relief pitchers?" Wolfson asked. Their proximity to the ballpark almost required baseball analogies. Wolfson had collected dozens in his day.

"They are lawyers from EmpiBank," Jackson said. "Since the death threat was made on Empi's employee, they have an interest in seeing that justice is done."

"The *alleged* death threat," Micah cut in.

Wolfson nodded. Then he mused, "Alleged death, or alleged threat?" It had come to this: parsing hum-drum legal phrases for hidden meanings. "So Mister Jackson, tell me about your case. Be brief, but tell me what you aim to prove."

The stenographer waited while Jackson rubbed his nose. "This is a case," Jackson began, feeling sharp and high, his moot court juices flowing, "about a repeatedly deficient employee threatening to kill his supervisor who disciplined him. This death threat was conveyed by means of interstate communications, triggering the anti-terrorism law to which we cite."

"I ain't deficient," Jack whispered heatedly to Micah. Wolfson glared at both of them.

"Our citation to that statute is not frivolous," Jackson said, almost convinced. "It is not simply a question of some domestic hothead falling into the net of a newly-passed law. The name he used, to make the threat, has a meaning we will make clear in this trial. The name he used -- and uses still -- to distribute for profit proprietary information of the company which he has stolen is also relevant--"

Jack couldn't contain himself. He thought of the dumpster, of the coffee-stained docs Janet was too lazy to shred. "I didn't steal *noth*ing," Jack said out loud.

"Mister Bender, you can't speak now. Your lawyer goes next. Take notes to show him, whatever you want to do. But no more outbursts. Are we clear?"

Jack nodded while shaking his head "no" like a bobble-head doll. Kurt was taking notes. Everyman behind closed doors. Wolfson was a trip -- *him*, Kurt wouldn't trash in his web reports. And least not yet.

"You will hear," Jackson continued, "from the target of this death threat, the manager of EmpiBank's much-needed branch in the West Farms community. She will recount for you the events that led to the defendant's suspension. She will describe how she knew where the fax came from. And then--" Jackson turned back, gesturing at George -- "you will hear from the employee of the Kinkos store from which the fax was sent. He will identify the man who faxed the threat. The statute will be satisfied in full. The defendant will be convicted and serve the mandatory sentence which his anti-social acts require." Jackson paused.

"Very eloquent," Wolfson said. "Mister Levine--

"I'm not finished," said Jackson. "Your Honor, this defendant got an Adjourned Contemplating Dismissal disposition of a previous case, a generous deal to clean up his act which he went ahead and broke. We'll be reinstating--"

"Objection," Micah said standing up. "His prior, in this case an unrelated misdemeanor charge, can't come up in this trial."

Wolfson leafed through the file. Here it was, Number 21-38-003. Perhaps that *wasn't* gravy, on this loser's tie. "I'm a judge, Mister Levine," Wolfson said. "I won't allow this previous charge to prejudice me in any way. Though I agree, I don't see how it's relevant."

"It will be at sentencing," Jackson said.

Jack thought of the Irish cop-whore that night on Boone; he thought of Zalie then he thought of running. Right out the door; straight to the airport or a Rent-A-Wreck™ place. Micah, perhaps, read his mind. "Take it easy," Micah whispered to Jack. "The judge knows this is all bullshit. It's going to be okay."

Easy for you to say, Jack thought. He turned around and glared at Janet Peel. Janet saw it and pointed; the Empi lawyers wrote on their pads. The third man wrote nothing, but thought: what a freak show. It was Mudnick, up from Baltimore on the Acela train to make sure that EmpiFinancial's proprietary methods were sufficiently safeguarded. Chuck Stewart from Security had briefed them in Jackson's office, but hadn't come back to the courtroom. Something about domestic violence, Mudnick couldn't remember. Empi's juice was overseas now. This was a sideshow.

"Okay, Mister Levine -- can we have your opening statement?" Wolfson thought this one would be better. Civil liberties and sticking it to the government were two of his last remaining pleasures in this robe. Since the death of his wife he'd made a list. He made many list but each one grew shorter.

"Certainly, Judge. I want to begin by apologizing for my client's shows of concern. It's not easy to take, being accused by not only an aggressive prosecutor like Mister Jackson, but by the largest bank in the world, behind him. I'll say my piece now, since I doubt that they'll even meet their burden of proof. A single witness, shown a single photograph--" Micah paused and tried to laugh. He'd written an outline but now he'd gone off-course. Begin at the beginning, he reminded himself.

"Let me tell you about my client, Mister Jack Bender. He could be any of us. He went to work for EmpiFinancial in Charlotte, North Carolina. They told him it was affiliated with EmpiBank, which advertises nationwide -- nothing about high-cost loans, only credit cards and student loans and financial advice from cradle to grave. It's one of America's great brands, a Coca-Cola of finance, a Disney World."

Wolfson looks at him strangely. You don't have to go there, he seemed to be saying. Stick to the fax.

But Micah had a plan. "Jack was promoted to branch manager in Charlotte. They must have liked his work, it seems fair to assume. Their only complaint, they noted in his file. Jack expressed concerns about the way they sold credit insurance. It didn't help the borrower, he said. Empi wrote this down as if it were a heresy." Micah paused. He and Wolfson should be able to laugh at the expense of the Catholics.

"They didn't burn him at the stake," Micah continued. "In fact they recruited him to help open a *new* Empi office, in the West Farms Mall here in The Bronx. Jack relocated, like a model employee, and helped to set the office up. He was the branch manager -- the branch founder, really. Their only complaint was that he wouldn't push credit insurance as aggressively as they wanted. Jack had a conversation with one of Mister Jackson's witnesses--" Micah turned back, gesturing -- "Miss Janet Peel, right there. He suggested to her that they cancel the credit insurance on a particular loan."

Micah turned back to Wolfson. "A loan to Bertha Watkins, a loan for a bed. Five thousand dollars for a bed, a very nice bed I'm sure--" as if he hadn't seen it -- "but nevertheless, just that: a bed. A loan officer, who is on our witness list, made the loan. Miss Gina Sunday. We will subpoena her if we must, about this loan. She told Bertha, Miss

Watkins, that she had to buy insurance. And after that happened, Jack told Janet Peel, let's cancel. And that's where his problems began."

Jackson looked back at the Empi lawyers, who were glaring. Jackson stood up. "Your Honor, I must object. This has nothing to do with this case. It's simply an attempt--"

"It's an opening statement," Wolfson said. "I let *you* talk about prostitution, said I'd keep an open mind. Same on this. Go on, Mister Levine. But try to be brief."

"Thank you, Judge. As I was saying, after Jack spoke up on insurance, his troubles began. They targeted his office for an audit. Jack was upset. Any problems they would find would only be those he was ordered to do. He was upset --" Micah lightly planted this seed, the human defense to the whoring charge in case it was needed -- "and he felt he'd be a scapegoat. When the audit occurred, he was not present." No reason to say where Jack *was* at the time: awaiting arraignment on the prostie rap. You took your clients as you found them. With their hands in their pants and jism on their tie if that was the case.

"Please get to the point, Mic -- Mister Levine," Wolfson said.

"I am, Judge. The audit was conducted by a man who as fate would have it is now in the courtroom with us." Micah turned. "Keith Mudnick, from Empi's home office in Baltimore."

Fuck, Mudnick thought. He should have stayed back in Action Jackson's office with Chuck.

"I want to make sure he'll be available as a witness," Micah continued. "Could you ask him, Your Honor?"

Wolfson shrugged. His court was like the Twilight Zone™ -- you came in to observe but you'd end up spilling your beans on the stand. "Will you be?" Wolfson asked.

Mudnick looked at the lawyer, no succor there. He stood up. "I only, uh, came up for the day," Mudnick stammered.

"Can you return tomorrow?"

Mudnick thought of the dogshit audits gathering dust on his desk on St. Paul's Place. "I'm quite busy, uh, Your Honor," he said, almost saying Your Excellency.

"It's important," Micah said, to Wolfson not Mudnick.

"Try to be here," Wolfson said. "Or I'll issue a subpoena." He turned back to Micah. "Two minute warning, Mister Levine. It's scintillating, the story you're telling. But I want to start the witnesses before lunch."

"As do I," Micah said. "To make a long story short, Miss Peel convinced Mr. Mudnick to suspend Jack Bender, for his lack of obedience on the credit insurance. We will show, with expert testimony, that selling credit insurance on items such as a bed is predatory *per se*." The rhyme again with Shah-Day and Zah-Day, Micah thought; a Latin phrase that made Jackson sick. "We will explain terms like insurance packing, loan flipping, the designation of document forgers as 'Mister Light.'" Micah was proud of his attention to detail. He'd pinched his leg while Bender'd droned on but now it would bear fruit.

"In sum, Your Honor, we will show that Jack Bender was a whistleblower, a complainant about corporate fraud who was fired for his efforts. Since then EmpiFinancial has done everything in its power to railroad my client, to intimidate borrowers with whom he's had contact, even to convince the otherwise reasonable District Attorney of our fair county to charge Mr. Bender with terrorism, under a statute that runs counter to decades of First and Fifth Amendment jurisprudence--"

"Okay, Mister Levine, you've got my attention. In an opening statement you couldn't ask for more. I usually take a break now but we're already late. Mister Jackson, put on your first witness. Tee it up and let it rip."

White men and golf, thought Jackson. Though he got in eighteen holes up in Westchester whenever possible. Empi had its own golf course in Armock, he'd heard. If he nailed this cracker those greens would be his.

* * *

White boys were a joke, Candida was thinking. Marcos' arms were are hard as steel chains. Why he wanted to know about her father she wasn't sure. Kurt and his cruelty; Kurt and his pornographic mind. Kurt had been good, in his way. But like her girlfriends said, he would never settle down. That had been fine with her but the zygote never stuck. Kurt thought it was her, she felt sure: old eggs awash in a pharmaceutical cocktail from the supply closets of Metropolitan Hospital. Marcos knew none of this, had never seen her cry. She could start over. He could get a college degree with his benefits from the Department of Defense. Her mind was racing forward, drinking venti lattes in the Starbucks on 99th Street. She'd already offered to pay, in support of Marcos' service to both of their adopted country. I love a man in a uniform, Candida thought, some punk rock song Kurt put on Stewart's stereo in her apartment, some hateful analogy between love and anthrax. He hated himself, Kurt did, with that Wheelock schtick. This Marcos was a man and she might let him prove it. The coffee was blasting away at the remnants of depressants; the juices were starting to flow.

46. The Snowman Tees It Up

First up for Empi was Janet prissy Peel -- Kurt wondered if she had a nickname, something about bitter fruit. Jack called her The Clam but it didn't quite fit. Who screamed the name Janet when the workday was done, when the liens were all filed and even the springs of the Rent-A-Center couches grew silent? Kurt wished he was a sketch artist, with his easel in the corner where the floor boards bent from water's leak. He could try to bring a digital video cam tomorrow, see if wacky Wolfson would let it slide.

"Good morning, Ms. Peel." This was Wing Tsai's moment, the actual work of the case: getting the evidence in like building a railroad tie-by-tie. They'd practiced this twice, the second time breaking off repeatedly for Jackson's cinematic directions. Ingmar Bergman on coke. Cries and whispers and still Wing had no read on lifeless Janet. Did she really fear for her life? Had she? Wing had no idea.

Janet took the oath, the kick-off "so help me God" in a strange monotone, her eyes fixed ten feet over Bender's head. The baby-napping fiasco had taken its toll. If they cut her loose after Wolfson ruled, she wouldn't work at HomeQuik, not as long as Jack was there. She'd done Mary Kay; she'd gotten a pitch from Advantage Marketing Systems. The many flavors of the Ponzi scheme, or the term they preferred, "network marketing." She was getting too old to start again at the bottom. She'd watch their back and they better watch hers.

"Ms. Peel, where do you work?"

"EmpiFinancial. I am a District Manager. I have been with the company for seventeen years."

"What are your duties, as a District Manager for EmpiFinancial?" They'd gone over this again and again. "Just that you supervise," he'd coached her. "We'll take the story from there."

"I am in charge of six branches. Three in Westchester, two in Queens, and this new one in The Bronx. I heard the defendant's lawyer say that he started the Bronx office, that he was the founder or something."

"Ms. Peel--" Wing tried to glare; it didn't come off.

"It's not true. *I* started that office. They brought him in just to run it. But he messed everything up."

"I was getting to that," Wing said. Jackson would say that he wasn't controlling the witness. But this lady had an axe to grind. She was grinding her teeth and Wing saw her mascara like powder, the inklings of a clown somehow -- bad luck to think that so he cut if off. "Tell us about Mister Bender, your experience supervising him up to the date of his suspension."

"He didn't know what he was doing. They brought him up from the Charlotte office. He would talk fast, honey this and honey that, but his paperwork was never in order. When the branch got audited--"

"Let's slow down, Ms. Peel. Since the defense is trying to say he was a model employee, walk me through the paperwork that you mentioned, and how Mister Bender's was not in order."

"We file daily reports with Home Office -- shelf space, it's called. Every one of my other offices turns them in on time. With Jack it was always a day late and a dollar short." Janet liked clichés, especially street-smart ones from movies. She'd taped An Officer and a Gentleman and watched it until the tape was frayed. She could channel Debra Winger. Wing was nonplussed. He wanted to cut this whistleblower crap off in the bud. Maybe the phrase was "nip," but that also meant Japanese, at least some people said. "How late would his paperwork be?"

"Two day, a week -- it was never on time. Home Office noticed it and they came up to audit." Janet watched as Jack whispered in his lawyer's ear. She pushed forward. "The day of the audit Jack didn't even come in to the office. Later we found out that he'd been arrested for hiring a prostitute--"

"Objection!" Micah said loudly, pushing Jack back with his hand. "Hearsay."

"We have judicial records on that, Your Honor," Wing said.

"No foundation," Micah countered.

"Calm *down*," Wolfson sighed. "As I said, I'm a judge, I won't let myself be prejudiced. For now I don't care why Mister Bender wasn't in the office that day. Pick it up from the audit results. And let's get to the fax. Please, let's get to the fax."

"Yeah Your Honor," Wing said. Micah sat down. His objection had essentially been sustained. And Jack'd already given him a nice tidbit for cross. About a friend of his, an acquaintance really, who'd ignored his advice because he had no balls.

"Did Mister Bender fail the audit?" Wing asked.

Janet began saying yes then stopped. "He got a Four," she said, adding, "not good."

Wing considered asking again about failure and decided not to. The lady was pissed enough that she would have said yes if she could. So why *did* he get fired, Wing wondered. This case sucked but he'd get the blame.

"So who decided to suspend Mr. Bender? The defense has suggested that you--"

Micah cut in. "He's leading the witness."

"Withdrawn," Wing said. "Who decided to suspend Mister Bender?"

Micah could have objected again: no foundation yet laid that Bender had been suspended. This Tsai guy was a rookie. Micah almost felt sorry for him. Almost.

"Home Office did."

Wing waited for more but Janet'd clammed up. "Who in Home Office?"

"Mister Mudnick. Right over there."

Maybe they'll pay for a hotel room, Mudnick thought. Three hours down to Baltimore and then back up was ridiculous. The action wasn't in Times Square anymore but he was sure he could find it elsewhere.

"And who conveyed this decision to Mister Bender?"

"I did," Janet said. "He was drunk and abusive." Jack rustled, whispering again to his lawyer and glaring at her. "He knocked over a file cabinet and he, uh, he used profanity."

Wing wondered whether to ask. No. The skel was going to testify and it would come out then. "Did he threaten you? At that time, before the fax."

Janet nodded. "He said, and I quote, 'You'll regret this you bitch.'"

Wing waited a beat, to let the hum-drum threat sink in.

And you will, Jack thought. They'll toss you out like they tossed me and you'll be selling your bony white ass on Boone Avenue and no one will stop. Jack smiled at the picture, some boozed-up Ricans in a low-rider having their fun with her. Micah stared into space. People say bitch everyday.

"And what happened next?" Wing asked. This was the main scene, the first link in the chain that would hang Jack Bender, or at least subject him to sodomy.

"I got a call that night," Janet said. "Or three calls, really. First from the New Rochelle office, then from Jackson Heights. Then finally from West Farms in the Bronx."

Wing held up his hand. He'd told her this: let him ask questions, answer them one at a time. Had to pace this right. Levine was an asshole who'd pounce on any mistake. "What were the calls about?"

"That a fax--"

"Objection!" Micah said. This was too easy. "Hearsay."

"Not offered for the truth," Wing began and then stopped. He'd asked Jackson why they didn't have Gina What's-Her-Name, the one who got the fax at West Farms. She could say what she read, and that she'd called Janet. The Snowman was lazy, liked to set his ADAs up for a fall and keep his hands clean.

"Mister Tsai?" Wolfson asked. "I'm going to sustain the objection unless you re-phrase." CUNY wasn't what it once was, Wolfson thought. Or, the CUNY law school had always been crap. But City College back in the day had pulsed with IQ along with other hormones. He noted his nostalgia, the racist tinge, and looked out the window.

"Did you come to see a fax?" Wing asked, jumping forward in his script, like Fast Forward while Play on a VCR, the tape would fray but who cared, one time through was all it took.

"Yes," Janet said. "I went to the West Farms office and was shown a fax that said I should die."

"Your Honor, People's Exhibit A," Wing said as he'd been trained. He handed a copy to Levine and another to judge.

"Any objection, Mister Levine?" Wolfson asked.

Micah showed it to Jack. "It's bullshit," Jack said loudly.

"A *legal* objection," Wolfson said. "Not barnyard."

"No, Judge," Micah said. "We'll raise our points on cross."

"Very well. You may proceed, Mister Tsai."

"Could you read the contents of the fax into the record, Ms. Peel? Just the parts that are highlighted." They'd used florescent yellow ink. This shouldn't be hard.

"It's full of misspellings," Janet said. "I'd think you want--"

"Just read the highlighted sections," Wing said. The mistakes were part of the point.

"Okay. 'You are been robbed.' The bin is spelled b-e-*e*-n, no I or G. Then it says, 'Janet Peel is a bitch and a thief and she should die.'"

Janet stopped, tried to bring up tears as she'd rehearsed, couldn't get them to come, made her hands shake instead.

"Do you need a moment, Ms. Peel?" Wing asked solicitously and on cue.

"No," Janet whispered hoarsely.

Go back to acting school, Kurt thought. He'd seen better performances in his sixth grade play, The Importance of Being Earnest. How to describe this right, like Oscar Wilde who'd quipped when he emigrated to France, "I have nothing to declare but my genius." Peel had nothing to declare but her total mediocrity. It was screaming in her self-vibrating hands. Kurt had seen Candida do that, but Candida was better. Some of her shakes were real.

"How is the fax signed, Ms. Peel?" Wing asked.

"It's with cut-out letters, like from a magazine." She glared at Jack. "It says 'Tareek Noor.'"

"And did you come to learn what that--"

Micah said "hearsay" without standing up.

"Fine," Wing said. "We have an expert."

"Are you done with the witness?" Wolfson asked, knowing Wing wasn't, but offering the novice a way out, a graceful exit. He would let them jump straight to Kinkos without even a connector. It pained Wolfson to see such a half-assed show. The law was a whore but still it had its rules. This was like the free verse in a how-to-assemble manual for a plastic hibachi.

"Uh, no Your Honor, we have a bit more."

"Get on with it then."

Wing licked his lips, avoiding Jackson's glare, the lifeless kangaroo court of the Empi hatchet men. "Did you go to the police?" Wing asked.

"I did. I filed a complaint with the Forty Eighth precinct."

"People's Exhibit B," Wing said, repeating the ritual. The police report. Even Wolfson would waive the cops' appearance here unless necessary, given the need for security in the World's Most Targeted City.™

"No objection," Levine said helpfully. He was itching to shish kebob this shiksa.

"So I went to the Kinkos--"

Wing cut her off. "Please, Ms. Peel, wait for *me* to ask the questions." One of the Empi lawyers groaned. "Looking back at the fax, at People's Exhibit A -- what does it say at the top?"

"It says Kinkos," Janet said flatly. Multi-level marketing seemed more attractive all the time. "It says 718, too."

"What   did   you   do?"

"I looked on the Internet, to find which Kinkos it was."

"People's Exhibit C, Your Honor," Wing said.

Wolfson rolled his eyes. "I'll take judicial notice of the Kinkos web site," he said. "I'll even check it myself at the lunch break, *just* to be sure. Time's a'wasting, Mister Tsai. Let's get to the point here."

Wing felt weak, still holding the Internet print-out. "Which Kinkos was it?" he managed to say.

"The one on Webster Avenue. I went there with Gina--" she stopped for a moment, was she supposed to mention the missing tramp or not -- "and I talked to the guy behind the counter. He said that yeah--"

"Objection," Micah said.

"I agree," Wolfson said. "This is going to be hearsay. Really, Mister Jackson, I thought your office *prepared* the witnesses..."

Jackson, hearing his name, looked up from a fantasy he had. "We defend a whole county," Jackson said.

"God help us," Wolfson muttered, then winked at the court reporter. She smiled back. That prayer would not go in the record. "So are the People done with Ms. Peel?"

"Yes," Wing said.

"Mister Levine, she's all yours," Wolfson said. "But it'll be after lunch. I recommend the new café on Walton and 158. All the Yankees' beat writers go there. We're adjourned."

Janet looked around the courtroom, adrenaline and hormones pumping now for naught. "How'd I do?" she asked Wing, or Jackson really, at the table. She looked past them at her real audience, Mudnick and the grim-faced suits. Tupperware, cosmetics -- when you met the public's need you didn't have to worry. It'd be just another slippery corporate ladder to climb.

47. The Clam Bake

At lunchtime it was that Ernie Swanker dropped his bomb on Artful Homes, at a Rochester press conference which Basso scrambled to attend but too late. It went like clockwork: Swanker flew in at a quarter to ten, freshened up at a riverfront hotel, combing his hair down down

down his shiny forehead. At noon the local press, such as it was, assembled in the hotel's Genesee Ballroom. The senior law enforcement officer in the state had news. The buzz words on the day book wire were predatory lending with a side dish of Basso. Chilean Sea Basso with a glaze of nuclear North Korean kimchi.

Swanker heard the pop pop pop of the cameras; he took out his speech, triple-spaced in 18 point type. "I have come here today to put an end to a racket," he began. "It is a scourge that steals the deepest dreams of our hardest-working citizens. They rise to catch the morning bus--" he stole this from a reverend, finding the irony with Artful Homes' evangelistic pitch delicious like fish -- "and at the end of the day, the end of the year, they dream of their own castle. Homeownership. It's the bedrock of our system, the way we buy the people in." That was ambiguous. He'd need new speechwriters for the House campaign. "It's how people buy into the American Dream," Swanker ad libbed. He still had it. These platitudes would take him far he thought.

"Which is why those who steal those dreams must be called what they are -- terrorists. As surely as Al Qaeda struck at Wall Street's nerve, predatory lenders gnaw at the heart of our capitalistic system." Who *wrote* this shit? Swanker had delegated this, concentrating on the politics of Basso and his upcoming appointment with the Doctor Bonely Hair Loss Clinic. Chewing a capitalistic heart? He felt sick but pressed onward. Drum roll please.

"Today I've indicted the owners and directors of the shady lender known as Artful Homes. The only thing artful about these crooks is their come-on." You couldn't win them all, but that one he liked. "There's a class that they give, called Pathways to Freedom." He paused, looking up from the speech and winging it. "*Think* of that name for a moment. Think of the national equity on which it plays. It's almost subliminal. It uses our highest aspiration -- freedom, sweet freedom -- and the mythical concept of the path, the struggle, the long way home. And then what does it do?"

The reporters waited; some of them wondered if Swanker was high. He wouldn't be the first; he wouldn't be the last. Statewide pols came to Monroe to rehab. To practice their speeches in the Rust Belt. Swanker's needed work.

"They destroy those dreams! They obliterate them as surely as an airplane full of jet fuel and people. They slice right through, cutting beams and all support. They collapse the towers of our hopes, leaving behind resentment and racial unrest."

Damn Artful Homes is good, one reporter thought. Nine Eleven, over-used, soon got stale.

"It's only money, you say. But five hundred dollars here, five hundred dollars there -- these crooks are living like CEOs, while their victims struggle to pay the rent and the light bill. It's a crime, and I've indicted it as such." Swanker paused, holding the aura of the absent Basso in his hands like fish over a barbecue grill.

"This is a local matter, you say."

Who, a reporter wondered. Who said that?

"And I agree," Swanker said. "For now Artful Homes' artful scam has been limited to Monroe County. So normally, I wouldn't be here." He smiled, putting down the speech because this part he'd written himself, this part he knew by heart. "But I've *had* to come. I've had to come because the local authorities, the local District Attorney, has done *nothing* to stop this scourge. I know what you think -- we're all members of the Democratic Party, we watch each other's backs. Well we try. I prefer to. But my duty is to the people, not to the party. And when a local D.A. refuses to act, I feel I must. I owe the people no less."

Hands shot up, microphones were thrust forward. "You mean Basso?"

No shit Sherlock, Swanker thought. The phrase was his son's but he liked it. Sidwell Friends, the Quaker school in DC, was good enough for Clinton, for Kennedy before him and Cuomos yet to come. It was good enough for Swanker's brood. "Sadly, I do."

"Are you saying--"

"No more questions," Swanker said. "I have pressing people's business back in Albany. Copies of the indictment are on the table by the door. Good day."

Mother *fuck,* Swanker whispered on the way to the airport. Basso would be clawing out from the shit for weeks to come. There were nothing but blue skies ahead; nothing but a full head of natural-looking relocated hair, nothing but C-SPAN and full franking privileges. This would teach Empi to try to squeeze his balls.

* * *

The signless restaurant that Wolfson had pitched wasn't bad. Micah had panini, provolone and olive spread. Jack said it was crap but ate roast beef. Kurt tagged along, after vowing to keep any privileged talk off his web site.

"I could see that clam pissing in her pants," Jack said, doing a three-way with the metaphor, squirting Gulden's Deli Style™ on his blood-red meat.

"She seemed like a zombie," Kurt said. "Like her heart wasn't in it."

"What heart?" Jack asked. "That bitch is a good fucking Nazi is what she is."

Micah gritted his teeth, as the Holocaust tended to make him do. "So was your paperwork really late?"

"Fuck no," Jack said. "I mean a couple times yeah sure maybe. I made *money* for those pieces a shit. That was always the point with them. As long as you did the Shelf Space by the end of the month, if the numbers were good, they would RocoPolize your ass."

"No swearing when you testify," Micah said again. "*If* you testify." He'd gotten more hopeful that it wouldn't get there. He'd move to dismiss after Jackson's case was done. And Wolfson would grant it since he wasn't blind. This way Bertha wouldn't have to testify either. They could celebrate the win in the way that he had planned.

"And another thing," Jack said. "We wasn't alone, Janet and me, when she told me I'm suspended. Gina Fucking Sunday was there, smiling like the whore she is. She heard the whole thing. I wasn't drunk neither."

"I mailed her a subpoena but got no response." Micah said. "Do you know where she is?"

"I asked her to come to the dark side," Jack said. Micah raised his eyebrows. "To HomeQuik. But the frigid bitch said no."

Micah waited for an answer.

"I could go there tonight," Jack said.

"Or I'll do it," Kurt offered.

"Let's see if we have to. My sense is Judge Wolfson's gonna call the whole thing off."

"You're serious?" Jack asked.

Micah remembered the Wall Street disclaimer. "Past results are no guarantee of future performance," he said. "But Wing Tsai is a newbie and Jackson is high."

Can I quote you, Kurt thought. WatchCorp would be singing tonight, if anybody cared.

"Let's go." Micah paid the check.

"Fuck that clam for me," Jack said on the way back on Walton.

Micah thought of City Island, a dozen oysters after slipping Mrs. Morales a twenty to babysit. Oysters were an aphrodisiac. An *Afro-*

desiac in this case, he hoped. "I'll fuck the clam," he agreed, though the main clam he wanted was Empi. "I'll fuck the clam until all that's left is the pearl of truth."

* * *

Chuck had heartburn, taking Jackson to the woodshed once again. "If - you - fuck - this - up -you're -out -- you understand?" "This judge is a Commie," Jackson said. "That's what all the losers say. You better have this George kid nailed down or we're dead." Chuck thought about George: the well-behaved young black male the country said it wanted. Where had it gotten him? Photocopying white kids' term papers at midnight; delivering camera-ready commercial artwork and drugs in the canyons of Midtown. And now a perjury trap or something like it. No justice no peace, thought Chuck. "Just do it," he said. "Play the card and make it work."

* * *

"Are you ready, Ms. Peel?" Wolfson asked.

Janet'd brought her own lunch, ate it in the jurors' waiting room on the second floor after the Empi lawyers' prepping. "Yes," she said. Deny deny deny, she reminded herself. Yes or no, no more than that.

"Good afternoon, Miss Peel," Micah said, smelling shell fish, relishing the moment, the olive paste taste still in his mouth.

Janet didn't answer. She wanted Empi's eyes and ears to see and hear her refusal to cooperate. I'm a good soldier, she thought. An officer and a gentlewoman.

"Just a few questions," Micah said, the way he always started, a few simple questions that would put in you jail, make insurers pay for the long-concealed layers of old lead paint, for the broken sidewalk or the scalpel forgotten in the wound.

"Now Miss Peel," Micah began, "you've said you are a district manager, overseeing six offices--"

"Yes," Janet said leaning forward, eager for that to once again be the case.

"But currently, in fact, you're merely the manager a single office, the West Farms branch -- isn't that correct?"

"That's just temporary, I mean--"

Micah raised his hand and turned to Wolfson. "Judge, could you instruct the witness to answer simply yes or no?"

Wolfson nodded. "Ms. Peel, this is different than when Mister Tsai questioned you. When Mister Levine says 'isn't that correct,' in his inimitable style--" actually it was straight from TV, straight from Brooklyn Law School moot court -- "you're to answer only yes or no. You might *want* to say more, you might want to explain. But that's not allowed at this juncture. Mister Tsai will be able to ask you a final round of questions, so you can clarify and amplify at that time. Do you understand?"

Janet was angry, at these games and these tricks. The judge spoke to her in the same nursery school sing-song as to Jack. "It's just not *true*, what he's saying," she complained..

"Then answer no," said Wolfson.

Micah smiled. "It'll ask it again. At present, Ms. Peel, your only job function at EmpiFinancial is as the manager of the West Farms branch -- true or false?"

"True, but--"

"Okay," Micah cut her off. "You testified that my client, Jack Bender, was previously the manager of that branch, isn't that correct?"

"Until he got susp--"

"Yes or no, Miss Peel."

Janet glared at Micah. "Yes," she said, then slumped back in her chair.

"So it'd be fair to say that you *took* Mister Bender's job, then -- isn't that correct?"

"No it would not," Janet said, leaning forward again. "I was his supervisor. I saw the way he was running the office and it couldn't be allowed to continue, it just couldn't--"

Micah let her proceed just this far, then raised his hand. "So you were in *favor* of Mister Bender being suspended, isn't that correct?"

"Yes I was," Janet said, proud to get this in.

"So you got him fired and took his job," Micah said matter-of-faxly, turning to face the shattered courtroom, spinning back to Peel to ask his next question. This first foray was just to piss her off, to rattle her cage and make her willing to blurt out answers she thought would help her. Micah couldn't resist taking another jab.

"Since you've taken Jack Bender's job, Miss Peel, isn't it true that the office has been the subject of a negative article in the New York Post?"

Janet didn't answer. Micah feigned surprise, raising his eyebrows, watching to the desk, ignoring Jack's florid face, his attempt to whisper advice. "Defendant's Exhibit A," Micah said, handing a copy of the "Empi Cradle" article to Tsai, then another to Wolfson. The third copy he kept for Janet.

"Objection," Jackson said, rising and stepping in front of Tsai. "This has nothing to do with the death threat--"

"Credibility of the witness, Your Honor," Micah said. Wolfson was reading the article, pretending he hadn't already surfed all this on the 'Net.

"I'll allow it," Wolfson said. "For babies everywhere, I have no choice but to allow it." He smiled at his own joke then added, "Though its probative value has yet to be shown."

"Thank you," Micah said. Janet's face had turned red, a more even red than Jack's but brighter too. She held the article as far away from herself as she could. "Do you recognize this article, Ms. Peel?"

"I've seen it. It really has nothing--"

"And that's you in the picture, is it not?" Janet nodded. "Yes or no, Miss Peel," Micah said. "For the court reporter."

"Yes."

"And what exactly were you doing, when this picture was taken?" It was Micah's first open-ended question, but there was nowhere for the clam to run, it would split open and spill its sad vindictive juice from the stand. Micah relished these moments and thought of tartar sauce.

"I was doing a repo -- a repossession of a car that the customer was delinquent on."

"We'll get back to that, delinquency," Micah said portentously for no one. "But it's the *baby* I'm asking about, the baby in the car seat. What were you doing with a baby, Miss Peel?"

Janet stared over at Jackson, then behind him at Mudnick, the stern-faced twin towers of Empi. Were cruel fertility jokes allowed in this court? "I was returning her," Janet said plainly. Give it a gender; make her caring clear. Janet avoided looking at Jack. His shameful disease has spread to her. She felt it on her face.

"From where?" Micah asked. "Was it your baby?"

Janet glared, this second cheap shot at her soft spot. "When we repossessed the car, for some reason the workmen didn't fully check it out. They are, or were, independent contractors. The baby was asleep in a car seat in the back. We returned it -- her -- as soon as we realized. Along with the car."

"So you kidnapped a customer's baby, to collect on a loan -- isn't that correct?"

"No," Janet said. "It was a mistake. The workmen's mistake. The next day I cancelled--"

"But aren't you the branch manager? Aren't *you* responsible for what happens, especially on a repossession run in which you participate?"

Janet didn't answer, and Micah didn't push it. He was tapping the clam's shell to test it; it was open for business, ready to yield up Empi's accounting fraud secrets.

"Let's talk about delinquency," Micah announced, like this was a talk show, or he a psychiatrist -- his mother had wanted him to be one but he liked this better. Cross-examination was a chance for legal cruelty. Silence could be mean but this was more fun. "Since it's listed as one of the reasons that Jack was suspended, let's talk about it. What is POT Thirty, Ms. Peel?"

Janet relaxed in her chair. This part wasn't about her and it was easier. "It means thirty days late on a loan," she said. She turned the New York Post article over, print side down, to not look at it again. See no evil.

"And POT Ninety would be ninety days past due, isn't that correct?"

Janet nodded, then said, "Yes."

"Now, the compensation at EmpiFinancial is tied to how few loans your branch has that are POT Thirty, or POT Ninety as the case may be, isn't that correct?"

"Yes," Janet said.

"Objection," said Jackson. "Relevance." The shorter your spiel, the better your likelihood of success. It was easier too.

"We *are* going a bit far afield," Wolfson mused. "But for now I'll allow it, subject to reconnection."

Micah nodded in thanks, decided to jump forward in his question tree. "Are you aware of instances where EmpiFinancial employees have mis-applied payments from one account to another to reduce their volume of delinquent loans?"

Janet was motionless. It was a well known trick in Empi, and there were many more. Mudnick was shaking his head at Janet from the front row; the lawyers next to him were glaring, burning holes in the back of Jackson's head.

"You'll soon see the relevance," Micah said to Wolfson, cutting Jackson and Tsai off before they could object.

"Please answer, Ms. Peel," Wolfson said. He'd traded a few stocks in his day, back when he still cared about the future; he'd read more recently about Enron and WorldCom. This might be grassroots accounting fraud that Micah was probing, but it made the day more interesting.

"I've *heard* of that," Janet said.

"Hearsay!" Jackson yelled too loud. Micah stifled a smile. He could ask these questions on cross, could make Janet answer about what she'd heard.

"State of mind," Micah said, to nail the point home.

"Go on," Wolfson said. The judge was paying more attention, Micah sensed. This transcript would be golden. Kurt was thinking the same. EmpiCon: Kurt could see the headline now.

"And have you heard of Empi branches seeking payment deferments based on tornadoes and other weather incidents, when in fact none occurred?"

This was Mudnick's problem not hers, Janet decided. It was his shop that approved the bogus tornado deferments, always near the end of the month when the bonuses were being calculated based on reductions in delinquency month-to-month. "Yeah I've heard of that," Janet said. "But that's not why we--"

"We'll get to Jack, don't worry," Micah said. "Just as you did. But first, please tell the court what an R.B.O. is."

Janet looked over at Mudnick, who was scribbling furiously on a yellow pad. He didn't hold it up to her. No message, no way out. "Refinance Balance Only," Janet answered.

"Meaning rewriting a loan with no extra money out to the customer, but to make the loan *appear* to be performing, while adding points and fees and other new changes to it -- isn't that correct?"

"You could describe it that way. It's really a favor to the customer, to help their credit history--"

"And it benefits the Empi employee, because it reduces delinquency and gets them a bonus, isn't that correct?"

"It could do that."

"And the borrower ends up owing more than they did before the RBO, isn't that correct?"

"Usually."

Micah smiled. "More like, always. But let me ask you -- is this what you understand by the term 'loan flipping,' which Empi has been accused of?"

"I think that's what they're referring to. They don't really understand our business." Janet was looking at Kurt; they'd told her he was the one behind WatchCorp, that web site they'd had to block from all the browsers in Empi, adding it to their NetNanny™ list along with porno and gambling and job-search sites. The Internet bred dissension. She could understand China, censoring the whole shebang, if she thought about it.

Fuck yeah, Jack was thinking. Let these fucking bastards swing in the breeze. He turn and grinned at Mudnick and his yuppie guard dogs. He wanted to say, Clint Eastwood-like, "Aren't cha sorry you didn't pay me my severance now? You're going down, you sleazy bastards." Jack wondered what they'd be willing to pay him now, to call off the dogs. But it might be too late for that. Micah was still barking.

"*Okay* Miss Peel," Micah said, feeling he'd gotten his bennies out of this case already. Bertha should have seen this. He still had to clear the poor fuck's name. "Now we'll get to Jack, or really to the fax you say you received, since there's no proof that Jack sent it." Micah paused, waiting for an objection that he'd shoot down with glee. They hadn't even tried to connect Jack to the fax in their questioning of Janet. That would ride on the boy George, who still wasn't back in the courtroom. Maybe he wouldn't come back -- if so, case closed, case dismissed, Cracker Walks Free and Micah-Snake make *mucho dinero* with Janet's admissions of loan flipping. He could imagine the cases already. With the loan files Jack had -- wherever he got them from -- Micah could cold-call at least a hundred Empi customers, make them aware they'd been ripped off and could sue. He could throw some more cases to Lorraine, start charging a referral fee. The cracker was a red-faced gold mine, in his stupid spotted tie. Micah cut to the chase.

"When you went to the Kinkos, did you take a photograph?"

"Yeah, because--"

"And you took only *one* photograph with you, isn't that correct?"

"We knew it was--"

"One photograph, yes or no?"

"Yes."

'We'll be hearing from another witness, George Wilson," Micah said to no one in particular. "Is he the person you spoke to at the Webster Avenue Kinkos?"

"I think that's his name." Janet knew, but there had to be a trick here somewhere.

"And you showed him that single photograph, isn't that correct?"

"Yeah and he said--"

"Hearsay," Micah said. "We'll let Mister Wilson speak for himself." Micah turned and walked back toward Jack. The cracker was making faces at the Empi trio in the front row. Let him have his fun, Micah thought before spinning back at Janet. "One question I forgot," he said.

Janet had started standing up, feeling the sweat on the back of her thighs, her polyester skirt stuck between them and the fake-leather chair -- now she sat back down. This bastard.

"When Home Office, as you call them, came to audit the West Farm branch, that was because of a *government* inquiry, isn't that correct?"

Janet was tugging at her skirt, trying to remember what she'd said before lunch, and where she'd sat in the jury waiting room. Who knew what scuz they left on those chairs. She looked at Mudnick but he was no help. "Uh, I'm not sure," Janet said.

"Let me help you," Micah said. "This morning, you said--" he looked down at his legal pad, though he knew this trick by heart -- "that Home Office noticed that Jack's paperwork was late, so they came up from Baltimore to do an audit."

"Yes," Janet said, relieved. "That's what happened."

Micah nodded, drawing the moment out. "But didn't you tell my client that the reason for the audit was that the Attorney General of New York State, Mister Ernest Swanker, had requested documents about the West Farms branch, and credit insurance more generally?"

"I, uh, I might have said--"

"Did you say it or not? Yes or no."

"I think I did say that, yes. There were a lot--"

"That will be all Miss Peel. Thank you for your candor."

Kurt's pen was flying to write this all down. Now Swanker's name had surfaced in the case and all bets were off. He wouldn't have to mention the nanny business, just the Q and A between Micah and The Clam. That Swanker'd been looking and then he backed off. A few blind quotes from the Riverdale terrace and bango. Kurt wanted to rush up to Fordham right now, write and upload, e-mail the stuck-up financial press and show 'em what they were missing, scoops that were the fruits of dogged pursuit of global corporations. Another world is possible, like the World Trade Organization protesters said. The anti-globalization movement would syndicate his Internet screeds and he'd become a minor pop star, like that No Logo quasi-hottie or the farmer from France with his battering-ram cheese wheels. *Moi no loco*, Kurt thought in Franglish.

"Is your next witness ready?" Wolfson asked Jackson and Tsai.

"He's been waiting in my office," Jackson said. "We'll go get him now."

"Ten minute recess," Wolfson said. Wolfson's contempt for Swanker was only partially envy. Maybe old Ernie'd have to come testify and bite the hand that fed him, or one of the hands at least. Wolfson no longer needed Empi or anyone else. Twelve more years and a casket. But Swanker needed Empi. A perjury trap for that prick might be just the trick.

48. Of Color / *De Colores*

The Empi team, including Jackson and Tsai, rushed out of the courtroom and into the elevators. Micah, Jack and Kurt stood in the hall. "You ripped the clam a new asshole," Jack gushed, slapping Micah on the back. Then he got more serious. "They're gonna drop the case, right?"

"They won't drop it," Micah said. "But as soon as the kid from Kinkos is done and they rest their case, I'll make a motion to dismiss. And I think Wolfson will grant it."

* * *

Thirty feet from them, through layers of false marble, rotting plaster and lathe -- some rats' nests and decades old wiring -- Wolfson was surfing the 'Net. Was Swanker chasing Empi or nor? One Wall Street Journal article said he was. A second one, mostly about a Securities and Exchange Commission investigation of insider trading in Empi's stock, implied that he wasn't. There was a Reuters story, from just a few hours ago, that mentioned Swanker and Empi. But Empi's name was near the bottom, some overview of the predatory lending issue. Swanker had declared war on Artful Homes, a company Wolfson'd never heard of, and on the Rochester District Attorney, natch. Swanker was shooting the privately-held guppies in the barrel and letting the great white shark swim free.

Wolfson would have liked to tell Micah: "Don't let this Swanker thread go. I'll dismiss every objection until there's enough in the record to pull that weasel into the case by his thinning black hair and make him squeal." Wolfson regally poured himself a Chivas, steadying his nerves for the Kinkos witness. What a mundane drama, he thought. A Greek tragedy in a strip mall. It was an appropriate case for his declining years. He would have joked about it with his wife, if she hadn't been dead. Who did he have to joke with now? His best and last friend was Chivas, his conversations now with books. He heard a rat in the wall and he no longer cared.

* * *

In Jackson's office Chuck was prepping George. "You'll get what we promised if you stick to the script," Chuck told him. "Bender's a racist, we both know that. And his lawyer acts slick 'cause that's his gig -- charming juries of color in the Bronx County court. But you know who his friends on the weekend are. White folk like him. Most of 'em Jewish, like the judge. Facts are facts, though, my brother -- am I right or what?"

It was like "isn't that correct," a phrase to box you in, in this case to an absurd race solidarity in defense of a loan shark. "I hear you," George said, which wasn't untrue. He'd heard the pitch, he'd read the script. The show must go on. They headed back to Wolfson's courtroom.

* * *

"Good afternoon, Mister Wilson," Jackson began. It was time for the big boys. Wing Tsai looked like he was about to cry. There was the race card, too: Jackson and George, two brothers representin' in a white judge's court in a county of color. *We are the future*, Jackson wanted to shout. Hear us roar. "Now there's two separate things that the court needs to hear. First about the faxing, then what came after. Do you remember that woman--" he pointed at Janet -- "coming into the Kinkos store in the time that you worked there?"

It was leading; it was typical Jackson, but Micah let it go. The one-photo line-up was all he would need.

"Yeah," George said. "She came in one night 'round eleven, said a fax had been sent from the store."

"Was it this one?" Jackson handed George a copy, flashing it to Micah and saying "People's A."

"Yeah. That's what she showed me."

"And the number at the top, that's the number of the Kinkos?"

"Yep," George said.

"Okay," Jackson said. The first link was made. Now to jump over the second one, the suggestive display of a single suspect's photo. "And do you see in this courtroom the person who sent the fax?" Jackson asked.

George hesitated. It wasn't as simple as this. But this is what they wanted: otherwise, they said, Levine would tear him up. "That man," George said, pointing at Jack. "At least that night, you know, right after it happened, I said it was that man."

The "at least" part wasn't in the script. But the kid was an independent thinker. Surprisingly, to Jackson at least, the kid has a conscience. They could deal with this. The I.D. had been made.

Micah was snapping his fingers, eager to rip this I.D. to shreds. "Ask him about the photo," Jack whispered.

"On cross," Micah said, shh-ing him again.

"Now we *expect* the defendant's lawyer to try to confuse you about photographs," Jackson said, flashing his pearly whites, feeling it, the preemptive strike his staff had drafted.

"He's testifying, Your Honor," Micah cut in.

"Questions, Mister Jackson, questions," Wolfson said. This jackass was no better than T'Sigh, and he had less excuse.

Jackson moved on. "Did photographs *help* you remember who it was, who sent the fax?"

"Uh, yes," George said then stopped. What did Jackson want?

"I mean, they con-*firmed* to you that it was the defendant who sent the fax. But you knew it alright, right?"

"Objection as to the form of the question," Micah said.

"You know what I'm saying," Jackson said, a street phrase pronounced with full articulation, directed at Micah, or George, or Wolfson, who knew. A wasted mind is a terrible thing to watch.

"That first night, the lady from EmpiBank showed me a photograph," George said helpfully. "And I pretty much recognized it. I mean, it was a blurry picture. Then later you all showed me a better picture, like a close-up. It was in color so I could see, like, yeah, the white guy's face was red. It was the same guy. There ain't many that look like him, come into that Kinkos store."

"The same guy who sent the fax?"

The same guy as in the driver's license picture, George thought. That was all he really knew. The part about the red may have bled in later. He nodded then said, "yeah." The guy had called him "yo" so it was only fair.

"Okay then," Jackson said. He still had it. The motherfucking cracker was nailed, identified and motive shown. Now the extra kick in the balls. "Did Mister Levine, the defendant's lawyer, contact you before this trial?"

This was easier. It was all true, and fully rehearsed with Chuck. "Yes he did," George said. "He called my new job, Megalopolis Messenger Service. He asked them to send me to his office on Morris."

Fuck, Micah thought. The kid had changed sides, was about to sell him out. He couldn't really object yet -- this first hearsay would buy him thirty seconds, tops -- so he got ready.

"And what did Mister Levine *tell* you when you met him?" "Hearsay," Micah said, knowing it was weak. He wanted to say , "Attorney client," or some other privilege. But he represented the cracker, not this kid. Fuck and double-fuck. Now he was glad Bertha wasn't here. Let her still picture him as Perry Mason from the re-runs, with dark eyeliner and burning black eyes. Sensuous and always smooth like a moot court Billy Dee Williams. A cross-over between Benny Goodman and Luther Vandross. Dave Brubeck but cooler. He felt a chill.

"It's your own words, Mister Levine," Wolfson said. The Chivas had made him mellow. He was thinking of Swanker but this might be interesting too. "Go on, Mister Wilson. What *did* Mister Levine tell you?"

"He gave me money," George said, just as he'd practiced, the four short words. "He gave me two twenty dollar bills and said he hoped I'd help him."

Micah objected but he couldn't say why. That day he'd had no witness, and he couldn't testify since he was the lawyer. His mind whirled. Maybe Lorraine could take over the case, and put him on the stand to deny it. This had ethics complaint written all over it. The forty bucks were a tip. That's what he'd say.

Wolfson shook his head, stared down at George. Witness tampering was as low as you could go. He'd heard that Levine was a snake but this was even lower. "Say that again," Wolfson said.

"He gave me money," George repeated. "Forty dollars to say that I made a mistake, that it was someone else who faxed it."

"You're sure on this," Jackson said, a statement rather than question. "We need to be totally sure."

"Yeah I'm sure. I bought some CDs with it but the more I thought about it, the more I knew it wasn't right. That's why I'm tellin' about it today." Another scripted line. Levine had tried the whistleblower card for the cracker -- now the whistle was being blown on him, or in him, and it was loud.

"That's all I have," Jackson told Wolfson. "Except that when this trial is done, we'll be asking you to refer Mister Levine to the disciplinary committee."

Wolfson glared at Micah and shook his head. "Your witness, *counselor*," he said. "And this better be good."

Micah wanted to ask for a break but it wouldn't look right. His law license might be on the line here, for forty stupid fucking dollars. He forgot about Jack for the moment, about the fax and the photo I.D.. "Mister Wilson," he began, "we need to nail this down."

"He's threatening the witness," Jackson chimed in, enjoying the desperation of this smart-ass, enjoying twisting his scrotum on each misphrased question.

"We need to *clarify* this," Micah continued. No possible confusion about crucifixion. "When you came to my office, what's the first thing I said to you?"

George thought back. He'd said he'd try to trick him, that's what he remembered. So fuck him anyway. "You offered me a soda."

Micah nodded. Code Red should have been a tip-off, somehow. "And after that?"

"You said, 'I wanna be up front.'" George said it prissily, mimicking Micah.

Micah regretted the phrase, how it sounded now. "And after that -- did I tell you I was Jack Bender's lawyer?"

"Yeah. You said--"

"And what did you tell me? Think about it before you answer. Because my secretary was there, and she remembers." Micah was playing the scene back in his mind: the fizzy red soda in his Brooklyn Law School mug, a witness for some parts of the conversation and not others. Would George remember what was overheard and what wasn't? Micah hoped not.

"We talked about the pictures. About whether I was sure."

"Correct," Micah said. It was a confirmation not a question, but Jackson was too cocky and coked-up to notice. "And you told me that you *weren't* sure, isn't that correct?"

George thought of the soda too, the woman who poured it, not half bad-looking she wasn't. She was there. "I said it might be him, it might not, it prob--"

"So you *said* that it might not be him, that's your testimony, right?"

"Yeah I said that. But the more I think--"

"But that's not what you said just now, with Mister Jackson. You didn't *say* that you had any doubts at all. You think that's fair to the defendant?" It was a question Micah had never asked before on cross, but it came out. Micah sensed something in the kid that might respond to this. The kid probably had been arrested at least once, or would be -- he must know what shit a lie could cause. Micah was desperate.

"Look it's a long time ago," George said. "We had like hundreds of people come in to that Kinkos. No way I can say for positive sure it was that guy. But it think it was."

"You *think*," Micah emphasized the word. "And isn't it true that the District Attorney's office sent you a photograph, again a single photograph, of my client?"

"Yeah they sent me one. It was better than the first. That's what made me surer it was him."

Micah turned to Wolfson. Fuck the rules. "Judge, I'm going to be arguing that this was prosecutorial misconduct, coaching the witness to identify my client."

Wolfson smirked. "You'll be *free* to argue that, Mister Levine. But not now. Do you have any more cross-examination?" He better, Wolfson thought. Forty dollars wasn't much but it still was bribe, at least to a McJob street kid like Wilson. Wolfson was on the verge of deeming Micah scum. And by extension his client. Never a dull moment in this court, unlike at Wolfson's widower's home.

Micah caught the implication: if you don't shake the kid off the bribe story, your client loses and you give up your law license, for a year or forever. He had one more point to make for Jack, zealous advocate that he was. "Mister Wilson, isn't it true that my client came into the Kinkos, after he'd been arrested based on Ms. Peel's complaint?"

"I don't know when it was," George said. "But yeah, he came in and asked if I was sure. He came to Mega--"

"Let's keep it to Kinkos. Since he came in to talk to you, isn't it possible that *that's* why you recognized the photo the District Attorney sent to you?"

George wanted to say no but how could he? "Sure it's possible," he said. "A lotta things are possible."

Levine glanced briefly at Wolfson, as he would at a jury. Reasonable doubt, remember that, he wanted to say. But Wolfson was glaring. This bribe shit was a bitch.

"Now you talked about forty dollars," Micah said. "Remember that you and I weren't the only ones there -- remember the soda." He stared into George's eyes, wishing he'd brought his secretary to court to rattle the kid a bit more. But she was in charge of the braindead babies today, the slip-and-falls, the whole empire of negligence that now hung mootly in the balance. "Did I ask you to *do* anything, anything at all, for the forty dollars?"

George thought about it. It was implied, he'd thought. Though the guy woulda given more if he was serious. Forty bucks in The Bronx ain't shit, really. Neither was the witness fee that Jackson was paying, or the two hundred bucks from before. The rest was all hot air. "No," George said. "You didn't straight-up ask me to do anything."

Micah took another chance because he had to. "Did you *think* I was asking you to do something for the money?"

George was about to say, you asked me not to come. But that had been earlier, before the soda even. He'd replayed this with Jackson, again and again, but he'd stuck to that timeline, that sequence. "Not really," George said. "I mean shoot, you and your boy wish I hadn't a said it was him. But for forty bucks it wasn't like I was goin' away."

"In fact," Micah said, suddenly strangely grateful to the kid but still on the warpath, "didn't I tell you, right at the start, that I'd give you a tip? For coming up to The Bronx? Didn't I tell you that?"

George nodded. "You did."

"Doesn't your company say that customers can't choose which messenger they send?"

"Yeah they do."

Micah wanted to ask, or really to say, that he'd mentioned the tip to the dispatcher. He'd subpoena him if needed. For now the kid had backed off enough. They could file an ethics charge but he'd have a defense, the same reasonable doubt he was raising for Jack. This was enough: no reason to take another fucking chance. "Thank you, Mister Wilson," Micah said. Inscrutable if he hated the kid or not. Enough that George couldn't tell. George started standing up.

"Re-direct," Jackson announced.

Kurt was transfixed. He'd had the story written in his head -- Peel admitting loan flipping, and that Swanker had been on the case -- and then this. Micah was fucked, it seemed clear. Spinning it as a tip was a neat trick, but didn't remove the stain. Jack could go to jail, probably would. And Micah the Snake'd take down his blinking signs. Have *You* Been Hurt? Micah had. And so Jack had too.

Jack was just glad that his stake-out of Mega hadn't come up. He knew he'd pissed this black kid off, but not like this. Micah'd offered a bribe on his behalf? Go for it. Cheap bastard had kept it at forty and that's why they were fucked. Both of them now.

Jackson was whispering at the railing with the Empi lawyers. Three heads were better than one: two and a half in this case but only one could re-direct.

"This is *your* case, Mister Jackson," Wolfson said from the bench. "Unless EmpiBank is the government now." He was still pissed at Micah, but the Snowman getting his marching order from Empi was too much. Corporate ventriloquism made Wolfson sick.

Jackson walked toward George. "Mister Wilson, when *else* did you see the defendant, Jack Bender?"

"He came to my job," George said, remembering the yo. "After his lawyer gave me the forty dollars. He was like hiding behind a car. He bum-rushed me as I went into the messenger center."

"Did he try to intimidate you?"

George almost laughed, that this white yo bozo might actually scare him. But they'd rehearsed this. "He was like sweating and shit. He talking about stringing up, something like that. That he had a daughter down south, that he had to--"

"He said he'd string you up?"

"Sump'm about stingin', yeah, he used that word."

Jackson looked up at Wolfson -- didn't all the Jew lawyers claim to be for civil rights, to have been in Freedom Summer, bus rides and voter registration? Threats of stringing up were the slam dunk. And one more: "Didn't Mister Levine say that you shouldn't come--"

"*Obj*ection!" Micah screamed. "This is re-direct, not cross. No leading questions allowed."

"He's right," Wolfson said. "You can't try to remind Mister Wilson what was said. He remembers or he doesn't. Do you?"

"He asked if I'd be comin' to the trial, yes sir he did."

"Then he gave you the money."

"That's the way it happened."

Jackson nodded, said to Wolfson, "That's it." Meaning, that's it for Levine. That's it for Jack Bender. Walking back to Tsai he grinned at Mudnick and the other more important two. They'd flipped the script but still gone yard. How did that guy on ESPN do the homerun highlights? "Say hello to mah little friend" -- yep, right up Bender's ass, Fishkill special.

"Your Honor," Micah said, "I need to do a supplemental cross."

Wolfson wavered. This wasn't the procedure. "Why?" he asked.

"There was new material on re-direct. I have a right--"
"Keep it brief," Wolfson said. The law license of a lawyer, even
of a snake like Micah, deserved some respect. The last clear chance to
protect. "Go ahead."

Micah stood in front of George -- he'd like to hit the kid in the
face, then he saw him as a slightly older Duwon, a Sega Genesis slacker,
a kid who probably still had a momma, one who'd taught him right
Micah hoped. "What I did was ask you if you were *planning* to testify,
isn't that correct?"

"You said, 'are you gonna go.'"

"And what did you say?"

"That yeah, I guess I got to."

Micah nodded. He could do this open-ended or closed. Open
would be better. If it worked. "And what did I say?"

George remembered. Straight was straight. "You said, 'okay
then.'" George stopped, to let Micah cut him off.

"Thank you," Micah said and meant it. He wouldn't leave the
poor fuck swinging in the breeze, swinging and stringing though the
cracker was a racist, Micah knew. Just not that kind.

"When my client said 'stringing up,' was he referring to you? Or
to himself?"

"He said they were tryin' a string *him* up. That they set him up,
what with the lady only showin' me one picture that first night."

"And that's all she showed you, isn't that correct?"

"Yeah. One."

Here's goes the ballgame, Micah thought. "And as you sit here
today, George, as you think under oath about the whole thing, there's one
thing we need to know. Can you be sure -- are you sure beyond a
reasonable doubt -- that it was my client, Mister Jack Bender, who sent
that fax, People's Exhibit A, that night?"

George stared back at Micah, then over his shoulder at the sad
white rapper with his baby in Charlotte. "No I can't say that," George
said. "Honest to God I can't be sure."

Micah's body relaxed; he heard a car's horn honking from down
on the Concourse. "That's all I have, Judge," he told Wolfson. Jackson
stood up, asking for another round of re-direct.

"That's it for today," Wolfson said. "Mister Wilson, thank you
for your patience, and for your honesty. You're done here. Good luck
and God speed." Wolfson really did wish him the best, this hapless

black teen caught up in Empi's mess. It was like he was setting George free, though of course he already was, in most ways.

George thought it was weird, this dying old judge whose breath smelled of booze thanking him for changing his story. Token perjury. He'd jump the turnstile if no one was looking. Mega'd turned off his MetroCard for the day. George walked right past Jackson, who was muttering something about debriefing with Chuck -- fuck that Uncle Tom, George thought -- straight to the stairway and down, three steps at a time, to the Concourse. This court shit was doper than TV. If the student loans came through, hell, who knew, maybe *he'd* go to Brooklyn Law School. He wouldn't represent crackers but he wouldn't be Jackson neither. Maybe *he'd* be a judge, not boozy, not white -- he'd put the screws to both sides like it was supposed to be done, like Zeus or something, like Thurgood Marshall kicking ass and taking names. George walked through Yankee Village to the D Train stop, through a maze of two-by-fours to the platform and laughed. The law wasn't white and it wasn't black either. It was gray; it was brown; it was mulatto yet still of color. It was worth looking into if the student loans came through. He jumped the turnstile and ran onto the express train just leaving.

49. The Clipboard / The Good Samaritan

The crash course was over and Gina was free. They told her to relax between now and the test. All that could be crammed in had been. Well almost. "Sleep well, even have some wine," the trainer said. The implication was: have sweaty animal sex, unleash hormones and other chemical agents that will keep you cool and relaxed while the clock of Series Seven's six hours inexorably ticks.

Gina was in Bryant Park, a Ground Zero for yuppies since it had been reclaimed from drug dealers during Rudy Giuliani's reign. When she arrived the park's paths were crowded. They'd roped-off the central lawn: a postage stamp of green surrounded by faceless glass office towers, an outmoded Debt Clock ticking away on Sixth and 43rd -- who *cared* about the national debt now that there was a War on Terror to be fought? Suddenly there were billions for SmartBombs, other billions to bail out the airlines, cash settlements for victims as far back as Oklahoma City. Gina for once was hungry. She scanned the storefronts on the park's perimeter: the graceful white curving-up of the Grace Building, expensive cafés incongruously spilling out the back of the public library.

On 42nd in smoked black marble was the spotless store of a Franco-British sandwich shop. Gina'd read about it, in a highbrow magazine whose lifestyle she aspired to acquire. Mange Moi, it was called, shortened for Americans with short attention spans to simply "Mange." The article she'd read recounted in detail the marketing meeting to decide on a nickname. "*Mange*," the French word for eat, was thought to too possibly connote mangy. But Moi would be mispronounced, moy like soy sauce, vaguely reminiscent of the Vietnam War, Hanoi and Ho Chi Minh. *Mangy*, then: in italics it worked, better than "Eat Me" at least.

The cooler was stainless steel; the sandwiches exotic and expensive. There were sun-dried tomatoes, sure. Also Thai chicken in a tortilla so green it looked moldy. Gina went Italian: salami and mozzarella on a thin baguette. This was a taste of things to come, when she passed the Series Seven. Bain had good taste. Together they could laugh at the world from the fenced-off balcony of the public library's main branch. Those lions were known worldwide and she too was an opportunistic and optimistic feline. Back in the park the ropes around lawn had been removed. A wave of yuppies, like immigrants on some border or tax-bracket, washed out onto the grass, throwing down blankets and ice chests. They showed movies in the park, old romantic movies from the 1950s, Cary Grant with overhanging Hitchcockian threats. Vinny liked Bruce Willis; Vinny'd watch snuff films if he could. Gina found a frail-looking chair, just vacated, and sat down. There was garlic mayonnaise on this sandwich -- eye-o-lee, the black teen behind *Mange*'s counter had called it -- and it was good. Gina's future was bright. The movie began at dusk, with some advertising trailers than only whet Gina's appetite more. There was nothing like this in The Bronx: no eye-o-lee, no picnicking yuppies, no classic movies for free at the heart of the world. It was almost like sex, the way the hormones were released. The homeless were gone and Gina had commodities down. She was ready.

* * *

Wolfson's rocket docket singed a hole in Micah's plans. The government's witnesses were almost done: only the expert on the meaning of Tariq Noor remained. Then it'd be Micah's turn. That the cracker should not testify was axiomatic. There'd be WatchCorp Kurt, to denounce all Empi's practices; if all went well there'd be Bertha, to describe the bed loan in all its surreal detail. But what about the bed loan's maker? Micah had a subpoena to serve and music to listen to. Micah needed to relax. His law license was on the line, for forty lousy bucks.   Steely Dan's smooth cynicism might call this savage anxious snake.

Kurt was hot to write, but helping Micah subpoena a loan shark was too good to miss.   They drove in silence to the half-Italian zones, an apartment building like any other.   "She's in 3D," Micah said, handing him an envelope and a clip board.   "Get her to sign for it or at least write down that she took it.   If no one's there, slip it under the door and write that down too."

Micah watched as Kurt disappeared into the lobby, then turned up the A.C. and the CD player.   The same Steely Dan; a slower song that mentioned Fordham Road.   The Bronx was famous in movie and song, but no one wanted to live here.   Bertha had mentioned some multicultural suburbs: Mount Vernon, Roosevelt on Long Island, Maplewood in Jersey.   To Micah these places were death.   Long waits at commuter rail stations, the professional classes lamenting in euphemisms the ghetto-ization of their towns.   Micah *liked* the Bronx.   Not only the juries but also the vibe.   He and Kurt were not so different, perhaps.   The kid might make a good investigator.   But having tasted the freedom of his own obscure web site Kurt would never submit.   Watch him fuck up the service of process, Micah thought.   He turned up the volume and closed his eyes.

The building was at the cusp of ghetto and middle class: the mailboxes weren't broken but the space beneath the stairs smelled of piss.   It was a walk-up.   Apartment 3D was at the end of a hallway with a flickering light.   Kurt felt for a moment he should have those cardboard sunglasses: 3D like three dimensional, full tenement Sensaround.™   He steadied the clip board and knocked on the door.   To hand over papers and say "you've been served" was one of his more accomplishable dreams.   There were footsteps, heavy and coming closer.   Then an eye in the peephole.

"What the fuck you want?"

"Uh, is Gina Sunday there?"

The door flew open.   A guy in a sleeveless t-shirt with his hand coming forward.   "Who wants to know?"

Kurt jumped back, changing his grip on the clip board, ready to swing it.   "Got some papers for her, that's all."

"Well she don't *fucking* live here no more.   Gimme that."

Vinny grabbed the clip board.   "They suin' her ass?" he asked. "You from Empi?"

"It's a case. It's not against her."

"Should be." Vinny took the clip board back inside the apartment and slammed the door.

"Hey, I need that," Kurt called through the peephole.

"Tough fucking luck." Kurt hear the tearing of paper, the footsteps receding from the door. They said The Bronx was dangerous; black and Hispanic, they implied, *mucho peligro.* But it was a white guy, the dregs of the dregs, who'd stolen his clip board. He knocked on the door until the guy told him to fuck off.

"Where's the clip board?" Micah snapped out of reverie of young southern girls in tight capris. Hapless Kurt stood empty-handed by the passenger's side door.

"She's moved out. Some guy, must be her ex, grabbed it from me and locked the door."

"No forwarding address?" Micah asked. Kurt didn't answer. He asked Micah to drop him on Fordham Road. Stuck in traffic he wondered if Micah really had offered to bribe the Kinkos kid. To get the cracker off for forty clams was good business. Micah was singing along to the radio. Micah was In the Zone, Kurt thought. But which zone?

* * *

The frying of The Clam was still Jack's focus. Empi trying to fuck him with the fax would expose all their ripping and packing, the jamming of insurance down customers' throat, the kidnapping of babies, all the sleazy bullshit they did in Charlotte and here. But none of it seemed to matter. He could be back in jail by next week or maybe sooner. It was time to get Plan B ready, the flight down to Charlotte, some quick double-talk to Diane then a life on the lam. He channeled George Raft, "you won't take me alive," as he walked past the dealers on Olinville. They looked him up and down, but no more than always. He thought of a rap song, "I'm close to the edge," and about Kinkos George trying to string him up about stringing. What a web we create. If he'd wanted to say lynching that's just what he woulda said. You had to walk on egg shells, more so up here than in Charlotte. Things were more relaxed in Bubba-Land, and probably more so in Mexico. He thought of that truck stop and its bumper stickers, "South of the Border." One if by land, two if by sea: should he fly or rent a car? That was the question. Live free or die, that was easier to answer.

* * *

Kurt was whispering to himself the previewed diction of his update -- "the Attorney General's name arose in testimony yesterday," never name the fucks, let 'em try to sue you for libel -- as he approached the Guzmans' house. The basement was locked. Inside on his cot Marcos had left a note. "Don't worry about Candida's father. I took care of his ass but good." Mother fuck, Kurt thought. Didn't they teach you in the Army not to admit anything in writing? He thought of the thin kid from Frisco, captured with the Taliban just before the prison riot that killed the Yank interrogator. Jihad Johnny, the tabloids called him. Why had the kid pleaded out to twenty years? He thought of the red room, redder now perhaps, short-eyes papa impaled on the boiler's valve. He'd mentioned to Marcos that he wanted to see the guy fucked up. He hadn't given money, just the idea. Still. Candida probably raised the stakes. He thought of tearing up the note, then put it in his pocket. All the world's a stage, and every stage is a plea-bargain, a trading tit-for-tat. Would he flip on Marcos and blame it all on him? He didn't think so. But to throw out documentary evidence made no sense -- that's how Micah would put it and on that score the snake was correct. Kurt needed to go to Queens and see for himself.

There was a bus from the zoo that went over the Whitestone to Flushing. From there the Seven Train, the midnight played-out streets to Candida's house of horrors. No blood on the stairway but the door to the red room was open. Marcos must think this is Kandahar, Kurt mused, Mogadishu or some other Wild West where you leave out your victim for pride. To get caught here would be -- what was the word? -- incriminating. He peaked around the door frame, saw a set of shoes and feet by the side of the boiler. The machine was rumbling but still he heard a groan. Assault with a deadly weapon, he thought. Attempted murder but not the whole hog.

Maybe he should shout upstairs that an ambulance was needed, then hit the road. Or maybe he should finish the job off. The weird ominous thoughts he'd had of the red room -- the need to atone to Candida by striking at the cause of her jonesing for sedatives, the Original Ass Fuck that set her arc in motion -- they faded away. Candida had a new man now. He'd played drunken matchmaker and now paramedic at midnight.

"*Ayuda me*," the man was groaning. "Help me please before I die."

These words woke Kurt from the loops of his thoughts. Like Juicy Fruit he could double his atonement: the rapist fucked and then assisted. The call of a man in distress -- something about the cry of a drowning woman heard from a bridge, something he'd read, very literary-- made the moment red and real. Life, like art, imitated fantasy. Kurt looked behind the boiler. The super from Hell had a broken jaw, hanging at an awkward angle with teeth through the cheek. There was blood on his t-shirt. He was curled up like a fetus, his face against the waste oil box. "It'll be okay," Kurt told him, kneeling down. "I'm going to call an ambulance and I'll ride to the hospital in it with you too."

The EMS team was salt and pepper, like a formula comedy with gurneys and machines. They didn't ask who Kurt was, only told him that the guy was stable. At Woodhull he waited on a plastic bench with a woman whose kid had swallowed dish washing liquid. The TV played Jerry Springer, again and again like a festival. For once Kurt could relate. Finally a nurse came out.

"He's lucky, your friend. His jaw is broken and a half-dozen ribs. Fifty stitches in his cheek but that's about it."

"Is he conscious?"

"He's doped up but--" the nurse paused. Probably as lucid as he ever was. She led Kurt in.

Candida's father was propped up in a bed at thirty degrees. White bandages covered half his face. "I'll leave you two," the nurse said. Kurt suddenly thought how easy it'd be to stab the man and run. Even after Nine Eleven security was lax.

"Who - are - you?" Candida's father asked, wincing as he shifted further away on the bed.

"I'm the one who found you," Kurt said. "What happened to you anyway?"

The man looked suspicious, at least his right unbandaged eye did. "I got mugged," he finally said. "Big Mexican jumped me from behind."

"Did he take anything?" There was another question Kurt wanted to ask -- the only question, really -- but he'd approach it indirectly. Let the bastard think he might know why he took this beating.

"I didn't have nothing with me."

"Are you going to call the cops?"

The man shook his bandaged head. "Fucking illegals," he mumbled. "They'd never catch his ass anyway."

Kurt wondered if Marcos had stated his reasons, before or during administering justice. Probably so. Otherwise the guy'd be calling for police.

The nurse came in, with two uniformed cops behind her. The radios on their belts were squawking as the nurse spoke. "Looks like it was all done by hand," she said. "No marks of a bat or metal or anything like that."

One of the cops, white with a Hispanic name on his badge, glanced down at Candida's father. "Nice work," he muttered, than louder: "*Señor*, we're here to take your complaint. Do you speak English?"

"I no want to complain."

"We gotta file a report. Rules and regulations." The cop turned to Kurt. "You know what happened?"

Kurt shook his head. "I'm just the guy who found him."

"Well don't go nowhere. We need your statement."

Kurt went out to the hall, looking for the soda machine and then the streets. No one had his name -- except Swanker, he realized. Bring it on you fucking Nannygate bastard, Kurt thought. A house of cards was falling and not how he'd planned.

50. Hostile Lap Dance

"Mister Jackson, we're ready for your next witness."

Wolfson was chipper. In his silent house, in his silent way, he'd burned up the 'Net last night. He turned the sound on his computer down. He now knew more about the Tarek Nour advertising agency in Egypt than he'd ever planned. Also some references to a Tarek "Ricky" Nour in a 1960s rock and roll band in Cairo -- The Mass, the band was called; they practiced in the Gezira Club and at Number 3 al-Fardous Street, Zamalek. Probably unrelated, Tarok was the name of a tribe in Nigeria; uncapitalized, there was a Slovakian card game called tarok. Wolfson jotted it all down. But what did it mean? He hoped to find out today. And to get Swanker's name in the record as many times as he could. "Mister Jackson, time's a'wasting."

"Uh, Your Honor, the People rest."

What the fuck, Wolfson thought. They promised a connection to terrorism and now this? "It's not my job to tell you how to present your case," Wolfson scolded Jackson. "But you haven't even *purported* to meet the elements of the terrorism charge."

"The evidence of the threat is in the record," Jackson said. "We'll tie it to each element of the statute at closing. For now, all we have is another exhibit."

This was a new low, even for the Snowman. Wolfson glared down from the bench. "No exhibit without a witness on the stand to authenticate it," he said.

"We believe this is an exhibit that speaks for itself, Your Honor," Jackson said. "People's D." He handed Micah two piece of paper stapled together, then gave a copy to Wolfson. It was an affidavit from some flunky within the Time Warner OnLine empire, reciting that the screen name Jackal was registered to a Jack Bender of Olinville Avenue, The Bronx.

"And so what?" Micah asked.

"We'll make that clear in our closing," Jackson said, using the royal we. "Here's a clue -- the New York Post article you introduced as Defendant's Exhibit A quoted 'a source who calls himself the Jackal.'" Jackson smiled brightly. Empi for some reason wanted to make this connection -- between Jack and the Jackal it wasn't too hard -- and he was happy to oblige, for the rewards that were sure to come later.

Wolfson shrugged and looked over to Micah. "Mister Levine?"

"At this time, judge, we're making a motion to dismiss the indictment. All they have is a garbled identification, by a witness who yesterday essentially recanted--"

"He didn't recant," Jackson interjected.

Wolfson raised his hand, stopping both of them. The case against Bender was shaky. But after doing all this research Wolfson was in no mood for the let-down of dismissal. "I'm going to deny that motion, Mister Levine. For now. You could renew the request after you've presented your witnesses. Though with this build-up, I'm *sure* eager to hear Mister Jackson's closing." Wolfson glanced at the court reporter, knowing the sarcasm wouldn't come through in the transcript. But the name Swanker would. He'd ask questions from the bench if that's what it took.

Micah was still staring at the screen name affidavit. He'd counted on some Tariq Noor fireworks to eat up the morning. Bertha was in the front row, though. He could put her on the stand -- rather than the many other more comfortable places he'd like to put her -- and dig around into Empi's predatory practices. What *was* this Jackal bullshit? And then it emerged, from the part of the collective unconscious that network television news had left like residue in him. There was some terrorist legend, Carlos the Jackal, dying in a French jail. Something about planes, Black September, smoldering storefronts. They were grasping at straws. Bender was what he was but Black September was beyond him. Jack was a red-faced April, innocent almost, a force of nature. "This is you, right?" Micah whispered.

Jack nodded. Those prying fucks. "There's gotta be a law, against them givin' up your name--"

Micah shook his head. The Nine Eleven statute gave prosecutors the same unlimited access to internet service providers as to libraries, with no notice to the target or his or her lawyer. "Don't worry about it," Micah said. "Ever heard of Carlos?"

"Carlos Santana yeah sure," Jack said.

Micah called to the stand his Black Magic Woman, hearing the song in his head -- "gonna make a Devil out of me" - and glad they didn't yet impose license or copyright fees on such flashbacks. Consciousness is unfathomable and more to the point unmeasurable, at least for now.

"Mrs. Watkins, good morning."

He'd coached her on this: no Bertha, no Micah. "Good morning yourself, Mister Levine."

"Are you a customer of EmpiFinancial?"

"Yes I am."

"Tell us about it."

Bertha told the bed saga: how Gina Sunday came in to Sicilian Furniture with her pennies a day insurance come-on, how the loan was at twenty five percent and wouldn't close, Gina implied, unless she took insurance too.

"Please say that again for the record," Micah said.

"She said if I didn't take the insurance, I wouldn't get the loan. At least I wouldn't get it then."

Micah nodded somberly. He could lay the groundwork for a class action on this hard-selling of insurance, as well as on the usurious interest rates. "Do you know what the prime rate is, Mrs. Watkins?"

She'd been told that very morning in the Court House Deli. Something about Alan Greenspan and the world being run by and for bond traders. "Under six percent," she said.

"Objection," Jackson cut in. "Not in this witness' expertise."

"I'll allow it," Wolfson said. "People in the South Bronx just *might* be more knowledgeable than you think, Mister Jackson."

Jackson glared at him. "We don't call it the South Bronx anymore," Jackson said. "We don't allow outsiders to define us." Then he sat down.

"And did you complain, Mrs. Watkins?"

"I shore did. I went back up to the West Farms Mall and that's when I met your client." She pointed at Jack. "I told him they wasn't no better than the Mafia and he didn't say nothing. Then he said--"

"Hearsay," Jackson said, on firmer ground this time. He wanted this Klansman on the stand, this low-rent piece of shit that Empi had a hard-on for. He could pull the fat out of the fire here, he felt sure, get this dumpy fuck so confused he'd plead out just like that hippie kid from California. Not Jihad but Plea-hod.

Wolfson smiled, too openly rueful. "He's right," he said to Micah. "Is your client going to be testifying?"

"We don't think that will be necessary," Micah said. By think he meant hope.

"Then proceed without the hearsay."

They tried -- Bertha explaining that though she'd recently stopped payments on the loan she'd already bought the damn bed three times over -- but it wasn't the same. Bertha knew that Jack had turned over a new leaf, had renounced credit insurance and seen the light -- but only from Micah. More hearsay. Micah needed to get into the record the cracker's first toots on the whistle and there was only one way. Mudnick was here, as Wolfson had commanded. So he'd be next. "Nothing more, Mrs. Watkins." He smiled broadly with deep lustful meaning. The bed was in; it was *on* that he wanted.

Jackson stood up. "What Mrs. Watkins said has nothing to do with this case," he said to Wolfson who shrugged. "But for the record I just want to ask -- did anyone *make* you take that loan, Mrs. Watkins?"

"They said--"

"Did anyone pull a gun on you?"

Bertha glared. "No sir they did not," she said.

Kurt thought of the basement and of the relativity of coercion; he thought of Candida and her Empi muscle. He pictured her father in Woodhull and wondered what he'd told the cops. Marcos wasn't here. Milly could come and testify about the gunshot but what would that prove?

"You signed the documents, right?"

"Yes."

"And you got the bed, isn't that correct?"

"For   five   thousand--"

"That'll be all. Thank you for your time today, Mrs. Watkins." Jackson turned back to his table, nodding at Empi's two lawyers like, I did your business, I defended your hard-lending bullshit now promote me. It was a democracy, sure, but Empi's support was not without consequence.

Bertha stepped down, shaking her head at this Uncle Tom defender of loan sharks. Bertha rarely voted -- she'd voted for Jesse, and for Dinkins the first time -- but she reminded herself to vote None Of The Above in the next D.A. race.   This guy was pathetic -- Colin Powell without the Horatio Alger story -- and a cokehead to boot, if what Micah said was true.   It usually was, at least about work.

"We call to the stand Keith Mudnick," Micah announced.

Mudnick rose slowly, hung-over and reticent, wishing he'd had more coffee at the Holiday Inn on 42nd Street.   He'd charged the room to his company debit card, listened to Rudehart's instructions conveyed by Chuck then hit the streets of Times Square.   No more peep shows, barely a lap dance to kill off the night.   He'd ended in a Stingfellows™ on Eleventh Avenue, grinding his groin into the buttocks of a part-time student at the Parsons School of Graphic Design.   Luckily he'd brought another pair of suit pants.   When they sent you overseas the action was hotter and less regulated.   First, this.

"Mister Mudnick, are you employed by EmpiFinancial?"

"Yes."

"You are an auditor, isn't that correct?"

Jackson stood up again.   "Objection as to the form of the question.   It's leading, and this isn't cross-examination."

Micah nodded: easily enough fixed.   "Withdrawn.   What is your job title, Mr. Mudnick?"

"I am a supervisor."

It was frustrating, trying to do direct examination with a tight-lipped bureaucrat.   The key was to get him to show his colors.   "And what do you do?"

"Supervise."   Mudnick smiled down from the witness stand, thinking of Bangkok or at least what he'd heard of it.

Okay then, Micah thought.   "Tell me about predatory lending, Mister Mudnick."

Kurt looked up, at this sword so quickly unsheathed.   Micah must have his reasons.

"I don't believe it occurs," Mudnick said.   "At least not at Empi."

"Move to have the witness declared hostile," Micah said to Wolfson.

Wolfson nodded.   "Mister Jackson?   Anything?"

"I disagree, I mean we disagree, that predatory lending so called has anything to do--"

"The motion is granted," Wolfson said.   "Continue, Mister Levine."

"Thank you.   You're an auditor, isn't that correct?"

Mudnick looked back at his handlers. This wasn't unforeseen but it was moving too fast, like the Parsons girl last night. This city was all business.

"Please answer, Mister Mudnick," Wolfson said.

"Yes," Mudnick said.

"And serving function did you have occasion to review my client's employment file at EmpiFinancial? Yes or no."

"Uh, yes."

"Defendant's exhibit B," Micah announced, handing pages to Jackson and then Wolfson and Mudnick. "Mister Mudnick, have you seen this document before?"

"I might have. I mean, there are a lot of computer systems at the company so--"

"Isn't it correct that the entry on the first page, the one you're looking at, says that Jack Bender doesn't want to sell insurance?"

Stupid the way they wrote that, Mudnick thought. And why hadn't they erased it after they fired him? Sloppy Monstro. "Yes," he said.

"And at EmpiFinancial that's considered a *bad* thing, right?"

Mudnick exhaled. "We want to make sure that our customers are offered all of the products that they might want. So if an employee says he's not comfortable with one of our products, yes, that might become an issue."

"Isn't it correct that Empi employees are paid bonuses based on how much credit insurance they sell?"

"That's *part* of the way employee incentive compensation is calculated," Mudnick recited. "But it's not an overriding factor." That was the company line, this reference to riding. Mudnick thought again of the Parsons girl and her inexorable grinding, of the percentage of this month's paycheck that went down that dancer's drain.

"Oh but isn't it." Micah pulled another stack of papers from his accordion file. "Defendant's exhibit C," he said, handing sets to Jackson, Wolfson then Mudnick. "This document is called Quick Plan Rocopoly, is it not?"

"That's what it says."

"And is it fair to say that it reflects how quarterly bonuses are awarded within Empi?"

Next he'll be pulling out the Rocopoly board, Mudnick thought, the laminated poster that ripped-off the board game Monopoly™ in order to incentivize employees to max out their customers. "It's one way that's calculated."

"And what does it say there in the second column?"

"You can read it."

"I'd rather that you do it. Just the part that's highlighted."

Mudnick rolled his eyes. "Insurance sales," he read tonelessly. "Premium dollars per thousand."

"So would it be fair to say that an employee *has* to sell credit insurance, whether the customer asks for it or not, in order to receive a bonus?"

"Most customers find it useful--"

"Answer my question, Mister Mudnick. Can an employee get a bonus if he or she doesn't meet the so-called 'qualifying level' of insurance sales?"

"No," Mudnick conceded. "But credit insurance provides peace of mind to--"

"Since you've been present in the court room, I assume you heard the testimony of the previous witness Bertha Watkins -- isn't that correct?"

"Most of it," Mudnick said. He'd been thinking of lap dances until he heard about the bed, and even after.

"So you heard her say that the loan was conditioned on taking insurance--"

"We dispute that," Mudnick cut in.

"But given how Empi compensates its loan officers, you'd have to admit that it's foreseeable that employees would say or do whatever they have to, to put insurance in loans -- isn't that correct?"

"Objection," Jackson said. A question that long, there had to be something wrong with it.

Before Wolfson rules, Micah moved on. "Explain to us, then, how having credit insurance on that bed was *helpful* to Mrs. Watkins, or provided her peace of mind as you say."

Mudnick thought about it. There was only the stock answer. "If she were to become disabled, or God forbid if she were too die, she could know that the debt she'd incurred to buy the bed would be paid." Mudnick winced as he recited it. If Empi had its own Arlington Cemetery he was earning himself a grave plot there.

Micah smiled. "Cold comfort to the dead," he said, then quickly continued before Jackson could object. "The idea, and tell me if I'm wrong, is that she pays for insurance so that if she can't pay on the bed loan, EmpiFinancial won't come and repossess it."

Mudnick chewed on his lower lip. "That's just about it," he mumbled.

"In your experience, Mister Mudnick, does EmpiFinancial go out and foreclose on beds?"

Mudnick searched the hung-over data base of his mind. "We take a security interest in the collateral, sure, so legally there's no question that we could--"

"Does EmpiFinancial make UCC filings to record its security interest on beds and other household goods?"

Consumer law bastard, Mudnick thought. Nineteen sixties outmoded hair-shirt. "No," he said.

"And as I asked you before, does EmpiFinancial foreclose on beds? And if so, what do they do -- hold *yard sales* to recoup what they're owned on the loans?"

"Argumentative!" Jackson shouted.

Outlandish, Wolfson thought. The biggest bank in the country was driving its profits with bed loans. "Answer the question, Mister Mudnick. The first question, not the part about yard sales. Unless, of course, that is company practice."

"It's not my line of responsibility in the company," Mudnick said, directing it to Wolfson, avoiding eye contact with Micah and the Empi lawyers.

"Perhaps we'll hear from someone who *does* know about this," Wolfson said. His stomach was rumbling, the movement of bowels and not hunger. "We'll take a break, then allow Mister Jackson his cross -- unless you have more, Mister Levine."

"I might."

51. Series Seven

In the hallway Jack wanted a cigarette. His relationship with nicotine went way back, including chaw and, for a time, roll-your-owns. Earlier he'd seen the butts in the courthouse stairway, right under the No Smoking signs. But first this to Micah: "You've got these cocksuckers on the run. Ask him about the insurance tracking forms. 'Trackin' for packin',' we used to call them. Ask him about the scripts they use to sell the fuckin' products. They print the shit on mouse pads and make you use it. Closed file closing they call it."

Closed casket funeral, Kurt thought. Kurt wanted to call Marcos. Or maybe he didn't.

"C'mon kid let's grab a smoke," Jack said. He opened the fire door and pulled Kurt through.

Micah was just as happy to be left alone with Bertha. "You did great," he told her. "Sorry about the hearsay bullshit."

"You think he's going to lose?" Bertha asked, gesturing toward the now-closed fire door.

"They have a shaky I.D.," Micah said. "But I can't get a read on Judge Wolfson anymore. The business about the forty dollars, I think he's pissed off." He'd told Bertha about it, dressing it up as pure slander.

"You could sue 'em for that, right?"

He'd made it seem that way. "I might just let it go," Micah said. "My first duty's to my client." In case the walls had ears.

Up in Jackson's office the shit had hit the fan. Chuck was on his cell phone to Rudehart. Mudnick listened in.

"Yeah... They almost got him to answer... You mean *now*? I can get those wheels in motion but I mean-- Okay, I understand." Chuck handed the phone to Jackson. "He wants to speak to you."

Jackson nodded and he listened. These phones got smaller and smaller every day. They were supposed to make you look jet-set but this was straight colonial. "If that's how you want it... It could be joint, right?... Look, I'll ask him but--" Then a series of yes yes yes. The last one, after Jackson had pushed Stop on the phone, was a sarcastic "yes *sir*." Things didn't look good, Mudnick thought. He could travel to Bangkok on his own dime in a pinch. They trooped downstairs, each with his own instructions.

* * *

"Mister Levine, if you have more questions for the witness--"

"That won't be necessary," Jackson announced.

"How so?" Wolfson asked.

"We are withdrawing the case at this time," Jackson said. "And we'd like Your Honor to order that what's been said in the case can't be reported, even on the Internet." Jackson was staring at Kurt, who was sniffing the nicotine smell on his fingers.

Motherfucker, Jack thought -- I'm free.

"We'll be refiling the terrorism charge in federal court," Jackson continued. "For that reason we want a protective order--"

"We object," Micah said. "Jeopardy has already attached. They can't start a prosecution and then pull back when they see--"

Wolfson raise his hand. "This is most unusual," he said. "You're free to dismiss the indictment. And the issue of double jeopardy is probably best addressed by the federal court, *if* in fact you re-file that charge." Wolfson paused, looking down at the court reporter. "The record here should reflect that Tarek Nour, at least in the public record, is nothing more than an advertising magnate in Egypt. Perhaps he played music once, if his nickname was Ricky."

Micah had found these articles and stifled a laugh. Then, "This is prosecutorial abuse, Judge. They tested their case out here, didn't like what they saw. Now they want to try again. We'd like you to rule on the double jeopardy issue--"

"No such luck," Wolfson said. "They haven't filed any second case yet so the issue's not ripe." It was the fruit, damn it, that made his stool so loose. "On the request that I preemptively block speech, I'll need briefs. I'm not in the business of prior restraint."

"We'll provide them," Jackson said, thinking of the Empi lawyers and their First Amendment tricks. "But we'd like a temporary injunction until we're heard on the issue."

"Who is it, exactly, that you're afraid of?" Wolfson asked.

Jackson didn't answer. The Empi lawyers looked down at the floor.

"We're done here," Wolfson said. The court reporter stopped typing on cue. "This was pathetic," Wolfson added. "Mister Bender, I want to express my apologies. On the other outstanding charge, just so you know, I was going to impose John School if anything. A class on why frequenting prostitutes is bad, for them, for you, for the future of our country. Do you have a daughter, Mister Bender?" It was George's stray line that had started this chain of thought rumbling.

None a your fucking business, Jack thought. He started unloosening his tie, looking up at Wolfson, saying nothing. John School -- it was probably a slide show of diseased dicks like over-ripe bananas; scared straight by limp rotting meat.

"My client is understandably distraught," Micah finally said. "But since there's no adjudication here, the ACD's still in place. No need for John School." Micah's heard of it -- not slide but big screen video, and yes of penises eaten by gonorrhea, testimonies by reformed prostitutes, graphs about AIDS. It would have gone right over Jack's head anyway, Micah thought.

Kurt had jotted down ADD -- attention deficit disorder - rather than ADC, Adjourned Contemplating Dismissal. The Jackal should be happy, Kurt thought. Though the threat of the federal case was a drag. He'd have to upload before Wolfson ruled on their First Amendment brief. Make the shit moot and archive it forever. No recalls or prior restraints on the 'Net: Pentagon Papers forever, or at least until Armageddon. And maybe after, if sufficiently mirrored.

"Do *not* leave the jurisdiction, Mister Bender," Jackson hissed as
he turned to go. "You're on notice. You too Mister Levine." The Empi
team retreated grim-faced. Chuck was directing the real traffic upstairs.

* * *

Gina was in Hour Five-of-Six of the Series Seven. The anxiety
she'd felt while answering the first two hundred questions had passed,
she felt like a wave after it had crested and crashed, the final smooth
flowing toward the shore, reflecting the azure of the Blue Sky Laws.
Market structure, options, variable annuities: she knocked down each
topic like a chip shot, like a tip-in gimme putt. She'd been reading up on
golf as well, acquiring the patina of hobbies she could use to attract
clients. That house in Greenwich, she'd get it yet. She thought of
leaving with ten minutes to spare, not checking her work, just pushing
Complete and having the computer grade it right then and there. But she
might one day get referrals from these drones who surrounded her. She
looked at her watch, the freckle on her wrist -- she was never surprised
that men liked her, if she were a man she'd like what she saw too. Bain
was waiting by the phone; this she knew.

A Dialogue Box™ popped up and said, "Please wait a moment
while we calculate your results." It was airless, the smell of sweat and
fear and greed all mixed as the mainframe whirled and concocted
individualized grades and ratios. She needed One Seventy Five, that's all
she needed: seventy percent. Anything beyond that was gravy. This
morning at the check-in desk at the Comfort Inn the clerk had tried to
hand her a stack of messages. She'd shaken her head. No distractions,
no blasts from the past to screw up the first day of her new life. She'd
memorialized each step in her Planner. It was coming to a crescendo,
this Power of Positive Thinking. The screen flashed its verdict; she
smiled and walked to the door. In the hallway she speed-dialed her cell
phone.

"I don't know what I did wrong," she said, a smile on her face.

"You can take it again," Bain stammered. "I'll help you more
this time."

Gina's façade cracked. "Like I need it. I nailed that sucker.
Drop the dime and let's go to dinner."

Bain let out a whoop, happy for this hard-charging filly and
happy for himself, pulling a new dream from the shell of the old. His
written notice he'd already prepared. He could e-mail the sucker to the
H.R. department. But instead he went to the Equities Desk. The old
man, his disavowing partner in crime, took off his head-set and accepted

the print-out. "I'm fuckin' *out* of here," Bain said. "If they fuck with my severance I'll spill the beans."

"They won't," the old man said. "You got your new gig lined up?"

"Goin' out on my own. I got the hunting license and I'm taking half my book."

"Take every freaking thing you can get your hands on," the guy said. "But tell me one thing. Who tipped you?"

"A little bird," Bain said. His new chick: the one with the Series Seven and the itch in her pants.

* * *

When Bertha got home -- she took the bus because Micah was celebrating with his still-jumpy cracker of a client -- she found Shaniqua crying in the hall with Mrs. Morales. It brought back in a flash the fatal night with Penny, her Penny Zade: the same look of shock on Starquaisha's face, Duwon in the kitchen punching the cabinets and screaming about The Man. The kids were alright. So what could it be?

"They took your fucking bed," Duwon shouted. "I opened the door and they pushed right in and took the shit out piece by piece. I'd like to *kill* them bastards."

"Watch your language," Bertha said by force of habit, turning into her bedroom and seeing the floor boards with their dust bunnies, the comforter and sheets piled on her rattan chair. They'd repo-ed her bed, like Duwon had said. The white weasel from Empi'd hemmed and hawed until they got the chance to show they meant business. "I'm gonna call Micah," Bertha said, to herself more than Duwon. "He'll sue 'em and make this whole thing right." He'd better, since he'd said she could stop paying. She'd put as much of the money as she could to the side but it hadn't been easy.

"Your *bed*, mamma," Starquaisha said.

"*Abusadores*," Mrs. Morales added. "I tell them they must wait 'til you come home but they say no."

Bertha dialed Micah's cell.

They were eating panini in the nameless fancy storefront, drinking beer this time too. Micah was riffing on federal law to Jack who still looked concerned. Micah answered his phone with a cocky hello.

"What? You're sure? They'll pay for this, I swear they will." He added, "Baby." It was in all the doo-wop songs that Bertha liked. It slipped out and Bertha let it go.

"They went and took her bed," Micah said still holding the phone. "To show that the insurance had value," Kurt deduced like some English detective on public TV. "I told ya they're sleazy," said Jack. "And I should know. Ya gonna sue to get it back?" "I'm gonna check out the paperwork first," Micah said. Maybe without a bed, at least for tonight, Bertha'd come and stay with him. She had let him call her baby but it might only be the shock. Post-repo stress disorder. With the right expert witnesses... "I gotta go," Micah said, tossing two twenty-dollar bills on the table. "You guys need a ride?" He didn't mean it and they knew. "Go get the bed back," Jack said. "If ya need me to testify when ya sue 'em, jes say that word."

Kurt had wanted to testify but now was time to write and upload. He was a reporter of sealed court proceedings, an Iago who procured busted lips and cheeks in the basements of Queens. He was there and yet he wasn't there. Kurt's hatreds were virtual, his role secondary like Great Gatsby Nick. He was haunted by FOCO, vulnerable to his addictions. But he could say it now: he was not Nicaraguan and that was okay. He was Kurt Wheelock of the anti-globalization Wheelocks, a raceless tribe yet to be born, exposing predatory lending and its variants where- and whenever. Things could be worse.

* * *

Jack took the Two Train to Pelham Parkway, still loose from the three beers he'd had after court. In the station he used his credit card in the MetroCard machine: fifteen bucks for eleven rides which meant one was free. This would be the one. As the train passed West Farms he laughed madly, seeing the dumpster overflowing on the asphalt behind. The dumb mother fuckers, he thought. The docs Micah'd used had all come from there; so had the leads that were fast making HomeQuik rich. Ehrenreich had begrudgingly given him the week off to clear his name. He'd take the rest of it and maybe more.

On the way from the El train Jack bought another beer. Fuck it he was a free man for now. The federal shit might be just a threat. He guzzled from the quart bottle, in the paper bag it came in. The block was as full as ever, the birth and employment rates both high. They always tried to fuck the underdog. Like Bertha The Loi-ah Watkins, trying to help him in court and losing her four-post mobster bed in the process. He'd help Micah with that, and the shyster would rep him in the federal court if it happened. Then Zalie, maybe legit with visitation. He felt like a man in a beer advertisement. Maybe he'd get himself another car, find a hunting ground for whores in a Free Trade Zone somewhere. Maybe even a girlfriend -- hell maybe even a second wife. He felt boozy and reborn.

He saw the fat man and the wild-haired teen and they saw him. Jack considered greeting them, maybe buying what they were selling just to throw it in the garbage, just to contribute to the economy and show that he could. But the two ducked across the street as he approached. They thought he was Charles Bronson -- a bitter angry white man ready to explode. They were wrong. It was party time now. A carnival of underdogs in mid-afternoon.

Jack double-locked his apartment door behind him, using the chain, looking forward to looseness. The pressure'd built up and could now be released. He was gonna change Internet service providers, drop the Jackal name like Micah'd said. But before he did he could drool on Arab porn, erase once and for all the bookmark to the story where Tariq Noor played white slaver in a way only the written word could convey. Jack signed on. When it said "*You*'ve got mail" he shouted back "Fuck you!" He finished the beer, laid his wallet open on the desk in case he chose to live it up and pay for porn this time, the real crazy stuff they wanted your credit card for. He'd gone to the ATM and had two hundred bucks in cash. He studied the bills while the browser opened. Andrew Jackson with more hair than he deserved. Over the White House In God We Trust. Micah'd said that, though he hadn't mentioned God. "The truth will out," the Snake had promised. Dumb animal luck, thought Jack. Only the good die young.

In the hall he heard voices, whispering which was rare. Usually the people in this building shouted -- "you get your ass back in here!" and other threats less practical. But now there were whispers, and right outside his door. There was a metal sound, like a rat's squeak but almost constant. The screw in his door lock was turning! The threads behind the bolt got shorter. They were taking off his lock like he wasn't even here.

Jack was about to yell "leave my fucking door alone" when he recognized the whisper. "Don't cap his ass right away," the voice said. The one who'd demanded his files the day he got fired. The fat fuck who turned all the young boys out, first playing look-out for cops on their banana-seated bicycles, then delivering the product then finally accepting payments.

"When they pay us the second half?" the other voice said. Wild-hair or who knew. Jack backed away from the door, picked up his wallet and went to the bedroom. There was no time to pack and what the fuck did he have here anyway. The fire escape gate squeaked when it opened. The airshaft was full of garbage bags, and a foot-high inflatable swimming pool that the super's daughter used. It was for Zalie he was saving his skin -- he reminded himself of that as he climbed down the fire escape. A woman on the second floor shouted "Pervert!" Jack flipped her the bird and unhooked the ladder, let it slide down to the concrete with a clank. As he climbed down rung by rung he looked up. The fat man's head was out his window. "The punk's running," Jack heard the fat man say. Jack clawed over the garbage bags to a passageway, out to the street and toward the El train as fast as he could run. In his mind there was Zalie and nothing else. There was nothing else.

Part Three: The Rate of ExchangePesos a Day

52. Fight or Flight

Gina's eyes were closed; she stood by the uncurtained windows and felt Tom Bain's lips kissing up her right inner thigh. Let him have it, she thought. And let *me* have it. All of it. The lifestyle, the dream -- not Tom Bain's manhood however it would end up being. That had been Vinny's claim to fame and what of it. She was Series Seven now. She was an Achiever;™ she would deserve everything that she'd get from here on in. "Don't rush," she told Tom. Bain mumbled something back and slowed down. Behind her the night sky was dark and starless without the hint of a plane.

Jack's first stop was the Guzmans. WatchCorp Kurt was there, talking with Milly out on the stoop. "It's the Last Innocent Man," Kurt said. "The exonerated one."

"They're tryin' a kill me," Jack blurted. "I'm gettin' the fuck out tonight."

Kurt tried to calm him down. "It's probably just a push-in robbery. Why do you think--"

"They were talkin' about cappin' me, about getting a second payment. Look it's my fucking life we're talking about. I want you to tell Micah what happened. And here's the keys to my apartment. Once I'm gone you can have it."

Death threats while the offer was made was full disclosure for sure, but it wasn't the world's strongest endorsement. Kurt needed a place so he took the keys. "Where will you go?" he asked, knowing he'd heard that line near the end of a half-dozen movies, not caring because here what the hell else was he supposed to say?

"I'll call you," Jack said. "I'll call you and not Micah so it can't be tapped or traced. You can tell him I had to go, but don't write none a this 'til I tell ya."

Kurt didn't answer. The fear in the Jackal's eyes was real. Kurt jingled the keys and decided he'd wait. He thought of Candida's father with his teeth-torn cheeks. Fight or flight. The cracker was a force of nature, a hero in his way, a swashbuckler with a comb-over and the prematurely red face of an alcoholic. Kurt had fifty bucks and he gave it to Jack. "You might need this."

Jack pocketed it. "Take care a yourself kid," he said.   It felt
scripted but that's how Jack left, down Park Avenue to Tremont, over to
Third to catch the bus.

"*El es loco*," Milly said in the space between trains.

"*El es un heroe*," Kurt said, not caring how stupid it sounded:
Jack was a hero, at least in WatchCorp's world. Perhaps in several others
as well.

Jack'd checked this shit on the 'Net: Sun Blue Airlines had no-
frills seats to Charlotte. Because of the growth of banking and
evangelical religion, NASDAQ and NASCAR, Charlotte had become the
hub of various second-tier airlines. The flights went there all night,
leaving people with two and three hour lay-overs in the sports bars of the
Charlotte-Douglas International Airport. What was international about
it, Jack could never figure out. He was fleeing back to Bubba-land like a
frightened kid might ran back to his momma, trying to get back in the
womb or however that Austrian prick had put it. The BX 15 bus came
quickly at Tremont, rumbled through the half-lit ruins of Third Avenue,
past Sicilian Furniture with its mesh titanium gates that allow glimpses
of whorehouse furniture complete with white fake marble fountains that
would flow soothingly in your bedroom all night. The bus crossed the
Harlem River, swung around corners of junkyards to 125th Street. This
was a transfer Jack didn't relish: fifteen minutes in front of an abandoned
building, a guy in a wheelchair panhandling the truck traffic preparing to
roar over the Triboro Bridge to Queens.

"Hey buddy you got a dollar or somethin'? It's for somethin' to
eat, I swear on my dead brother's grave."

Jack nodded, looked both way, and gave the wheelchair guy a
dollar. Maybe the guy could walk; maybe it was all a scam. But Jack
needed good luck, good karma, the reciprocal nature of the nighttime
skies. Finally the M60 bus came and Jack used his MetroCard again. He
looked out the window at the towers of Midtown, out over the roof of a
mental hospital they passed. They looked like toys: a roof cut at 45
degrees; the Empire State Building still lit red white and blue at the top.
The bus descended into Queens, Greek restaurants and then a cemetery.
They were trying to kill him -- Jack whispered it to himself. The three
other passengers all worked for the airlines. There was a thin blond
stewardess with breasts that didn't move -- implants, Jack figured -- and
two black guys dressed in mechanics' uniforms. They passed row houses
with yellow taxi cabs in front. This is where the hack drivers lived. A
man in a turban was out on his lawn in flip-flops, spraying his small

piece of lawn with a hose. American dreamers, thought Jack, eeking out their livings driving blow-hard impotent businessmen from place to place. Finally they reached LaGuardia Airport, the ring road past parking lots and the stand-alone terminals of the larger airlines. Sun Blue didn't even have its own counter: it shared one with AmericaWest and some outfit called National that had flights to Vegas.

Jack knew more about home equity than the technology of surveillance, but he'd heard of Carnivore and so he paused. Maybe they could check his credit card receipts and see where he'd gone. He counted his cash: two hundred plus the fifty Kurt gave him. Sun Blue was cheaper at night, to avoid entirely empty planes. Jack paid cash; he sweated while they looked at his driver's license. Was he already on some watch-list, his data entered in by Jackson or Empi to prepare for the federal terrorism charge?

"Have your bags been in your possession and control the entire-"

"I don't *have* no bags, lady."

This was part of a profile: one-way tickets and no baggage to declare. "What's the purpose of your trip?"

None a your fucking business, thought Jack. "To see my daughter," he said. The woman smiled and handed him a boarding pass. "Gate A18," she said. "Have fun with your daughter."

A soldier who looked about twelve preened in combat boots and an M16. They made Jack take off his sneakers, swabbed them with a Q-Tip and watched a small machine. "You may proceed." Jack slipped his sneakers on and off without untying them. He bought a triple-decker burger to eat on the plane and waited by the gate. First the First Class then the women and children. It made him think of the Titanic. They frisked him again then he sat in 17F by the window. It pulled from the gate, rushed headlong toward Shea Stadium and rose. Again the Empire State Building; a loop over The Bronx with its prisons and waste transfer stations, the Cross Bronx at a standstill, the view south along Manhattan isle and then the clouds.

* * *

Bain and Gina were on their second fuck of the night. The first had been too fast -- even Bain would admit it -- but there was time. Bain liked to drink, thinking it made him a more creative lover or at least more hungry for it. But it made his hardness less than it should be. Gina seemed pleased; she moved lithely on the cool white sheets. She had more body hair than he'd imagined. He liked it, the primal ooze of this Series Seven cooze. "You can go for it now," she said in his ear, the message that he'd performed his job, he'd met his quota, it was all gravy now. Bain picked up his pace, closing his eyes and let his mind roam where it would. For a moment there was that Nicole Nour chick, the image of her ass in the air over a table in a Chinese restaurant. This made him feel less and not more. He changed channels, seeing Elizabeth now, the way it always was, that single night in the Science Center at school. They'd snorted cocaine -- it was the only time she'd taken it that he knew of -- and it unleashed something in her, Sappho and not Emily Dickinson, she'd said the word dick (another first) and called for it faster and harder and deeper like a porno tape. That night he'd been at the top of his game, impossible to come, a vicious reaming without cease. Pure Wall Street. He channeled that energy now, but with none of the self control. He felt a feeling like liquid rising in his thighs. "I'm close," he muttered.

"Let it go," Gina said. He felt himself squirting and heard her moan as if on cue. His body froze, the pinnacle moment reached and questioned. He'd moved heaven and earth for this, his first (or second) taste of the pie that he'd have as his staple for the foreseeable future. Was this all there was? Ten seconds of pleasure and then the timeless numb? Yes, he thought, this is all there is. What more else could there be? Be careful what you wish for -- he pushed the thought from his mind. The hair in her pits was maddening even after release. "I think this is gonna work real well," he said. Gina didn't answer.

* * *

Second-tier night riders, bleary-eyed gamblers returning from Vegas awaiting connecting flights, a clean-up crew almost entirely African American vacuuming up the ticket stubs and Cheese Puffs: it was a bleak scene at night in the Charlotte-Douglas International Airport yet Jack despite himself felt at home. He could take the CATS Number 5 bus -- the Charlotte Area Transit System not the Broadway play -- but why? He would need to be mobile and Charlotte's bus system sucked. He went to Dollar Rent-a-Car. The clerk had bright blue mascara and explained the intricacies of Tennessee's car rental statute. It was cheaper, she fast-talked, to get insurance rather than not. "Fuck it," said Jack, "whatever's cheaper." She required a credit card and Jack fought then said what the hell. By the time they found him, if they found him, he'd be gone.

None of the Interstates, not even the Billy Graham Parkway, were extended to the airport. Jack drove in along Wilkinson Boulevard. It was the Hall of Fame for shock absorbers and body work, peppered here and there with strip clubs and package stores. Charlotte loved cars, and cars or at least their accessories loved Charlotte back. The heir of the Gunk fortune, also known for Liquid Wrench,™ had endowed the symphony.   It was a Mecca to race fans -- not pigment but NASCAR, the enormous speedway drew more visitors even than Six Flags Over Jesus and here Down South that meant something.

Jack pulled into the lot of the Midtown Square Mall, looking up at the skyscrapers built since he'd been gone, the absurd football stadium with the Swedish name at the end of downtown, the jughead ramps of Interstates 77 and 277. It was too late to call Eric Taylor, especially since he'd probably only reach his ex, Maggie, who was sure to be drunk. It was not the time to make his play for Zalie. By the Greyhound station on lower West Trade there was a TraveLodge with balconies.   His Olinville escape made Jack prize these secondary means of egress. He paid with his card, parked the faceless rent-a-car in the back by a dumpster, and set off walking through downtown.

The city called itself cosmopolitan but there was nobody here. Tryon was empty in both directions -- the Mint Museum as pathetic as ever -- except for an all-night Kinkos on the corner of West Third. Jack laughed, thinking of faxing and fucking and now the final F, fleeing. On East Trade he stopped and read the bronze plaques for the first time, something about Stonewall Jackson, munitions for the Confederacy, even the old Rebel flag.   These people are shameless, Jack thought, remembering Mr. Cromartie and his fruity urging to Go North, Young Man. Or was that Go *Down*, Young Man, or something to do with Moses?

Even the bus terminal was empty -- the Burger King shuttered, the city closed up tight like Southern belles might have been at one time. The rich lived in Myers Park; Eric Taylor lived in Dillworth, a step up from the dump on Camden Road in south Charlotte he'd used to rent. Who knew where Eric lived, now that he'd left Maggie and taken up with the skank as Diane said. Jack could find him tomorrow at work, at the EmpiFinancial on Fairview. He needed something hot to eat; he need a friend but he found neither. He bought three bags of Combos,™ a range from nacho cheese to pepperoni pizza flavored, and a twelve pack of beer for his night in TraveLodge. The Gastonia college radio station was less Bubba than most; Jack turned the clock radio up and drank until numb. It was a time to plan like Stonewall Jackson.

53. The Patriot / Tracking the Douche Bag

Marcos bashed on the door. Kurt had it double-locked. "Open up, yo, I got problems," Marcos said. Kurt put on his boxer shorts and opened the door. He expected to see Candida but Marcos was alone. "I shoulda killed that fucker," Marcos said. "Only a pussy tells tales."

"He knew who you were?"

"Yeah somehow he did. The cops came to Candida's place last night. She kept 'em in the hall and I stayed under her bed. But they're gonna figure it out, soon as they ask the doorman there about the big Mexican who's been stayin' with Candida. I was wearin' camouflage."

"A lotta people do that now, Kurt said. He added, "I'm sorry," to cover a multitude of sins.

"Hey I'm the one who did it. I did it for *her*, dig?" Marcos paused. "That's a hot shit woman, dynamite even when she's on drugs. Don't know why you dissed her, b. But your loss is my gain."

"She told you?" Kurt didn't spell it out, in case she hadn't.

"That you hit her? Shit yeah. That shit happen, man. But sometimes you lose somethin' you might want back one day."

Kurt relaxed. The d.v. brotherhood, the *La Vida* he'd read about in Oscar Lewis but never quite found. Candida wasn't it. Her madness was too conscious. "Is she still pissed?"

"Yeah. But less so now." Marcos smiled, then grew solemn. "The fucked up shit is, now I got the cops lookin' for me."

"You could tell 'em why you did it," Kurt said. "If they catch you."

"That won't work, you should know that. I thought you were a lawyer and whatnot."

"I'm just helping Micah." Kurt wondered where Bender had gone, remembered the set of keys in the pocket of his shorts on the chair. "That guy--"

"The cracker--"

"He says they tried to kill him last night. He came here pissing in his pants, gave me the keys to his place." Kurt paused. "When the shit dies down I could move up there, leave you the basement, you know."

Marcos shook his head. "I'm not stupid. I'm too young to go to jail."

"What're you gonna do?"

"Re-enlist -- what else? They'll ship my ass back to Bagram, or maybe Baghdad this time. North Korea. You know, the whole axis of evil."

Kurt thought about it, at least Marcos' piece. "What about Candida?"

"I don't know, man. I figure if she takes up with some guy while I'm gone then so be it. My moms wants me to marry *una mehicana* anyway. Out in L.A. probably so I could visit *her* moms."

"Look, I'm sorry," Kurt said again.

"Stop that shit. I did that shit myself and had fun doin' it. I kicked him in the balls too, as hard as I could. He won't be ass-fuckin' nothin' for a good long time." Marcos laughed at the thought of it.

"Yeah but what you said about the Army," Kurt said, remembering.

Marcos shrugged. "Wherever you go you could do fucked-up shit. And least this way you *might* be killin' the right people. I mean it's like you got protection -- they tell you you're doing the right thing, everybody says you're a hero so maybe you are."

"Just watch your ass out there," Kurt said. "You're gonna tell your mother?"

"Yeah, right now. I'm takin' the bus today, tonight, as soon as I can."

"You told Candida?"

"Not where I'm goin' but she knows that I am. She held off the cops for me, man -- that's deep."

It is, Kurt thought: she almost *called* them on me. "You need anything?"

"Nah, man. In the Service it's all taken care of."

Kurt saluted before he thought the better of it. Marcos laughed and saluted back. "Been nice knowin' ya," Marcos said. "If you stay around here keep your eye on my moms, and on her moms if she comes. *Mi abuelita*, that's someone I'm gonna miss."

* * *

Jack woke early and took his belongings, all in his pockets, down to the Rent-a-Car. Eric Taylor'd be at Empi, at least until the repo field calls started. Jack gunned the car into the strip mall, stripping the gears in the shift to reverse, thinking of West Farms. Inside the shit hadn't changed: the Rocopoly board was still on the wall, the Trackin' for Packin' charts, the scripts on the mouse pads, the whole nine.

"The prodigal," Eric started, with his good Baptist upbringing.

"I'm not here for long," Jack said. "But I need a coupla favors."

"Shoot," said Eric.

"Not here." They went outside.

Empi shared the mall with Trojan Labor and a payday lender. There was also a coffee shop. Jack recounted his tale like Odysseus in the Duncan Donuts. Eric's eyes got wide. "Mother fucker," he said again and again. A lady with glasses like the B-52s glared at them. They might have come from Athens, Georgia. The New South was hip, in its way.

"So here's the deal," Jack said. "I don't wanna tell her I'm goin' on a trip, nothin' about that. Jes that I'm back in town for a while, stayin' at your place and I want Zalie to visit for the day."

"You know she never liked me."

That was true. "If I say I'm stayin' with anyone else she wouldn't believe it. You know how she is." Eric nodded. "And if I say a motel, she'll smell kidnappin' -- milk cartons an' the whole nine yards." Jack paused. "You really left Maggie?"

"Yeah. Life is too short, ya know what I mean?"

Jack knew.

* * *

Micah got the fax, that his client Jack Bender should not leave town. It was signed by a federal judge. Micah'd spent last night considering the bed's repo from all angles except the one he'd really wanted. Bertha hadn't agreed to stay over. "I'm not a school girl no more," she said. "If we're gonna do this we gotta do it right." He was looking through the Daily News real estate ads when the fax came through. "Well it's finally happened," he told his secretary. "I have a client charged in federal court with terrorism." He was proud in a way, thinking of Clarence Darrow, some unionists charged with a political bombing, some strange European word, "attenta" maybe that was it. The cracker was a fall-guy but he needed a defense. And Micah was ready. He'd get a new suit at Moe Ginsberg and give 'em hell. Braindead babies be damned; full speed ahead.

* * *

Chuck'd been to Olinville by now -- the super had fixed the lock on Jack's door and refused to change the cylinder or key, since the rent had been paid through the end of the month. Chuck shorted the Ricans since they didn't do the job. Show me the body -- wasn't that what *habeus corpus* meant? Rudehart knew I.T. and began the search. Credit card records were easy to get, if you worked for EmpiBank. The last five purchases -- they came in on a half-day delay -- including a MetroCard. This too Chuck knew, through his friends still on the job. They could track any MetroCard through the system, just like E-Z Pass on the bridges to Jersey.

"He took the M 60 line," Chuck told Rudehart. They both knew what that meant. The Train To The Plane™ was a bust: no subway went anywhere near LaGuardia Airport. And so this bus, from Columbia University east on 125th into Queens and LGA.

"Check the airlines," Rudehart commanded. Whether they'd give the information to the FBI fugitive-from-justice team or use it themselves could be talked about later. Like everything else, including the presidents of several small countries, it'd be Sandy's decision.

* * *

Eric and Jack drove up to Jack's old house -- he was still paying the fucking mortgage so no need to walk on eggshells -- and parked in the black asphalt driveway. Diane's car was there, with duct tape on the right rear blinker. Her Shoney's shift was at night. She might still be asleep, then get up and fuck up and say goodbye to Zalie in a haze and go back to bed.

"Wait here," Jack said. "You're like a prop -- I just want her to see you, make it look like an everyday thang. Then we go to the ATM, right?"

Eric nodded. Jack'd helped him in his hour of need, or many of them. Eric had been closing loans and packing insurance like a mother fucker. So he could afford it.

Jack still had the key but he knocked. The door opened; a face he knew -- a face he would do anything for -- looking out at him through the screen. One of her two front teeth had fallen out but it would come back soon, Jack quickly told himself.

"Daddy!"

"Baby!" Jack opened the door, picked Zalie up, still in her pajamas with the dog's heads on the end of the toes. The TV was on, set to cartoons. From the bedroom there was some banging around. Jack heard Diane shhh someone -- what the fuck? -- and then she came out, wrapped in a towel that barely reached mid-thigh. Her hair was loose and still winged like Farrah Fawcett. She wasn't looking half-bad except that he knew.

"Why din you call?" Diane asked.

"I thought a surprisin' you and I guess I did."

"This ain't yer house no more."

Jack shrugged. "But this shore is my daughter." Diane didn't answer -- she kept glancing behind at the bedroom door which she'd closed -- so Jack continued. "I'm back in town, stayin' at Eric. I'm gonna take Zalie out for the day, down to Six Flags maybe--"

"Oh yes Daddy, let's go there, I ain't been there since the last time you took me--"

"Haven't," Diane and then Jack corrected in unison. Jack almost laughed and Diane was smiling. It was like one crisp apple in a barrel that had gone bad.

"We gotta get the court to decide on visitation," Diane said. "Ya can't jes show up here whenever ya feel like it."

"Soon enough," Jack said. He meant: never. "Go get a change of clothes," he told Zalie. "Your bathing suit and stuff."

"Ya gotta bring her home by eight," Diane said.

Yeah -- Two Thousand and Eight, Jack thought. "Whatever," he said. "Eric's in the car outside." Might as well use the prop since he brung it.

"Don't he got to work?"

"He's takin' a sick day."

"I hope yore not plannin' to have that skank go with ya--"

"Nah," Jack cut her off. Zalie came out with her Mickey Mouse book bag.

"Ain't it great that Daddy's back?" Zalie asked, the TV as much as anyone else.

"If anythin' comes up I'll call," Jack said at the door. Zalie was already running toward the car.

"Nothin' *better* come up," Diane said.

Jack turned away and smiled. He even muttered "I loved you," emphasizing the D but so soft she couldn't hear him. If you're gonna be a fugitive, you might as well go whole hog. It might as well be for something you care about. He got in the passenger's seat next to Eric. "Back to the mall," he said. "But first the ATM."

* * *

Kurt had a job: to tell Micah what was up. The cracker'd taken flight. There was The Eagle Has Landed; there were steps small and large, Buzz Aldron and all that crap. This was more mundane but it should be said in person. Kurt took the BX 55 to the corner of Bergen, walked the vendored streets toward Lincoln Hospital.

"They filed," Micah told him.

"He's gone," replied Kurt, then explained the cracker's tale.

"Paranoid fuck -- it was probably just muggers," Micah said.

"He said they were talking about a second payment."

Micah paused and considered. What would he tell the court? "We never had this conversation," he told Kurt. He could bluff that the cracker had gone into seclusion, witness protection, a religious retreat. Let them prove he was out of compliance with the order. Maybe Jack'd left before the fax came in. Micah hoped so. Bedless Bertha would know what to do. "And don't write this," he added to Kurt.

"I know," Kurt said. It pained him but he did. This was a prior restraint he'd have to live with.

* * *

When next installment of credit card data came through, it had a hit. "The douche bag is in North Carolina somewhere," Chuck announced. "Mecklenburg -- like some German place."

"That's Mecklenburg *County*," Rudehart sneered. He knew it from bank litigation against the Tryon twins. "It's Charlotte. Call our people down there and let's get on it."

54. Powder Puff / The Donor Zone

The shit of it was, should he fly or keep the car? To fly you had to show I.D.. They typed your name in and then anything could happen. He would just keep the Dollar car, let 'em charge him by the day not knowing where it was. Eric shouldn't know either. Jack maxed out his credit card, cash advance as far as it would go. Eric withdrew five hundred from one place, then another five large from another.

"Why we need all this money Daddy?" Zalie asked.

"It's gonna be fun," Jack said. "You'll see."

Eric drove them back to the strip mall. "Too bad I can't show you mah new woman Lynda," Eric said.

"It'll have to keep," said Jack. Typical Bubba shit, Eric thinking with his dick.

"If they ask me what do I say?"

"Diane's gonna talk anyway. Say I came askin' a favor but you didn't know nothing. You did the favor but you didn't know why." Jack thought some more. "You thought I was stayin' at the TraveLodge, came home on vacation that's all you knew."

Eric smiled. "You're some piece a work, Bender."

The last thing Jack told Eric was: "Get outta Empi 'fore they drain you dry." Then Jack and Zalie pulled out onto Interstate 85 toward Atlanta.

On the highway to Greenville Zalie told him about school. As they crossed into Georgia she asked, "Are you shore we can get back by eight?" It was time to tell the truth. What could a six year old girl understand, Jack wondered. That he loved her. That she was all he cared about. That he had to run and she must be with him. If guns were ever drawn he'd drop her at a police station, point at the blurb on the milk cartons' side and be gone.

"Daddy's got problems," he finally said. "There's some bad people up in New York who want to hurt Daddy. So we're goin' on a trip."

"I *like* a trip," Zalie said. "But won't momma be mad?"

Jack didn't answer for a mile or two. "We'll call her, I swear we will," he finally said.

"I don't like her new boyfriend," Zalie said. Jack started to question then stopped. He knew it'd be pretext. It'd all come out anyway. They were going coast to coast, with nothing but time to talk and play the license plate game. He'd teach her all the states and even how to add the numbers, play Blackjack Twenty One when the traffic got too heavy. For now the road was open. They could get to Montgomery or further then sleep.

* * *

Before Diane was even worried two guys in suits were at her door. "Is he in there?" the bigger one demanded. Diane thought of her new man, gone to check up on the second shift at Shoney's.

"We're looking for Jack Bender," the shorter one said.

"He was here this mornin'," Diane said. "He took our daughter Zalie down to Six Flags."

The men called Chuck on the cell phone. The cracker'd gone to an amusement park? Typical. They asked Diane another question: "Where's he staying?"

She gave them Eric's name and where he worked. But they already knew that.

* * *

Swanker wasn't full unconscious but he was under the knife of one of Doctor Boneley's disciples. Incisions were made in his Donor Zone; hair follicles were removed intact. He'd given a false name for the procedure. No way his insurance would pay so what the hell. He'd seen the tabloids run before-and-after photographs of various pols. The uncomfortable questions: where did you get it done, why did you do it, do you think the voters are so shallow. *Fuck* the voters -- he was doing this for him, for his sense of self, to keep the chippies tightly in orbit until his kids were old enough for him to make the leap. If it came to that. The cuts weren't painless however. "You don't got morphine?" he asked through clenched teeth. "Or laughing gas?"

"Those are controlled substances, Mister Smith."

To maintain an ego at the top of your game was not easy.

* * *

As Jack reached Alabama, in The Bronx Milagros was crying. Not uncontrollably; not like a soap opera or *novela*. But her son was putting himself again in danger's way. "And what about your *abuelita*?" Milly asked. "I thought you were going to visit her."

"I have to go," Marcos said. He hadn't told her why. "I sent her a quarter of my check before and I'l keep doin' it."

"I know you do, you're a good son, a good grandson. It's just that we'll all miss you. You barely got back and already you're going."

"We're at war, Ma," Marcos said. "When duty calls the men gotta go."

She knew it was something more but it was his life; he'd have to learn to be a man. "I'll send you photos," he continued. "Over the Internet like before."

"Okay, *m'hijo*," she said. "*Que Dios le bendiga*."

* * *

Jack pushed on past Montgomery. It was dark now and Zalie was asleep. They'd need clothes at some point. Maybe he'd get a glue-on beard, or shave his remaining hair like a skin head. The border crossing he knew best -- the only one he knew when you came right down to it -- was in Tijuana. He'd return this piece of shit car out there and they'd just disappear, the concrete walkway over I-5, the metal turnstiles, the whorehouses and the curio shops. Most people spoke English there, if only to hawk chicklets. Zalie'd feel at home. He passed an exit for Brooklyn and it made him laugh. Cromartie'd said Go North and he had. Now he was pressing South like a dick into pussy, like a knife through butter and all of them clichés. Mobile was a beautiful place. He remembered the abandoned shanties he'd seen, and the no-name hotels by the highway. He'd say his name was Doe and he'd pay in cash.

In the room they had cable: ESPN but also the Cartoon Network and that's what Zalie liked. He went to a gas station across from the motel and took four po' boy sandwiches from the freezer, heated 'em in the microwave until the plastic bags popped. He looked at the stack of newspaper as if he might see his name in them then turned away. Zalie was watching the Powder Puff Girls, transfixed. "Don't you think we should call momma?" she asked when the show was done.

"Tomorrow," Jack said. "It's late now and we don't want to wake--"

"I know, her stinky boyfriend. Let's have waffles for breakfast tomorrow, Daddy. With syrup and bacon and even hot chocolate."

"I promise," Jack said. Zalie'd loved Waffle House since her first time in the high chair, throwing sausage links on the floor and then clapping. The room was too small to jerk off in and that was probably for the best. He studied the dog-earred Road Atlas that Eric gave him. Biloxi and Gulf Port; straight through Baton Rouge to Lake Charles, Beaumont, maybe Houston if he sped. He'd burn the engine right out of this rented piece of shit. That's what you paid for. No reason to say thanks while they were charging his card.

* * *

They rousted Eric from his bed just as he came down from his little slice of heaven. He wanted Lynda to stop dancing but on Empi's wages she said no. "And why'dja give that guy a thousand bucks?" Lynda asked. "Y'all faggots or somethin'?"

Lynda had the mouth that she needed to survive at the club. She wasn't the kinda piece you married, Eric knew. But the TV always showed people gettin' theirs, right here right now. He was doin' a porn star, that's what he told himself though she was only a dancer on Wilkinson Boulevard. Everything was relative. For the Bible Belt, Eric was the Marquis de Sade.

"Open the fucking door or we'll break it!"

He was their own employee, not the presumptively uninvolved ex-wife, so what the fuck. Chuck Stewart would be arriving in the morning and they wanted to have results.

"Yo, yo yo -- I just got that shit at Home Depot, leave it alone," Eric said. He was still semi-hard in his Y-fronts; he felt like he was on the Cops™ TV show, all that was missing were the cameras and the reggae music.

"Where'd he go?" the bigger one demanded. "We *know* you gave him money. So don't waste our fucking time. Just give it up: where?"

Lynda came out of the bedroom. She was naked, consciously so, and the guys liked what they saw. "How'd he getcha, sweetheart? You owe money to Empi or somethin'?"

Lynda didn't like that. She was a dancer not a whore. "Don'tchall need a warrant?" she asked.

"We're not the cops, honey. When ya work for Empi your ass is ours twenty four seven."

"Well *my* ass sure ain't," Lynda said, slapping it like she would at the club and heading to the bedroom. They stared at the red mark in the silence following the ass-slap's echo.

By this time Eric had remembered the script that Jack'd given him. "He's at the TraveLodge," he said. "He came down on vacation to see his daughter."

The shorter one hit Eric in the stomach, once but hard. "Vacation," he said to the other, shaking his head. Then back to Eric who was now doubled-over. "Your friend's in deep shit, not only with us but with the law. We're tryin' a *help* him, but there's nothin' we can do if we can't find him. So let's try this again -- where the fuck is he?"

"I swear to God, TraveLodge that's all I know," Eric wheezed.

"Yeah well he shore better n' be there, or we're comin' back for a piece a that whore you got in there. I almost hope the fucker's not at TraveLodge."

"Me too," said the other. Then they left.

"That company's got you by the balls," Lynda commented.

Eric begged to differ but it didn't come easy.

* * *

Swanker lay in bed next to Carolyn, feeling pulsing under the bandages on his scalp. They called it an out-patient procedures and that was true -- if you liked to lie in agony in your own bed. Carolyn breathed slow and regular, a product of sleeping pills. "You're gonna look better," she'd mumbled before falling asleep. "Even better," she added, always diplomatic, stroking Swanker's ego, smiling her icy smile, thinking her unfathomable thoughts.

Swanker got up limp and limped down to his home-office. He'd already printed the hatchet jobs on Basso, the guy's pathetic defense of his work, some grumbling about grandstanding. What else exactly was the state A.G. to do? Work behind the scenes for the common good and just count on the voters remembering? What a joke. Micah surfed to the Wall Street Journal site, checked the closing bid-and-asked for the main stocks he owned. They were supposed to be in a blind trust -- but only the blind follow the blind, Swanker thought. He checked the Yankee box score -- another blow-out of a team with Double-A talent -- then clicked on his bookmarks to that WatchCorp piece of shit. Just to make sure that the site was still dead. It wasn't. His head started to throb while he printed and printed -- the story of Jack Bender's exoneration, full of typos and knee-jerk swipes at Empi. What bothered him was his name was there: some low level flunky from Empi had spoken the word. No mention of the nanny thing but that wasn't the point. This blackmailing punk was ignoring his threat. When his head and hair healed he'd fight back and with a vengeance. Carolyn had no fucking idea what a hard guy she'd married. A hairy hard guy now, not only on his back but on his forehead once again. The magic was back and Georgetown was calling.

55. The Abundance of Life

Like the crow of a rooster the Visa data downloaded at dawn. So the cracker had rented a car at the Charlotte airport. Rudehart called Chuck, reaching him at the gate at LaGuardia. "Go straight the fuck to the Dollar Rent-A-Car there. Tell 'em their car's been stolen and to put out an APB."

"I thought you didn't want the cops--"

"Okay scratch that." Rudehart didn't like to admit when he got confused. "For now. But you better find that bastard. Hiring those scumbags on Olinville was your fault and Sandy won't like it."

As Chuck stared down at the low-rise East Coast sprawl, Zalie poured blueberry syrup on her waffle stack. On the tip of her nose was a dollop of spray-on whipped cream from her cocoa. "I love you baby," Jack said and meant it.

"Let's swim today Daddy," Zalie said. "It's borin' jes bein' in the car all the time."

The road map showed state parks: there was one in Louisiana they could reach before lunch time. "You can sleep in the car," Jack said. "Least at first."

* * *

Diane had begun to worry -- her shift had come and gone, no sign of Jack or Zalie and she didn't even know where Eric Taylor lived now. Maggie would know, might know, but Diane was in no mood for an Oprah. She went to the Empi, past the losers lined up in front of Trojan Labor, and confronted Eric Taylor. "Where's my daughter?" she said loud, so loud the borrowers in getting their loans flipped looked up. She was too young to have any daughter that this Empi guy'd be fucking. So what was it?

Eric took her outside to the parking lot; the closing scripts could wait. "Look I don't know where he went, I swear on my gran momma's grave I don't. But there's somethin' I do know. He's in trouble, he's like runnin' from somethin'. These guys from Empi, not from aroun' here, they came to mah house las night--"

"Yeah they came to mine too. I told 'em he was stayin' with you 'cause that's what he tole me."

"He din say where he was goin'. But he's in trouble. And he's benn missin' Zalie, you know."

"Well now he's done up and took her. I'm callin' the cops, that's what I'll do."

"Give him some time," Eric said. "You know he loves her -- I mean, more than most a these men around here. More than most men period."

"It's kidnappin' an' I know my rights."

"He'll bring her back I know he will," Eric said. He didn't know any such thing. But some chances to pack insurance, to upsell these marks from sales finance to a sweet first lien, they were walking out the door. "I gotta go," he said.

Diane sat in her car watching the shape-up at Trojan. She'd give Jack 'til nightfall. Tomorrow morning at the outside. To set the cops on her own daughter, who knew what could happen. They shot first and asked questions later. She'd wait.

* * *

Not waiting -- sleepless with his scalp on fire -- was Swanker. He drove the car himself, over the Henry Hudson bridge, down the West Side Highway. If the woman that WatchCorp Kurt had hit would complain, he could have him in lock-up by lunchtime. He still had the address and number that his secretary got, the day of Nicole Nour's fax. He'd do this visit himself. What kind of name was Candida? Something to do with Voltaire, Swanker remembered from some boring theater class he'd taken. But this one was Spanish -- not black comedy but *café-au-lait* like that petty turn-coat Milagros.

Candida was staring at vials of pills. She'd lined them up on the soft-sanded grainy wood of her kitchen table, like chess men on a board. Revenge was sweet and so was her coffee. Neither however did the trick. She'd dramatized in her mind the kick in the balls that Marcos had delivered and described. Closing her eyes she felt rage, glee almost, like a banshee, kicking that bastard again and again at the root of his sin. But Marcos was gone now; she'd lied and said she knew no Mexicans, an Uncle Tom Latina, a wannabe white in her white-walled apartment. Marcos hadn't withdrawn, he hadn't played cheap and freaky like Kurt. She'd been with a hero. She'd supported the war effort. She was Rosie the Riveter with a board full of controlled substances. Then the knock on the door and the rush to hide the vials in her already-stuffed purse.

"How can I help you?" Candida asked insanely composed, ready to help Marcos again by denying she knew anything about him.

"I'm Ernest Swanker," the guy announced. She'd thought she'd recognized him but with the turban on his head it was hard to tell. "Can I come in?"

The vials were gone so why not. She offered him coffee but he shook his head -- very slightly, she noticed, as if the turban were a bandage and he'd had elecro-shock.

"I am a strong supporter of privacy," he said. "A woman's right to choose, a woman's right to decide how much to take, when to complain. But domestic violence in my experience is never cured by itself."

Candida wondered: how did this bandaged big-shot know? "I have no idea what you're talking about," Candida said. Could it be about Marcos? He'd beaten her father in the boiler room; that was domestic in a way.

"Come on now, I've seen the pictures. Kurt Wheelock. We know all about him. What I want you to know is that you'll have the support of my office -- you can file your complaint under seal and probably wouldn't even have to testify. It's important, though." He looked into her eyes and saw only black.

"That's behind me now," Candida said. "And I don't know where you get off coming--"

"He can be charged without your involvement," Swanker cut in. "You can be subpoenaed as a witness -- it's not the way we like to do things but it *can* be done."

"I want you to leave," Candida said. It might be a trap to get her to talk about Marcos. The slap was crap. Kurt had really pissed these people off though, she thought with some admiration. Not lust anymore but a certain respect.

Swanker wasn't leaving. "You only have to sign this affidavit," he said. "We'll take care of all the rest."

"You're upsetting me," Candida said flatly. "And it's not the right time." She paused. "I'm pregnant."

Swanker felt a vein under the bandage. "By him?"

"No," Candida said. She might be. Only time and the piss-on sticks would tell. Any baby of Marcos' would be strong and noble. She could teach it good English and get it in pre-school. She would love it to within an inch of its life. "Now leave."

* * *

The river was opaque and muddy, Zalie so cute in her prison-stripe one-piece. "You first Daddy," she said.

Jack had his boxers on. They'd be too revealing when he climbed from the river wet. He folded his pants on the knuckle-like root of a tree at the water line. Some Okies in a camper were frying breakfast meat not far away. "Here I go," Jack said and dove into the river. Opening his eyes under water they burned; it was dark and weird like a bad dream. He broke the surface, treading the muddy water. Something was trying to eat him. Fingers were grabbing his ankles and feet. "Ahr!" he screamed, swimming toward the shore. He grabbed the tree root but it was slippery and he fell back in.

"What's wrong Daddy?"

Jack clenched his jaw and shimmied up the muddy riverbank. "Don't go in," he told her.

The Okie -- the head of the Okies, the *pater familias* with a spatula in hand -- came over guffawing. "It's fulla fish, jes fulla fish," he said. "If you ain't expectin' it, it could feel like somethin' else."

Jack thanked the bastard, cursing all Bubbas at once and put on his pants. "We'll find a swimmin' pool, darlin'," he told Zalie. "I'll find us a motel tonight that has one, I swear I will."

Zalie was glum as they continued toward Houston.

* * *

Swanker's next stop was uptown, in the esteemed office of Bronx District Attorney Snowman. Jackson summoned Tsai but Swanker sent him out. "You're not wired, right?" Swanker asked. Surreptitious taping was a hallmark of the Bronx County Democratic Committee, which was the swamp that Swanker had arisen from, risen far above it he was glad to say -- no way he'd go back, not him, not ever. Jackson was just the kind of petty grifter that Swanker's father dealt with, to make arson charges go away.

Jackson raised his arms, offering a pat-down. Swanker's was the job the Snowman craved, the next step up for an enforcer of the law.

Swanker declined to frisk his colleague. He remembered a micro-scandal in Jersey, where the green right-wing governoress -- governess, he realized, would sound sexist even in thought -- had done a photo-op slapping the cuffs on some crack-slingers in Camden. There'd been a civil rights backlash, a measured one since that horse-farming ice queen still had power and money to dole out. "A lack of judgment," that's what they'd charged. She'd copped to it and paid what they charged. Who knew if Jackson would play that card on him some day.

"Let's just talk," Swanker said.   "From what I've read, *l'affaire* Bender was a cluster-fuck."

"Empi didn't have the evidence," Jackson complained. Swanker's French left him cold. "I mean I *tried* and all. Anyway they pulled the rug out from under me at the end and withdrew it." Jackson was deft though it often went unnoticed. His reference to rugs being pulled out was not unrelated to the bandages on Swanker's head. Black men can be bald, Jackson thought proudly, thinking of half the NBA. But for a white man it's death. Political death at least unless you're like Dick Cheney and just don't give a fuck anymore since you don't have to.

"This WatchCorp web site--"

"That hippie kid was in the courtroom, I tried to get the judge to shut him down but Wolfson -- well, you remember."

Sure: one of the last trickster Tribe Members wearing the black robes in The Bronx. "That's what I'm here for. I'll help you with a motion to make him seal the record. We can file the whole thing confidentially, under the terrorism statute with no notice to my *amigo* Micah Levine."

The way he pursed on the Spanish word made Jackson ask, "You deal with that sleaze?"

"Used to. Anyway let's get to work."

Empi had Swanker's balls in a vise too, Jackson realized. Out of the swamp and into the sauna. They could talk about succession later.

* * *

Houston would be as good a place as any. By the courthouse there were bail bondsmen and liquor stores, with a line of payphones out in front. Jack went through an Arby's drive-throw, getting Zalie a burger and himself ten bucks of quarters. Then he double-parked in front on the phones so he could keep an eye on Zalie. "I'll be right there honey," he told her, pointing at the phones. "If they come and say to move it I'll hang up. So don't worry."

"I wanna call momma," Zalie said for the sixteenth time. Then, as if of equal importance, "And I wanna swim. Like really swim in a pool or somethin'."

"We'll do that, baby, I swear," Jack said, meaning the latter. He wouldn't charge this call to his credit card: he was too smart for that.

After four rings WatchCorp Kurt picked up. "Where are you?" he asked, of course, what else.

"If I tole you I'd have to kill you," Jack said then laughed.

"Micah got a summons from the federal court, saying that you can't leave New York."

"Catch me if you can."

"He's worried," Kurt said.

"Yeah well I care about him too. Ak-cha-lee I wanna talk to him. 'Bout another problem I got. But I thought that callin' him direct might really put his ass on the grill."

Kurt had an idea: his phone in the Guzmans' basement was simple but it had a speaker phone function and two-line capacity. "I'll call Micah and you two can talk through this line," Kurt suggested.

Jack looked away from the car for a moment. "You're alright, kid, you know that?"

Kurt dialed Micah, talked through the secretary and got the Snake himself.

"They're not fucking around," Micah began. "They faxed me the summons. So far I'm bluffing them. But they'll want to arraign you soon and unless you can suggest a body-double...".

The Jackal was one of a kind, Kurt thought. Kurt could almost mimic his voice, but the way his comb-over fell, the distinct splotching pattern on his face and his gravy stained tie -- the Jackal was inimitable in his way.

"I got bigger trouble," Jack announced. "I told y'all about my daughter, right?"

"Oh no," Micah said.

"Yeah well she's with me. I mean it's her I've had in mind all this time, so what the hell, if I'm going down it's gonna be with her."

"Stupid," Micah said softly, more to himself than to Jack.

"You don't got any kids, right?" Jack challenged. "So what the hell would you know about it?"

Micah thought of Duwon and the girls, even Penny Zade to whom his only connection was considering her legal claim after her death. Enshrouded in regret like a second skin Micah asked flatly, "So what's your question?"

"What could they do to me?"

"They could charge you with kidnapping for starters," Micah answered. "Has the mother filed a complaint?"

"How the fuck should I know?"

Micah thought about it. "Gimme her number. Maybe I can keep her cool. But I'm gonna have to promise her--"

"Say whatever the fuck it takes," Jack instructed, watching Zalie nibble at her burger and play with the car radio. "Yore my lawyer, right?"

Yeah, Micah thought: I'm representing an accused terrorist who's also a kidnapper taking a minor across state lines. He counted the felonies. "You should come back," Micah said.

"I jes might do that," Jack said then hung up.

56. Milk Carton Days

Special Agent Susan Schtump played the tape again and again. "He's taken his daughter," she told the other members of the Privilege Team.™ "But the call into Levine's office came from The Bronx."

"Levine *did* tell him to 'come back,'" someone pointed out.

"That's just for our benefit," Schtump said. It was important to maintain this: under Attorney General Ashcroft's guidelines, they could only tap lawyers' phone if they decided, without any judge's review, that "a reasonable suspicion exists to believe that a suspect may use the communications with attorneys or their agents to further or facilitate acts of terrorism." Schtump read them all the guidelines again. "Let's get on the same page here -- that's still the case here, right?"

There were grunts of assent; there was silence. "Then let's raid the place where the call to Levine came from. And I'm gonna track down the wife. If she makes a complaint we can play dragnet on that basis. Motherhood and apple pie."

* * *

"I'm not comfortable with this," Wolfson repeated. Jackson was back for a second bite at the apple. Wolfson smelled Swanker behind it but had no way to prove it.

"The statute is clear," Jackson said, happy to see the old Jew squirm. Today there was no audience. Just him and the two Empi lawyers, who added some more citations to the brief Swanker'd drafted. Just an *ex parte* motion to get what Wolfson shoulda given the first day: no press, sealed file. Prior restraint the way it oughta be.

"I don't like to rule *ex parte*," Wolfson said. It meant while hearing from only one side. Wolfson thought of the Snake, tried to imagine what arguments he'd make. It wasn't the same, though. You couldn't at the same time be the judge and one of the parties. "If it's so secret, why are they here?" He gestured at the Empi hit men. "Why can a corporation be present while information supposedly about terrorism is discussed, but the defendant can't?"

"Don't ask me -- ask Congress," Jackson said. "We're prepared to appeal you, immediately, if you don't sign the sealing order." Wolfson thought about it. That's how he'd gotten this case in the first place: Birnbaum got blindsided. That was by Micah. It was time to channel Solomon, the old chestnut about the bisected baby. "I'm issuing two orders, then," Wolfson announced. "I'll seal the file, sure. But given the lack of evidence at trial, the eleventh-hour withdrawal of the case to take a second shot at this Bender in another venue, I'm gonna award attorney's fees to Levine. All his time on the case at the lode star rate. What are partners in the white shoe firms getting these days?"

Neither Jackson nor the Empi twins answered. Money was not their concern -- Micah's fee would be paid from interest and insurance premiums racked out of EmpiFinancial's customers. From the poor and their suffering, like all of Micah's money was. "The two orders go together," Wolfson continued. They knew what he meant: if they appealed the award of fees, he'd find a way to rescind his sealing order on some technicality, throw open the file to any bottom-feeding journalist casting around in the embers of dead cases for a story.

Wolfson thought of his empty house, his now-empty life, his corrupted nation. Maybe that was too grandiose. He had cut the baby in two and they just stood watching. Solomon need a good stiff drink -- Swallowmon, Wolfson joked to himself; Solomon hadn't had an erection in seventeen months. "I want these fees paid as soon as possible," Wolfson added. "Like, yesterday." Micah still had a chance to do something. Maybe he could save the baby. Maybe he could clone another one, from the half that Wolfson had carved for him.

* * *

It was two babies, in fact, of whom Micah was thinking. The cracker's Charlotte offspring -- Micah couldn't picture her -- and the case file that was Penny Zade, Bertha's busted dream, something deep deep inside her that he'd never be able to reach, 'specially endowed as he was. The cracker and his daughter were still on the table, calling in through Kurt from a payphone somewhere. Micah stared at the Charlotte phone number then dialed.

"Mrs. Bender?"

"That ain't my name no more."

"But you *were* Mrs. Bender once?"

"Yeah in a nightmare."

"I'm your ex-husband's lawyer--"

"Where is that bastard? He stole my daughter and I'm gonna call the police, the FBI or whoever you're supposed to call--"

"Calm down. I'm calling to tell you that your daughter's alright." Micah paused. He hadn't actually spoken to the brat, the rug rat, whatever it was that this Bender could spawn. He was only an emissary, bearing glad tidings to the place his client called Bubba-land.

"Where is she?"

Micah had no idea, but saying that would only get the rug rat's mother madder. "Jack wants you to know that your daughter's okay. He'll be bringing her back soon, you have my word on it." Micah grimaced as he said this; he would have crossed his fingers if he still believed in those rookie lawyer's tricks.

"Yeah well your word don't mean fuck all to me."

Whatever happened to Southern gentility, Micah wondered. The worst Rhett Butler said was damn. Anybody in The Bronx could say fuck all, and many of them did. "I'm an attorney," he said. "I'm an officer of the court."

"Don't make me laugh. He's late on the alimony and child support -- he ain't gettin' custody this a way. You tell that scuz bag he brings my daughter back now, right now, or I'll see to it he goes to jail for the rest of his miserable life. Down here that ain't pretty."

The miserable life part was at least more poetic -- accurate too, Micah thought. "Just give him a little time," he said. "Let me give you my number." He didn't want to, but it'd be better to give her a place to vent other than the FBI. He played the scenario out in his head: the Benders were white, sure, but neither blond nor upwardly mobile. As such they'd merit the side of a milk carton, if that. Unless there were some extant photos of the daughter in a g-string. He didn't ask. "You can call me anytime," Micah said. He hoped she wouldn't.

* * *

It was Sealy, though the beds were a knock-off; the selling point to Jack was the pool with its Astro-turfed terrace, the water slide that was open 'til ten. He sat on the loose elastic of a beach chair drinking beers from a brown paper bag by his side. Zalie was holding her nose in the shallow end. "Watch me Daddy!" she screamed each time before she submerged her head.

"That all was great," he said when she came up. There was no turning back now: they'd filed that federal case in New York, made him out to be a Goddamn Timothy McVeigh or something. He'd read about that crew-cut wacko who'd blasted OKC. Also his sidekick, the part about his getting a mail-order bride from Manila. Maybe he'd do that too someday, Jack thought. Zalie'd need a mother, to tell her 'bout tampons and who knew what else. Where he was going he wouldn't even need to use the mail: the females were desperate, half-blind at twenty from assembling Panasonic TVs. He'd read in some porno about the girls who disappeared in Ciudad Juarez. The mag had pitched it as a turn-on, but even for him it'd been too much. Maybe it was having a daughter that had mellowed him out over the years. Maybe it was this beer, or maybe all the beers before. He remembered a line that Mister Cromartie the fruit had written in big print on the blackboard one day: *Amor fati.* "Love of fate," he'd said it meant, the motto of that same crazy German. The kids in the back row next to Jack had another translation: I More Faggy. The English teacher's hunger for cornholing. Jack liked the German better, which was rare except with beer. He was drinking Bud now, but one day he'd go Dutch. Or maybe the dark one from Mexico in the short brown bottles. Short hairy women who'd know how to treat a gringo loan shark and his daughter right. He mused, half-hard, until the waterslide closed.

* * *

There were guns again in the Guzmans' basement -- legit this time, no warrant but an FBI shield and this female agent whose name meant fuck in Yiddish. "I am Special Agent Schtump," she told Kurt. "We need to know about the call you made to Micah Levine."

Kurt wanted to talk about attorney-client privilege -- he'd read enough about it -- but he wasn't a lawyer. There was a loophole, though, that even he saw. He could play client. "I don't have to tell you what I say to my lawyer." He wondered if this was really about Candida, or maybe Candida's father.

"One, that's not true, and two we're asking about *where*, not what," Schtump said tat-tat-tat. "You patched-in a call from here to Levine's. We could just get your phone records, you know."

"On what basis?"

"Providing material assistance to an accused terrorist," Schtump said with a smile. She memorized and recited these things not unlike an Empi loan officer. We're here to protect you.

"I don't know where any call came from," Kurt said, putting it all in the subjective and qualifying every noun open-endedly like Micah and TV both taught. "And I'm going to tell the phone company to notify me -- I mean Mister Levine -- if any request is made. We'll oppose it."

"You're just getting yourself in deeper," Schtump threatened.

But Kurt had heard that before.

* * *

They just might have stumbled on a purely domestic conspiracy, Schtump thought to herself on the Cross Bronx Expressway. The Jackal -- that's what they called him in the Bureau now, in the Joint Terrorism Task Force, the whole machinery that now required a purpose -- must have talked to his wife, because she refused to file a complaint. She said she might do it later and then she hung up. Something about Shoney's. Schtump wondered sometimes about the morals of the Americans she gave up her life and most weekends to defend. Where were they all going, on the gridlocked highway? Nowhere. And they'd kill to keep it so.

* * *

"We need to talk," Kurt told Micah. "And not over the phone." He'd developed a code and he hoped Micah got it. "Tomorrow at the single A version of Duwon's favorite place." He'd listened to Micah closely -- once a cult member, always a junkie, at least for a mentor.

"The kid--" Micah stopped. It was probably just Kurt's paranoia, but the "not over the phone" business he took seriously. Micah thought of the video arcade in Times Square. But the single A reference didn't make any sense. Then he got it. He surfed the Net and confirmed the time for tomorrow. WatchCorp Kurt should be a spy, Micah thought. Maybe he was.

* * *

Gina and Bain had learned a bit about each other's reactions: Gina liked 69 and Bain with his head for numbers wasn't complaining. It'd be time on the morrow to announce their partnership, at least the business side, to the world. What better venue than the loveless Arab bitch who'd gotten him fired? She'd done Heard on the Street™ once; she could do it again. "We'll go in person," Gina announced. "I can tell you like her."

"Lik*ed*," Bain said. "And only 'til you came along."

"Speaking of coming...".

* * *

Susan Schtump's profile of today's youth -- Duwon connoted African American but how different could they be? -- told her that this "favorite place" must have something to do with computer games, or maybe wrestling or rap music. Single A, single A: she wracked her brain. She commenced searching the Manhattan and Bronx phone books for entertainment venues with two A's consecutively in their names. There was a parlor for luxury ice cream but no variant with a single A. She vaguely remembered some double-A Danish philosopher, from her liberal arts run-up to Quantico -- then applying her profile she put it out of her mind. She expanded her scope to include comic book stores. It would be a long night.

57. Flatonia / The Crack of the Bat

The sun, rising in the East, touched the nation first near Lubec, Maine. Bain and Gina slept sheetless and in need of mouthwash, a dozen brands of which were for sale in the RiteAid downstairs. The dumpster behind Empi's branch in the West Farms Mall was full of social security numbers but there was no jackal about to harvest these prospects. The jackal was snoring on the shag-carpeted floor of a motel in Sealy, Texas. There was only one bed, a king-sized PosturePedic™ on which Zalie slept alone, scrunched up against the wood veneer bedside table with its Gideon's Bible. Mudnick slept the deep sleep of the drones in Lutherville; Candida slept well-drugged, perhaps for two, in her white padded walls on Riverside Drive. Kurt was awake, alone in the Guzmans' basement, wondering if the Jackal would call, ready to tell him not to do it again. Before meeting Micah he'd call Nicole, try to pitch her on terror, on his déjà vu with guns.

Milagros rose early too, as she always did. The mother of a soldier was supposed to be proud and in most ways she was. Marcos was kicking the Arabs back from what they'd done to New York. But had all the Arabs done it? And weren't Hispanics in The Bronx, especially immigrants, getting grilled by the INS, by *la migra*, just because they might *look* Arab? Milly preferred the Army's earlier ads, "Be All That You Can Be." This new "Army of One" slogan was sad somehow. How could one person be an army?

This morning she drank two cups of coffee before calling down to Kurt. He bounded upstairs, dressed already and with a wild look in his eyes. After some coffee he told her, "I'm thinking of running the story of Swanker. What you heard on the terrace, the W2 business, the whole thing--

"I don't know why you did not do that already."

Kurt did. And maybe it was time to confess. "Look, the woman who came here that day, with the guy with the gun--

"*El prieto?*"

Kurt nodded. Milly had a half-dozen words for African Americans -- *moreno* was another one; none of them were considered racist as Jack's term Knee-Grow was. "Yeah anyway, she was my girlfriend."

"This I thought."

"And she was mad because... well, some things happened and I ended up slapping her." Kurt stopped, waiting for Milly to say something: three Hail Mary's perhaps, some way to atone.

"This can happen," Milly said. "But if you love her you should not do it. She might stay with you but she will look elsewhere for love."

Kurt didn't answer. That was no longer his problem. "Anyway, Swanker found out, he says he has a photograph."

"You hit her hard?"

"Not really."

"How does he find out these things?"

Candida, Kurt thought. Or Empi. It didn't matter. "He said he'll use the photo against me if I run the story."

Milly nodded. "You must decide, then. You should speak with the woman. If she loves you it is not a problem."

Kurt thought of Marcos. Would Milagros be proud that her son had taken sloppy seconds with Candida, that he'd kicked her rapist father in the balls? "Are you worried about Marcos?" he asked.

"A mother always worries," Milly sighed. "It's like the way my mother worries about me, and I about her. Her house is falling down and she cannot buy the medicine she needs. I want to bring her North, but the pills are cheaper there."

Kurt thought again: if he made any money off this case, this scenario, this saga, he'd give half of it to Milly for her mother. The old woman had become real to him, wrinkled she must be, in a tin shack in a smoggy city massed on the border.

"What will you do?" Milly asked.

It was time to call Nicole, and then see Micah. "Something," Kurt said.

* * *

Micah stopped at his office and the news surprised even him. Wolfson had ordered Jackson's office to pay his fees and costs -- and the Snowman was offering to pay up as soon as Micah could certify his hours and meet with him. Empi must be paying, Micah thought. Wolfson had also sealed the case file. That was the quid pro quo. But money was money and this one didn't have that braindead baby smell. It would kill off the possible ethics charge from the Kinkos bribery too. He wanted to tell Bertha, in person, in her bedless bedroom.

Micah drove his Beamer east, filled to the brim with this news of fees and what it might mean. The piss smell in the hallway on St. Ann's didn't bother him; nor did Bertha's curlers nor the green lotion on her face. She called it a mask, though the bottle used a Q, like the Masque of the Red Death. Chromatics brought Bender splotched face to mind, and some worries. "I'm getting a fee," Micah announced. "I can doctor up my hours so it could be enough for a down payment." The idea that they'd together choose a place to start a life together struck Micah as romantic. He'd pay; she'd choose. In the ghetto but not of it.

"But that cracker, your client -- what's up with him? Are they really gonna put him on trial again?"

"They want to. They faxed me a summons and everything. But he's hit the road." Micah paused, wondering how this would strike Bertha. A man kidnapping his daughter was hard to defend. Especially to a woman who'd lost a daughter herself, permanently unless you believed in Heaven, which Micah didn't. He told her.

"That's fucked up," Bertha said. "Is the mother pressing charges?"

"She's just about to. Though my sense is--" Micah paused, wondering if this was too cynical even for him -- "that she cares as much about alimony as about anything else. Maybe it's that she knows Jack won't hurt their daughter. I mean, I don't think he would either."

Bertha considered this. She thought of Penny Zade, but not in any way that Micah could understand. It was intuitive; it was karmic. "You should use that fee to help them settle their problems," Bertha said.

This had not been Micah's plan. It hadn't occurred to him and why should it? He'd started referring all these slam-dunk braindead babies to Lorraine Thompson. He'd given up good money for this cracker already. Why should he give his fee? "Like I said, I'm thinking of it as our down payment on a house."

Bertha shook her head. "We could do that another way, if we're really gonna do it."

Micah waited. They didn't give away houses for free, even in the South Bronx.

"You could settle my bed case with them," Bertha continued. "And use some of *that* money to solve that little girl's problems. So she's not a football that everyone's chasin', parents callin' the cops on each other just to make a point."

Bertha was like Princess Di except she was offering to do it with her own money. For a southern cracker who'd supervised her bed loan in the first place. Micah's head hurt, and what his heart felt, he couldn't tell.

Maybe they wouldn't get a house after all. Maybe that wasn't what Bertha wanted.

* * *

Jack and Zalie were movin' on down the road, past exits for insane towns like Schulenburg and Flatonia -- grandiose names from this flat expanse of Texas along Interstate 10. They drove at the speed of the traffic, between seventy and eighty MPH but the air conditioning was getting weak. "I'm gonna take you to the Alamo, baby," Jack said, lighting a smoke and rolling down the window.

"How far is it to Disney World?" Zalie asked.

He'd show her the map tonight, let her see for herself that they'd left Florida far behind them. Maybe ask her then about Diane's new man. He'd gotten a bag of Cracker Jacks in the motel's gift shop in Sealy -- no more than a closet, really, with condoms and disposable cameras and a blue-haired lady boring the hell out of everyone with her militia-like rants against the sales tax. "You can eat some of this," he told Zalie. Whether they still had prizes inside he didn't know.

* * *

Kurt called Nicole from a payphone -- Schtump might already be tapping his line, he figured -- and he told her about the Bender case, and even what Rudehart had said on the terrace.

"You can *prove* this?" Nicole asked.

"There's a woman who heard it. She works for Swanker."

She said, he said -- the word of a maid against that of an ex-Treasury Secretary. "I'm gonna need more," Nicole said.

"I'm working on it," said Kurt. And he was.

The ferry to Staten Island was free. They'd used to charge a quarter, but it cost them more to collect it so they stopped. There'd been a terminal fire that was blamed on the homeless. Now the fast food joints with their neon pretzels were gone. The ferries no longer carried cars, but the boat Kurt took was one of the old ones, where you could stand outside on the bottom level and get splashed by the harbor's salty water, look back at the glass towers still standing at the foot of Manhattan. Only if you knew, only if you'd seen it before, would you notice the hole. The two buck teeth were gone, the infinite before and after: like Vesuvius or worse, the end of the post-Cold War era, that's what they all said. Hiroshima had killed fifty times more people. But they were yellow and they deserved it because of their country's foreign policy, that was the line. The investment banks were decamping to Jersey, to four-story buildings that were not shown on maps. Kurt saw the Statue of Liberty but couldn't see the flame. Speed boats with sharks' mouths painted on them jumped the waves. If Micah didn't get his code then fuck him.

Micah flashed his high beams in the far left lane on the Verrazano Bridge. Bertha's seeming selflessness might just reflect cold feet. Interracial coupling was still the big taboo. Salt and pepper detectives, no problem. But the Cosby's were all black. At first it had been the southern whites, terrified by the itch in their virgin daughters' pants. Now even the black groups opposed the portrayal of interracial love. Black man, white woman was seen as revenge. White man, black woman? It had the aura of slavery days, something about Thomas Jefferson, something that freckled Malcolm X had said. Duwon had probably read it. Duwon who loved the Yankees, some surrogate winners to identify with even though only two of their players, if that, were black. Baseball was Spanish now, even in the minor leagues. If he'd understood paranoid Kurt correctly, he'd be at the ballpark by the ferry for this ill-attended *beisbol* day game.

Micah took Bay Street to Richmond Terrace, parked his Beemer in the commuter lot by the ferry. There was a new orange brick plaza at the entrance of the Richmond County Bank ballpark.™ And there was WatchCorp Kurt, wearing ludicrous green shorts from the bottom of which the white fabric of his pockets emerged.

"I thought you'd get it," Kurt said.

"It's too cloak and dagger for me," Micah said. He could be picking up his attorney's fees right now instead of here with this kid.

"They're tapping your phone," Kurt announced.

"Who?"

"The FBI. They came to the Guzmans' yesterday, since that's where the call to your office came from."

Micah's mind was racing, from race to the Constitution. "Those fuckers," he said softly.

"C'mon, I already bought two tickets," said Kurt. At eight bucks apiece this was a junket he could afford.

They chose seats halfway up the right field line, no one around them, just the smell of frying meat from a barbecue pit by the foul pole. It was the Staten Island Yankees against Cal Ripken's Aberdeen Ironbirds -- the players were all in their early 20s, hungry for money that most of them would never see. The Ironbirds' pitcher was wild and it gave them time to talk. Mostly it was Micah, blowing off steam about the Sixth Amendment right to counsel, Fourth Amendment privacy, all of it moot and trumped by terror. "This is *fuck*ing outrageous," Micah said, as if anyone cared. A bonus-baby Yankee hit a lazy fly ball down the line; the right fielder dropped it and two runs scored. "They're a little rough around the edges," Micah remarked. "They should be called the Iron-Gloves." Ashcroft might have repealed the Constitution but they still had baseball and related wisecracks.

"You've got to oppose them getting the phone records on my line," Kurt said. "Otherwise they'll know where Jack called from."

Just what Micah needed: another client who couldn't or wouldn't pay. But he'd make that motion today, to protect Kurt's phone line and indirectly himself. There was precedent; there was tradition. "Have you ever heard of John Peter Zenger?"

"No," Kurt said. They were sweeping the infield dirt to the disco strains of the Village People's Y-M-C-A.

"He was a printer, accused of seditious conspiracy," Micah said. "The lawyers who represented him got disbarred."

"You're worried about that?"

"They tried to set me up with that Kinkos kid, right? Which reminds me -- you can't print, or whatever they call it on the Internet, anything more about Jack's case in the Bronx. Wolfson sealed it."

Now Kurt was outraged, citing his own favorite Amendment, the First.

"How could one fucking cracker cause all these problems?" Micah wondered out loud, speaking for both of them. He told Kurt about the fees and Bertha's idea. Kurt had an idea, or a debt, of his own. By the seventh inning stretch a plan had emerged and they left, Micah to make his anti-phone tapping motion and Kurt to play Voice of God to the Jackal. The Ironbirds were going down slowly.

58. Black-out Phil / The Markets Recap

The Alamo was a tourist trap: bulbous patriots from all over the South snapped digital pictures of themselves in front of its bullet-marked walls. "Remember the Alamo." Jack'd always heard that, from Mister Cromartie and even before, but he couldn't fathom why. Because we stole Texas and California from the Mexicans? Because for once we lost, like at the World Trade Towers? Maybe the Towers would be the new Alamo, and soon there'd be snapshots and postcards and new slogans in text books. Concession stands. There already were.

"This is *bo*ring Daddy," Zalie said. "It's too hot here and it's hot in the car. I wanna swim again."

They retraced their steps to the overpriced lot. The car started but the A/C sputtered then grew still. "Fucking Tercel," Jack cursed.

"I wanna go home," Zalie said.

He pretended he didn't hear. "It'll be alright baby. We'll keep the windows rolled down." And they'd drive through the night when it was cooler.

* * *

These brokers were shameless. Here was this bozo, the one she'd fingered for the SEC, pitching Nicole and the Journal on his new venture.

"Take out an ad," Nicole told him. "One of those tombstones -- 'we are happy to announce the opening,' you know the drill."

"I think there's a story here. Page One with the pen and ink drawing and all. I can see the headline in my head: 'Maverick Broker Turns the Tables on The Street.'"

He was ballsy if nothing else, this Bain. Nicole agreed to hear him out. Hunan beef'd be just the ticket.

* * *

Micah felt high from how fast he'd gotten an injunction against the tapping of Kurt's phone: he still knew how to judge-shop, how to strum the strings of Constitutional outrage. Now Micah told the Snowman he wanted the Empi twins there. Snowman said sure, why not -- the more he sucked up to them the higher he'd rise. But the shit about the four-post bed sandbagged him. "That's *not* what this is about," Jackson said.

"It is now," said Micah. "If you want me to leave this case alone I've got to tie up every loose end."

"What -- you want the bed back?" the taller of the Empi twins asked.

Micah laughed. "No. Triple damages and a commitment to stop--"

"We'll pay," the North Tower said. "But we're not gonna be changing what we sell or how we sell it." Paying was no problem. This was just the end-game Sandy'd foretold. For money even the dogs will dance: this was a cynical nugget Sandy had picked up south of the border. It applied up North even more than down there.

* * *

Micah'd dropped Kurt at 149th Street; from there Kurt took the bus up to Tremont, back to his basement. He just might move to the jackal's den on Olinville. But he had rent to pay before that, some way to atone, if only to the wrong party. He would pay it forward like that schmaltz movie said. He'd pay back Hispanics for the way he'd appropriated their suffering. He'd wheel and deal his Wheelock way, at least for now with his phone line certifiably not tapped courtesy of Micah's judge-shopping.

Jackal called in from Kerrville. "I'm goin' crazy," he said. "Did Micah talk to Diane?"

Kurt recounted their conversation, the emphasis on alimony. "Don't use your credit card," he told Jack. "Micah says they could track you that way."

"Yeah I know, I've seen movies. Look, I have an idea."

So do I, thought Kurt. "Shoot."

"There's a second copy of my credit card in my apartment on Olinville. It's at the bottom of the top drawer in my desk. I want you to go get it, and to use it right there in New York. That'll fuck 'em up."

Kurt liked the idea. But the Jackal had more.

"Use it to buy something for a little girl. Like a bathing suit or something. Go to a kids' clothing store but make sure they ain't got a security camera."

"Where'd you learn this shit?" Kurt asked.

It wasn't Mister Cromartie. Maybe that German he talked about, Beyond Good and Evil.

"Micah got a fee," Kurt announced. Actually it was two. "He told me to tell you he's gonna do something with it."

"Ain't that money mine?" Jack asked. He needed it.

"You'll get some. But here's how it's gonna work."

Kurt hoped that Schtump hadn't tapped his line already. Micah'd filed a motion with the federal court, by e-mail attachment like they allowed, basing most of his argument on the 1981 Upjohn case and Wigmore on Evidence: the attorney-client privilege is "the oldest of the privileges for confidential communications known to the common law." Kurt liked how Micah wrote, and how fast he moved. He was a Gene Ramos with none of the delusions of grandeur. Micah'd suggested that Kurt apply to go to law school, and maybe he would. But first this wheeling and dealing. It was in his blood.

"A quarter of it is going to Diane," Kurt said. "We'll get her to agree to joint custody so you're no longer, you know, a kidnapper."

"She'll do it for the money," Jack said.

Kurt winced and continued. "The rest we're going to wire. But not directly to you. There's gonna be a processing fee and it's gonna be steep."

Jack felt the tables turning on him, a smooth quarter turn counter-clockwise: he remembered standing in the strip mall saying, "Yeah it's like the Mafia -- so what?"

It all had symmetry, Kurt thought. And then he called Nicole.

"What I told you this morning, at least the part about the Bender case, you can't use it."

Like I was going to, Nicole thought. Bain's story had helped her put it all together. She might not run this one either -- they might not let her -- but at least she knew. She told Kurt because there was no one else to tell. "Remember my insider trading story?" Nicole began.

"Yeah."

"Turns out it was true, but not the way I thought. The broker, this guy Tom Bain, he did get tipped off about Swanker's aborted investigation of Empi. But not by anyone in Empi, or in Swanker's office, none of that. By a low-level loan officer! The one in my Guzman story. *She* knew that Swanker was digging around."

"Is that even insider trading?" Kurt asked. "I mean it was just a rumor, something an employee heard and passed along."

"The SEC's playing defense," Nicole pontificated. "They fucked up so badly on the big guys, and did nothing -- Bush, Enron, Cheney, WorldCom, you name it, even Empi -- that now they love to crack down on the little guys when they catch them."

"So this Bain guy's going down?"

Nicole laughed. "Quite the opposite. He's setting up his own firm, with the lady from Empi, Gina Sunday. They're gonna call it Bain Sunday."

Nicole caught herself, babbling more than was her style. She was a perfectionist but even she had to laugh when she found who Bain's source had been. Not Lena Jones, not the leaking brain of Ernie Swanker, but the lowly loan officer she'd trashed without even calling. The ways of The Street were at once mysterious and mundane.

"Why are you telling me all this?" Kurt asked.

"To close the books on all this bullshit." The Street only cared about what you actually produce, or claimed to. She was using Kurt as a toilet, blowing off steam in the only way she knew.

"The photo of Candida -- uh, Miss Azuela, you're gonna throw it out?"

"I already have."

"We should have a drink sometime."

Nicole laughed. The horniness and stupidity of men never ceased to amaze her.

* * *

Micah, feeling horny and heroic, drove to Bertha's again. It was dark already and the money had changed hands, or accounts at least. With Mrs. Morales doing the babysitting, he and Bertha walked ten yards or so into St. Mary's Park. Any further and they could be mugged; the worthy feeling would wash away just like that, just another white mark with a yen for the sweetest juice from this darkest of berries.

"You're sure you want to do this?" Micah asked. "I mean, the bed money is yours."

"Do it with your fee, then," Bertha said. "And whatever part of mine you have to use."

"You're really amazing," Micah said.

Bertha for once felt the same. The Snake had stood up to The Man. They were tapping his phone, like they did to the Reverend and the Panthers, all the way back to Frederick Douglass, an unbroken line of breaking the chain -- and he hadn't backed down. Arthur was one example, and she missed him still. Micah however had balls too in his way: pink and hairy, shriveling in the cold but balls nonetheless. Together they'd fight like hell for the living; this first skirmish was for the memory of Penny Zade. "I've seen a house for sale," she told him.

Micah smiled, forgetting for a moment the drug dealers and the four hundred year dynamic. "In the Bronx?"

"Yeah. Up by Arthur Avenue -- you know, the supposed Little Italy that's mostly Mexicans and Albanians now?"

"I know it well." It was one of the few integrated working class neighborhoods in The Bronx -- in New York City and the whole eastern seaboard maybe.

"It's on 183rd Street between Adams and Hughes. It used to belong to a tailor so it has a storefront, and five rooms upstairs. I was thinking--"

Micah could see it already: a home office, a tailor's shop with no blinking lights, no "Have You Been Hurt," no trolling for braindead babies like before. He'd be like William Kunstler, or like Clarence Darrow before him. The most maligned would seek him out, and he'd emerge from his love-den with his legal briefs in flames.

"There's a hospital right by there too," Bertha continued. "In case you need to keep doing those kind of cases for a while."

Negligence and malpractice right outside the front door -- what could be better?

"I love you," Micah said in the darkness, muffled by the elevated Two Train rumbling two blocks away.

Bertha didn't answer but she did.

* * *

Kurt was on that Two Train, heading to Olinville with Jack's keys in his hand. It was dark on the block; there were drugs as always but no more than in Tremont, a genteel crowd that drove up in cars and waited while the kids on bikes returned with their stash from the weeds of the parking lot. Kurt clocked it all then climbed the stairs to Jack's, expecting to see crime scene tape or the black guy from Empi -- but nothing. The key worked in the lock and Kurt went inside.

The credit card was where Jack had said. There were coffee-stained Empi documents and print-outs of porno. Kurt leafed through the docs, not without interest, finding here and there a fast food napkin. He figured it out: Jack's smoking gun files had come from the garbage. He'd been dumpster diving, getting his hands dirty literally to fight back at Empi. It was pathetic and it was noble. It was moot now, with Jack on the run. Kurt grabbed a beer from the fridge and turned on Jack's desktop computer. Half of the bookmarks were porno, including one about Islam. Was he a sleeper agent or just a sleeper? The next bookmark was a Star Trek site; when Kurt followed the link, a two word phrase was highlighted and it made him laugh, there in the half-light: Tarok Nor. It was a Goddamned orbital space station near something called Bajor. The Cracker Jackal was a Trekkie, as well as a wanker. Kurt wasn't surprised, nor judgmental, really, truth be told. There was space on Jack's hard drive. Kurt could install his web publishing software and continue WatchCorp from here. Everyone one else was getting paid off -- that's how Empi solved its problems -- but he would continue, his focus like FOCO, his addiction, this new American Revolution like the Zenger guy who Micah'd mentioned. Maybe he'd even sleep here tonight. But first he had to use Jack's card.

The Gap™ in Manhattan would surely be open, but he'd rather drive them crazy right here in The Bronx. On Tremont and Park was an all-night store named Phil's. It sold cross-bows and rifles, hunting coats and bathing suits. It was open all night since the last City black-out. As the night had progressed and the crowds had grown larger, store after store on this strip had been looted. Some had signs, "Black Owned Business," but it hardly mattered. People carted off TV sets and cases of liquor, a decade's supply of toilet paper and baking soda. Phil had drawn a line in the sand, a line on the corner of Tremont and Park. He'd stood outside with a double-barreled shotgun and screamed madly at the mob, "Come and get it you motherfuckers! You want my guns I'll give 'em to you, right up the ass!" Only his store had survived that night. And since then he'd barely slept. Phil Junior had mace but no video cameras. If you shot a shoplifter why leave any record? It was the perfect place for Kurt, the perfect ruse for Empi's dogs.

Kurt bought a nice one-piece suit for a six year old niece; he waited to see if they'd ask for I.D.. They didn't. As he signed Kurt added a new home address for Jack. 174th Street, at least the south side, was lined with apartment buildings. Kurt watched as the credit card charge went through. He could see this store from the basement window in the Guzmans' house. He'd stay there and wait; he'd follow to watch the end-game.

59. The American Dream / Of Mobility

At night amid the eighteen-wheel rigs with their radar the minimum speed was ninety. Texas was a nation unto itself: Odessa like Russia, Fort Hancock by the Rio Grande. Jack thought of the dead girls in Ciudad Juarez as they passed; they ate huevos rancheros in their honor in Las Cruces. With No-Doze™ he could make it to the Coast with no more stops. The truckers did it and so could he. It was an American right of passage but he wished he had speed. Real speed, benzedrine, whatever that shit was that Eric took to fuck all night or so he said. Crossing some Indian land Jack hallucinated Diane, how things mighta been if she wasn't such a cunt. He was a prick, maybe -- the lack of sleep, the rhythm of the broken lines, they made for self-reflection which was rare. After Eloy the choice came: due west on I-8 or north then west on 10. He chose the latter, not from any love of Phoenix. Like millions before him, La-La Land called. To show Zalie the veil of Maya, and maybe Universal Studios and the La Brea Tar Pits.

While Jack imagined Diane's face rising from the desert at the state line at Blythe, Rudehart read the Visa data-run and smiled. "That jackass is back," he said. "He's slunk back to the Bronx and he shouldn't be hard to find." It was time to tell Sandy that the fix was in. With all the accounting scandal crap, this Bender hunt had been good fun. All's well that bends well. They'd stretch this Southern asshole to the limit then break him.

There was no time for Armonk: they'd do it right here in the executive suite, the final debrief before snapping this Bender.

"It's about fucking time," Sandy said. "Some piece of white trash from Charlotte and we can't even find him."

"He's back in the Bronx. Dumb fuck bought a girl's bathing suit at a place called Phil's."

"He's a freak?" This, Sandy liked. The Empi Cradle photograph wouldn't stand up as disparagement in court, but a man might agree to even longer and more permanent silence to keep his cross-dressing in the closet. Might even blow his brains out in there.

"He stole his daughter," Rudehart reported. "It's a long story but it's going to end soon."

"It better," Sandy said. "With what I'm paying you it better."

Rudehart thought of Sandy's 232 million not counting stock options. Even if you expensed them it was an outrage. But everything was relative in this Rome. It was time for a funeral dirge; it was time for a chorus with masks. Chuck drove him to The Bronx.

* * *

The tour of LA. was a litany of death. "That's where RFK was killed," Jack whispered in front of the fenced-in Ambassador Hotel, his voice gone, his eyes bleary, the sunlight bright like an autopsy and fake.

"Who's RFK Daddy?" Zalie asked.

He explained, complete with Cromartie-isms. "And that's where Biggie Smalls was shot, right by that parking lot." It was right near the Tar Pits so they saw that too. Air bubbles roiled the black surface. In the rest room Jack threw up.

He'd thought he'd return the smoking Tercel to the Dollar Rent-a-Car at LAX. But why give them a lead? It was time for a last hurrah with this piece of shit Toyota. Jack was a wanted man already, unless Micah could fix that. He stopped in Santa Monica for a coffee -- the name of the place, Legal Grind, made him laugh -- then drove north with the four windows down on the Pacific Coastal Highway. "That's what we came here for baby," he told Zalie, pointing west at the water.

"Are there sharks?" Zalie asked. He didn't know.

He turned inland on Sunset Boulevard, up a hill past the golden domes of some Self-Realization™ racket. He pointed at Bel Air as they passed and denounced Ronald Reagan, Alzheimer's or not. The Chateau Marmont, fruitcakes of West Hollywood, and finally The Strip itself. He joggled one block north to the Boulevard: whores in the daytime and everyone looked foreign. He'd have to get used to that. He parked and let Zalie out to look at the stars in the sidewalk, sitcom heroes, lip-synching tramps with boob-jobs and an agent. At Vine they had a burrito. Their time was growing short.

Downtown was the skid row that Jack'd been looking for, along 5th Street south of Pershing Park. He found a street called Wall and laughed madly at the irony. "What are we doing here, Daddy?" Zalie asked, looking at the homeless guys with their shopping carts, their lean-tos against the gray metal fence of a junkyard.

"Take all your stuff with you," he told her. "We're going to go to Disneyland."

With twenty bucks it wasn't hard.

"You want me to burn it?" the dredlocked guy asked.

"Yeah. You can take the parts first." Jack's already taken off the license plates and scratched out the VIN. "Just burn the engine n' leave no trace. There's plenty a gas in the tank."

"You're fuckin' crazy Mister," the guy said. But twenty was twenty.

Jack and Zalie stood on Alameda Street and watched the black smoke then heard the explosion. "Cheap fucking car," Jack muttered. "Rent a wreck for sure." He looked down at Zalie, who looked excited and terrified at the same time. "C'mon baby," he told her. "We got a train to catch."

Union Station was just like in the movies, high-ceilinged and shady with black wooden beams and a rude lady at the Amtrak counter. She demanded I.D. and Jack bobbed and wove. Finally he slipped her an extra twenty and she shrugged. They had two tickets on the SurfLiner,™ straight down the coast to San Diego by way of Anaheim. The train was double-decker. It ran past cement factories and oil tanks and then reached Disneyland. "Okay baby," Jack told Zalie. "This is for you."

* * *

Chuck and Rudehart played show-and-tell with Junior Phil. What they showed were two hundred dollar bills; what they were told was the home address Bender had given when he bought the bathing suit last night. "It was for his niece," Phil remembered and said, to give value for value. That might have been a tip-off: but what else would a kidnapper say? Chuck saw the address on One Seven Four and he shrugged. If he'd have been Bender he wouldn't return to Olinville either. They got back in the car and Kurt, watching, flagged a gypsy cab to follow.

They drove east on Tremont, past discount stores and an abandoned movie theater, turned left down Southern Boulevard. "I'm surprised the guy was so stupid," Chuck said as he drove.

"I'm not," said Rudehart.

Chuck hung a left under the El at Boston Road. The address was an odd number. Which was odd like strange because the tenements here were all on the downtown side, their numbers even. The numbers got too high and so Chuck hooked a U. Kurt paid six bucks, two for a tip, and got out. He wanted to see their faces. Especially Rudehart. He pulled his digital camera from his backpack.

Chuck got it first. The cracker lived in Rent-a-Center? No, that'd be the store next door. The Empi-Fucking-Financial from which all these problems flowed. Chuck licked his lips and thought of his pension. He might even have wished the trickster cracker well.

Rudehart got out of the car, staring at the paper Phil'd written the address on. Rudehart gritted his teeth and his face turned red. It was a humid day in the West Farms Mall and the heat rose from the black asphalt. Kurt clicked away as Janet came out, almost curtseying like this were England.

"You stupid *bitch*!" Kurt heard Rudehart say. Self-criticism is always productive, no matter how late it comes.

* * *

Mickey spoke in a high-pitched voice but Minnie was hot, at least to Jack. Zalie squealed at Donald Duck. The scene was Americana and yet it wasn't. "C'mon hon we've got to keep moving," Jack told her and she didn't complain.

"You're the best, Dad," she said on the train, first time she'd contracted it that way, not Daddy but Dad. She was growing up and maybe he was as well.

* * *

Micah had the money; a faint echo of Empi, he had the power to solve and resolve. First was Diane. He was calling from Bertha's bedroom, with the door closed. It didn't take long.

"He *wants* to do the right thing," Micah said. "That what he's always wanted."

Diane doubted it, at least as to the past. But this lawyer spoke direct deposit; he knew joint custody and even had a contract faxed. "She's gotta come back in time for school," Diane said.

Micah dodged that, now that he knew Jack's plan. "Raising a child is a partnership for life," he said, thinking of Bertha who was out in the living room, wondering if her eggs still dropped. She still used tampons: that, he knew from the bathroom here. On 183rd Street over the tailor's shop, they'd learn each others' dankest smells, their deepest fears -- they'd name the house for Penny, Penny Zade the baby he couldn't save or represent.

"Have them call me," Diane said. She'd fax back the contract from Kinkos, West Third and Tryon, just as soon as the lump-sum alimony showed up in her account. But she wanted to talk to her Zalie. She had things to apologize for, amends to make.

* * *

The trolley from San Diego ran straight down the coast to the border. Chula Vista: Jack knew that it meant Pretty View. And so it was, these Mexican-American girls in their cut-off shorts, then the dry brown Imperial desert in which so many immigrants died. Jack was a reverse immigrant, a dry-back one might call him, since the border at San Ysidro was mostly a highway, a concrete irrigation bed that ran with raw sewage if anything in the hot half of the year.

They got off the trolley, facing a one-block strip of fast food joints and the concrete block command of the border patrol. The telephones on the other side might not be as Jack remembered. So he stopped in a *casa de cambio*, got twenty dollars in quarters -- they'd be good to tip with if he didn't use them all -- and dialed Kurt from a payphone on the trolley platform.

"You can patch into Micah again, right?"

"Nah -- he's here. They've bugged the line at his office. I'll put him on speaker phone."

Jack flashed back to the burning car on skid row and was glad for it. "So what's the deal?" he asked.

"I talked to Diane, everything's cool. You should call her. But she's agreed to joint custody, and no complaint to the police. The next part, you have to do the work."

Jack looked down at Zalie, who was reading the comics in the San Diego Union-Tribune. "Hit me," Jack said. Zalie looked up and punched him softly in the thigh. Jack wanted to cry out, how cute it was -- he wanted to tell Micah and Kurt but they wouldn't understand. He could hear it already, "ya had to be there." And here he was, on the border of a new life with a fistful of quarters. He fed the phone again.

"It'll go like this," Micah said. "I'm wiring three quarters of my fee--" he didn't mention Bertha's settlement though some was in there too

--"to a money-transfer place in TJ. You'll love this: it's EmpiBank, or the company they bought down there, NaraMex. It's in downtown, Avenida Negrete and -- what's this?"

"*Calle* 3A," Kurt said.

Jack wrote it down. "You're the man," he said like a beer commercial.

"You're splitting it," Micah said flatly.

"What?"

"You're splitting it with Milly Guzman's mother. Her name is Esmeralda. Milly is telling her to meet you at the EmpiBank, or NaraMex, whatever the sign says. Neither of you can get the money without the other's signature. It's fifty-fifty, kid. But you'll have enough to live down there for a while."

At first Jack thought fuck then he thought what the hell. He hadn't expected this money anyway and there were people poorer than him.

"How will I recognize her?"

Micah laughed, picturing the scene. "She'll recognize you. Hurry up -- you're supposed to meet her there in an hour."

60. BG&E: The Bill of Rights and Wrongs

The security on the border was only one-way. Jack and Zalie walked up concrete stairs and crossed a long overpass over the highway. There were guards in glassed-in offices; none of them came out. On the other side were a pair of metal turnstiles, the head-to-toe ones, squeaking as you passed through -- maybe they counted each turn, each revolution, to measure the southbound foot traffic. But there was no I.D. check, just a voluntary customs booth and then a chaotic mini-mall full of men offering two-for-one drinks. There were signs for Viagra -- "No prescription! Wholesale price!" -- and this Jack Bender liked. He didn't need artificial stimulus but the nights could be long here and if Bob Dole took it, and the Texas Rangers' first baseman, why not him?

"C'mon Zalie, Daddy's got to be somewhere," he said, adding, "Dad." They brushed off a dozen pitch-men and headed in on Revolucion, the street lined with two-story buildings with balconies, the sidewalks narrow, Jack's mouth dry. On Calle 3A he turned left, a sort of strip mall of white ceramic statues and there on the corner, a bank branch with a NaraMex sign and Empi's logo. How different from West Farms, Jack thought, and yet how not different.

"I don't think I like it here Daddy," Zalie said.

You will, he thought. You better. "It's nice further south. There's a place we're gonna go, Rosarito Beach it's called. Daddy went there was he was younger." He thought again of Viagra. "You can swim in the ocean and we'll call Mommy from there. Alright?"

Zalie pursed her lips but she nodded, ever so slightly.

"Daddy's got to meet a woman in the bank. This way we'll have money."

"Is she your new girlfriend?"

"No."

"I'm hungry," Zalie said.

"Soon," said Jack.

At the entrance to the bank was a hunched-over lady. She had on a black dress; her hair was gray but neatly tied-back.

"*Usted es el Senor Bender?*" she asked.

"Bender, yeah, that's me."

"*Que Dios le bendiga.*" They went into the bank, straight to a teller who had a nose ring and spoke English.

"It's a wire transfer," Jack said. "Bender and Guzman."

The computer beeped. "Two percent is for the transfer," the punk rock clerk said.

Those squeezing bastards, Jack thought then let it go. The clerk counted out a stack of bills, dealing them into two stacks like cards. "*La mitad es sua,*" she told Esmeralda. Jack saw the stack grow and no longer cared, even about the exchange rate.

"I'm hungry," Zalie reminded him.

"We can eat together," Esmeralda said in accented English. "Now we are rich."

They followed her back to Revolucion, turned north from Calle 3A to 4. "You will like this," Esmeralda told Zalie, leading them into an arcade-like mall, down some tiled steps to a windowless basement. It was called Café Especial and Esmeralda ordered *carne asada* for all of them. Jack ordered a tequila and a beer chaser.

"Where you are going?" Esmeralda asked.

"Rosarito Beach," Jack said. "I figure we'll find a place to rent down there."

"I think I find you one," Esmeralda said. "So they not -- how you say? -- reep you off."

Jack laughed, at the prevalence of this reaping throughout the world. Maybe it was the tequila and the lack of sleep. "I'd appreciate that," he said. "Somewhere near the beach but not too expensive."

"You know they film 'Titanic' there," Esmeralda said, making quote marks in the air around the name Titanic.

"Did it, like, bring money in or anything?"

"Not much I do not think," Esmeralda said. "Sometime I think that America, *el norte*, it is like the Titanic. It is crazy and dangerous. For now I stay here. That, and the price of medicine."

"I like that movie," Zalie said. Jack, not knowing what to say, finished his beans with a spoon, not a tortilla as Esmeralda and Zalie were doing.

"There is a bus from right near the border," Esmeralda said. "I take bus there also. I will show you."

"Where do you live?" Jack asked.

"It is called Maclovia Rojas. It is on a hill to the east. I could give you tour, if you want. Because you are tourists, right?"

"Something like that," Jack muttered.

"Let's go see it Daddy. I like this lady I really do."

And so they took the bus standing up, climbing a treeless desert hillside, the houses getting rattier and rattier as they went. "Those are doors from *Los An-hell-es*," Esmeralda said pointing. "We *Tijuanenses* use them for walls. They are door to the house where you keep your car."

"Garage doors," Jack said softly. They were wooden and here people lived in them.

"Here we get off," Esmeralda announced. They walked a narrow dirt road; shirtless children played soccer. Esmeralda's house was plywood and tin. She had a black-and-white TV that Zalie turned on, and an enormous poster of La Virgen de la Guadalupe on the wall. He who'd seen her had belatedly been declared a saint by a Pope who's hands shook. There was also a painting of a woman with huge breasts in a torn dress symbolizing the Mexican Revolution. Jack stared.

"In New York, you know my daughter?"

Jack turned and hesitated, remembering Gina ripping Milly and Amado on points, fees and insurance. He'd refi-ed them but not without cost. "Not well," Jack said.

Esmeralda nodded. "I will go use the phone of my neighbor. I will find you a place by the beach by tonight. Your daughter, she is very pretty. You are a good father I am sure of it."

"I'll try to," Jack said, using the future tense because he couldn't use the past. He had no use for the past at all, not anymore.

* * *

Micah called the Assistant U.S. Attorney for the Southern District. "So you tapped my phone," he began.

"I'm walled off from that," the guy said. "In case they overhear anything that's privileged."

Bullshit, Micah thought. But that wasn't the point. "My client," he announced, "has gone into exile."

There was silence; the phone on the other end was covered and Micah could hear but not make out the whispers. He felt at the center of a surreal diplomatic incident: a cracker defecting from a country that didn't want him anyway.

"You tipped him off," the guy said when he came back on. "We could charge you right now for providing material aid to a fugitive."

"He didn't need me," Micah said. "Anyway, I'm just letting you know. And I'm going to be moving my office. When I have a new number for you to tap rest assured I'll provide it, like a good American."

"We'll just get him extradited."

"Somehow I doubt that," Micah said. They didn't know where he was, and even if they did, Vinny Fox was playing leftist this year, since all his sucking-up to Bush had gotten him nowhere. Mexico had provide refuge in the past to guerrillas from Nicaragua, El Salvador and Puerto Rico. Why not now a red-blooded American like Jack Bender, a rebel without a cause, a loan-sharking political prisoner with a red schnoz?

"Tell you what," Micah offered. "If and when he re-enters the United States, I commit to tell you."

The guy scoffed. "That's not how we do Homeland Defense, Mister Levine."

There was something fascist in the way he said it, something pathetic and anachronistic, like Containment or the Domino Theory. "It's the best I can offer," Micah said then wrapped up.

* * *

Bain was schmoozing his book of clients; Gina was prepping for a seminar for EmpiFinancial refugees. Together they paid protection money to Elizabeth's Dad and fucked ever-ready like New Economy rabbits. Bain's theory was that each time they did it, Liz Dickinson receded further into the past, like Nine Eleven. That Liz had come out of her walk-in closet as a lesbian, in the end, was better for Bain's self-image. You had to be cocky to sell and that's just what Bain did, building their assets-under-management to one day buy their freedom. Gina, in a ritual, had burned her Franklin Cubby Planners; something about the road not taken that Bain chose to ignore. The Planner had served a function, like training wheels on a bike -- but now Gina was ready to race, sleek and with little to no resistance to the wind. Gina poached the Alphas from EmpiFinancial's northeast region and thus they built a team, paying nothing but commissions and circumnavigating the Ground Zero island of Manhattan in rented cruise ships once a quarter. Liz's father came twice to inspect the business and even he had to admit it was more cut-throat than he'd been able to muster. History, apparently, was an inexorably rising graph-line of progress.

Swanker still waited for the transplanted hair to catch hold, fetishizing in the painful interim the newest polling numbers. He cursed pattern-baldness and the powers of incumbency. But to remain the state A.G. was not so bad. Timing was everything: there were more cheap corporate pelts to amass, more nationwide enforcement actions to manipulate and take credit for. His wife Carolyn grew more brittle and more photogenic, all at once. Swanker dreamed of a Presidential run where this carefully constructed résumé would trump the Beltway gridlock boys.

Candida continued pissing on sticks; Marcos was bench-pressing two fifty and e-mailing her heartfelt soft porn each night. If the pissing came to naught they could try again when he got leave. The world was almost safe for democracy; a botox-infused newswoman had triplets and spoke of the wonders of the fertility arts so there was still hope. Candida's father got Alzheimers: a good revenge and even a blessing for him, perhaps.

Vinny pined and bought whores in Hunts Point feeling nothing. Gina, the one-who-got-away, would remain in his dreams. Blowman and Bernie carried their discredited road show to Asia, recycling it like pesticides long outlawed in the Land of the Free. Mudnick awaited his transfer to China while cleaning up after repos gone wrong from Sarasota to Sacramento. This was a business that knew no end: Empi improved each year in the science of plausible deniability. Lena Jones spun; Chuck step-n'-fetched it ironically waiting for his pension; Rudehart prepared for a weekend of speeches in Bohemian Grove. His dalliance in the world of the Bertha Watkins' had been beneath him. Now he spoke of the need for compassionate capitalism and, relatedly, a strong dollar.

Sandy Vyle listened to books-on-tape about cryogenics while preparing to be named CEO of the year. Empi's Anguilla tax-dodge was briefly debated in Congress but nothing was done about it. The markets, however, or pundits desperate for screen time, worked their own reformist magic. A clamor grew from the break-up of EmpiGroup into its constituent parts. "For national security," some faux-populist Republicans said. "To unlock the hidden value" was the market's rationale. Sandy would fight to keep his baby in one piece, so long as he lived. "From my cold dead hands," he'd intone as he slowly lost it. *Aprés moi, le déluge.*

The Snowman's habit grew worse; paradoxically he became a spokesman against the death penalty, a position forged on demographics and not principles but those saved by it -- those lucky enough to commit their murders in The Bronx -- weren't complaining. Wolfson sat at night alone in his house clinging to the Constitution and his dignity, and now to an oxygen mask which alone gave him peace. The Bender case remained sealed and the long arm of John Ashcroft looked elsewhere, at least for now, draping the marble breasts of Lady Justice in the American flag.

Lorraine Thompson taught CLE classes about infant death syndrome and birth defects, complete with Gray's Anatomy and a checklist for use in cross-examination of doctors. She'd inherited Micah's braindead baby practice and it remained lucrative.

Milagros was proud of what she'd done for her *mama*. The house in Maclovia Rojas had morphed from plywood and tin to stuccoed cinderblock. If and when pharmaceutical prices ever declined in El Norte, her mother would join them.

Micah and Bertha did it unprotected over the Constitutional tailor's shop on 183rd Street. Their bedroom -- and their life together -- was a shrine to Penny Zade. Duwon liked the neighborhood and began to do better in school. The girl swam for free year-round in the refurbished pool of P.S. 32. The Snake would pay to send the kids to Horace Mann, including the one to come, God willing. And Kurt, in Olinville, moved further and further out. His motiveless story would continue, online and off: the tales of WatchCorp Kurt. He was looking at predatory lending now in India and Kenya, and one day soon in Mexico.

* * *

The sun had turned the blue sea pink, then orange, then finally as red as blood or sangria. Jack sat in his beach chair, watching Zalie bodysurf in the knee-deep tide. The deal Esmeralda had gotten them had bought them time. There were the first stirrings of a mortgage market here in Mexico, the beginning of late-night TV ads for home equity and bill consolidation loans. Jack might soon join the game. *El Rey del*

Credito, the Credit King, he liked that name, though he might opt for Prince, and use as his logo the Jack of Hearts from an antique set of playing cards he'd seen while playing poker. He'd expanded his gambling to the mainstream too: he'd invested what he could with the firm of Bain Sunday and the returns weren't half bad. They seemed to know what the market would do a day or more before it happened. Even if it went down -- and it did -- you could short it, they explained. Gina'd done well hooking up with this Bain character, even Jack had to admit it. When she'd blown him off about coming over to the dark side at HomeQuik, he'd thought she was stupid, a high-falutin' hottie who'd stay trapped at Empi like The Clam Janet Peel. Live and learn.

Jack's checks-up on Bain Sunday had gotten less frequent. He still downloaded porn, though only late at night after Zalie was asleep. He'd gone down on a drunk co-ed from UC Davis; the over-the-counter Viagra had made it so he couldn't come at all. But it wasn't about that anymore; he didn't need to max-out every moment like Empi had taught him.

He was reading now, not just porn, but the books that Cromartie had pitched so long ago. He'd been right about that German -- the syphilitic fuck was *funny*, though Jack wasn't always sure that he understood what the jokes meant. If you're gonna be wrong, make it about something short. Jack best liked the epigrams in Beyond Good and Evil, the one he called BG&E like the gas and electric company in EmpiFinancial's hometown. Looking out at Zalie he was reminded of one; he wanted to get the wording right so he picked up his dog-earred book, the one he'd bought in the gift shop of the Centro Cultural up in Tijuana when they'd had an exhibit about native son Carlos Santana. Here it was, Number 153: "Whatever is done from love always occurs beyond good and evil."

Zalie justified all of it, this love he felt but couldn't explain. Mister Cromartie was dead. Jack had checked, the Charlotte Observer obit screamed AIDS between the lines. But Cromartie woulda been proud. Jack'd buried his momma; he'd buried his past. Zalie was his future. His future and his dreams were on hold. Nietzsche had something on this, too: "Either we have no dreams or our dreams are interesting. We should learn to arrange our waking life the same way: nothing or interesting." For now Jack drank beer in his comfortable loving nothingness. After years of loan-sharking he had time to reflect. Or not, if he didn't want to. There was another one from The Gay Science -- the title embarrassed him so he didn't bring it to the beach -- right at the end of Book Three: "What is the seal of Liberation? -- No longer being ashamed in front of oneself." Jack perhaps had never been, but now less so than ever. They'd tried to fuck him and he'd done what he did. He wasn't the one who was crazy -- though after the money had been wired and the fix was in, WatchCorp Kurt had asked him about Star Wars and called him a crazy motherfucker.

There was one in here that ol' WatchCorp could learn from: "Whoever fights monsters should see to it that in the process he does not become a monster." He'd e-mail it to Kurt like a warning tonight, when after tucking Zalie in he went online to read up on the progress of the War on Terror from which he'd had to flee. His name was still on a watch-list, though whether the rent-a-cops at the San Ysidro station would figure it out, so intent were they on flashing their M-16 and strutting south with Mexicans in plastic handcuffs, who knew. For now it was a witch hunt; Jack'd called it a Red-Neck Scare and Micah'd laughed. Jack had even read him an epigram: "Madness is rare in individuals -- but in groups, parties, nations and ages it is the rule." This rule applied to companies as well, they agreed.

He was fuckin' that black chick, Micah was. Well good for him. Jack'd like to get one; the race didn't matter. Interesting or nothing had become his rule so he pleasured himself. He was a single Dad on a Mexican beach. Life wasn't so bad -- you should leave life blessing it, as Nietzsche said of Odysseus, but not in love with it. Love Jack saved for Zalie. One day the two of them would go back to the Homeland. They would have to wait until the madness -- this predatory bender -- passed. And that might take awhile.